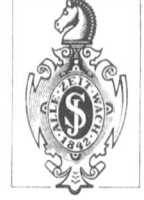

Essential Hypertension

Calcium Mechanisms and Treatment

Edited by K. Aoki

With 94 Figures

Springer-Verlag
Tokyo Berlin Heidelberg New York
London Paris

Dr. KYUZO AOKI
2nd Department of Internal Medicine
Nagoya City University Medical School
Mizuho-ku, Nagoya, 467 Japan

Library of Congress Cataloging-in-Publication Data
Essential hypertension.
Contains papers presented at the First International Symposium on Mechanism
and Treatment in Essential Hypertension, held on Oct. 23–24, 1985 in Nagoya,
Japan, as a satellite symposium to the Fifth International Symposium on Rats
with Spontaneous Hypertension and Related Studies held in Kyoto, Oct. 20–
22, 1985.
Includes bibliographies and index.
1. Essential hypertension—Etiology—Congresses.   2. Calcium—Physiological effect—Congresses.   3. Calcium—Antagonists—Therapeutic use—
Congresses. 4. Hypotensive agents—Congresses. I. Aoki, K. (Kyuzo),
1933–   . II. International Symposium on Mechanism and Treatment in
Essential Hypertension (1st:1985:Nagoya-shi, Japan) III. International
Symposium on Rats with Spontaneous Hypertension and Related Studies
(5th:1985:Kyoto, Japan) [DNLM: 1. Antihypertensive Agents—therapeutic use—congresses.   2. Calcium   Channel   Blockers—therapeutic   use—
congresses. 3. Hypertension—drug therapy—congresses. WG 340 E7853
1985]
RC685.H8E874   1986   616.1'32061   86-29688

ISBN-13: 978-4-431-68050-5   e-ISBN-13: 978-4-431-68048-2
DOI: 10.1007/978-4-431-68048-2

Typesetting: Asco Trade Typesetting Ltd., Hong Kong

Preface

This volume contains papers presented at the First International Symposium on Mechanism and Treatment in Essential Hypertension, which was held on October 23 and 24, 1985 in Nagoya, Japan. The meeting was an official satellite symposium to the meeting of the Fifth International Symposium on Rats with Spontaneous Hypertension and Related Studies in Kyoto, October 20–22, 1985. The Nagoya symposium was made possible by official grants from the city of Nagoya and Aichi Prefecture and the generous financial support of many companies.

The aim of the symposium was to provide a forum for presentation and discussion of recent advances in the area of essential hypertension, particularly with regard to calcium mechanisms in vasoconstriction and vasodilation in arterial vessels and the function of arterial smooth muscle. The role of calcium ions in the function of arterial smooth muscle has attracted a great deal of attention in the last two decades. The mode of action of calcium ions was revealed at the molecular level. The hypertension model of the spontaneously hypertensive rat has been widely utilized for research into the fundamental mechanisms of genetic hypertension, stroke, and cardiovascular disease as well as into therapeutic measures. New tools of calcium agonists and antagonists have become available to research into the mechanism, prevention, and treatment of essential hypertension at the molecular, subcellular, and cellular levels of arterial smooth muscle, at the organ level of arterial vessels, as well as at the total systemic level.

The authors here provide new findings, an overview of their own work, related studies from other laboratories, and their hypotheses in this field. I would like to thank the contributors for their excellent papers and all the participants for outstanding scientific achievements and cooperation.

The symposium was a success due to the endeavors of the Organizing Committee, Drs. Koichi Sato and Masahiko Yamamoto, and the dedication and expertise of Ms Yukimi Kuga (Takeda) and Ms Junko Ito, who took on most of the administrative load.

It is hoped that these proceedings will stimulate the discovery of hypertension mechanisms as well as preventive and therapeutic measures. I would like to thank the staff of Springer-Verlag Tokyo for their highly professional and skillful efforts in making this attractive publication.

October, 1986   KYUZO AOKI

List of Contributors

The addresses can be found at the page numbers indicated

Table of Contents

Introduction:
Spontaneously Hypertensive Rats

Discovery of the Spontaneously Hypertensive Rat

K. Aoki

Second Department of Internal Medicine, Nagoya City University
Medical School, Mizuho-ku, Nagoya, 467 Japan

Summary. This report deals with the discovery, development, and establishment of spontaneously hypertensive rats (Aoki SHR) by the production of a new apparatus for the measurement of rat blood pressure and selective inbreeding of rats with the highest blood pressure. In 1959, a reliable apparatus was produced for measuring the blood pressure of rats. To examine the accuracy of the new apparatus, the blood pressure of approximately ten Wistar rats from the Animal Center of Kyoto University was measured and a male SHR was discovered. The male SHR was mated with a female normotensive rat to obtain SHR offspring. The rats with the highest blood pressure were selected from the offspring and brother-sister inbreeding provided rats with spontaneous hypertension. All the offspring of the third and successive generations developed hypertension. The development and establishment of a strain of SHR were completed by 1963.

Key words: Spontaneously hypertensive rats—Establishment of SHR strain

In 1959, I joined the Department of Pathology, School of Medicine, Kyoto University as a graduate student. The research interest of the department then was the production of animal models of disease [1], including diabetes mellitus, endocrine diseases, obesity, arteriosclerosis, and hypertension. My interest was only in hypertension [2–5].

Discovery of a Spontaneously Hypertensive Rat

To measure the blood pressure of the rats, a reliable apparatus was produced by a modification of the tail water-plethysmographic devices of William et al. (6), Byrom and Wilson [7], Sobin [8], and Umezawa [9]. A plethysmographic chamber was made of a transparent acrylic tube with an exhaust pipe in the top of the chamber to let out the air [2–5]. The chamber, cuff, and rat holder were arranged in a box. Prior to measurement, the rat was warmed for 10 min in a box at 38°C. The tail of the rat was placed in the plastic chamber through the cuff in the box; the temperature of the box was 37°C. The plethysmographic chamber was filled with warm water at 37°C, and the blood pressure was measured without anesthesia (Fig. 1).

To examine the accuracy of the new apparatus, the blood pressure of approximately ten Wistar rats, which were kindly supplied by Katsuya from the Animal Center of Kyoto University, was measured. The blood pressure of the rats was

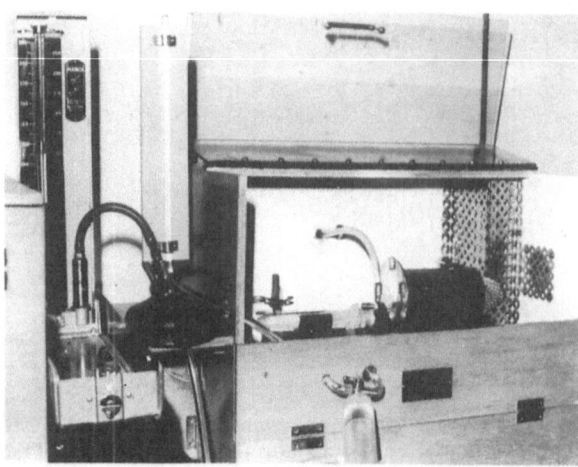

Fig. 1. Tail water-plethysmographic apparatus for measurement of rat blood pressure. The apparatus was designed and made by the author. After Aoki [3]

measured daily. Among these rats there happened to be a male rat whose systolic blood pressure was 150–175 mmHg at the age of 7 weeks. This hypertensive rat was the origin of the spontaneously hypertensive rats [2–5].

Development and Establishment of a Strain of Spontaneously Hypertensive Rats

It was possible to develop a pure strain of genetic (major gene) hypertensive rat by the selection of the genetic hypertensive rats and brother-sister inbreeding.

The male hypertensive rat was bred with a female normotensive rat whose blood pressure was 130–140 mmHg. The first generation obtained consisted of 16 males and 20 females from four litters. In normotensive rats of the first generation, the blood pressure was 108 and 138 mmHg in the male and 111 ± 3 and 131 ± 12 mmHg in the females at the age of 5 and 25 weeks, respectively. The blood pressure of the hypertensive rats in this generation was 115 ± 4 and 169 ± 13 mmHg in the males and 115 ± 3 and 156 ± 14 mmHg in the females at the age of 5 ad 25 weeks, respectively. The blood pressure of the hypertensive rats rose with age (Fig. 2). Hypertension was defined as systolic blood pressure over 150 mmHg. The incidence of hypertension in this generation was 75% in males and 37% in females at the age of 25 weeks [2–5].

The rats were selected from the first generation which (1) had developed hypertension at a young age and (2) had the highest blood pressure at the age of 10 weeks. The brother-sister inbreeding provided 20 males and 32 females in the second generation. In female normotensive rats of the second generation, the blood pressure was 111 ± 3 mmHg at the age of 5 weeks and 131 ± 12 mmHg at the age of 25 weeks. In hypertensive rats of this generation, the blood pressure was 119 ± 8 and 179 ± 14 mmHg in males, and 125 ± 12 and 167 ± 16 mmHg in females at the age of 5 and 25 weeks, respectively. The incidence of hypertension in the second generation was 100% in males and 76% in females at the age of 25 weeks.

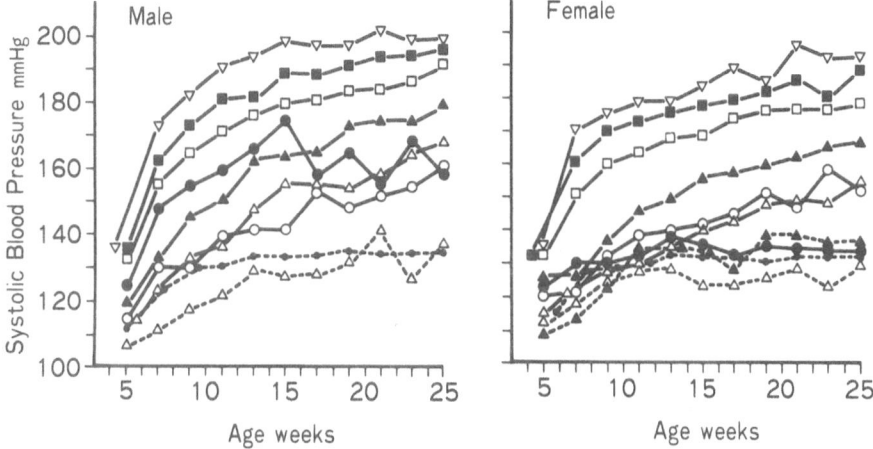

Fig. 2. Blood pressure in control rats and SHR in males (*left*) and females (*right*). There were
normotensive (--●--) and hypertensive (-○-) rats in the control group. A male SHR (-●-) was bred
with a female normotensive rat (-●-). There were normotensive rats in the first (--▲--) and second
generations (--▲--). Blood pressure of SHR is shown for first (-▲-), second (-▲-), third (-□-) fourth
(-■-), and fifth (-▽-) generations. After Okamoto and Aoki [2]

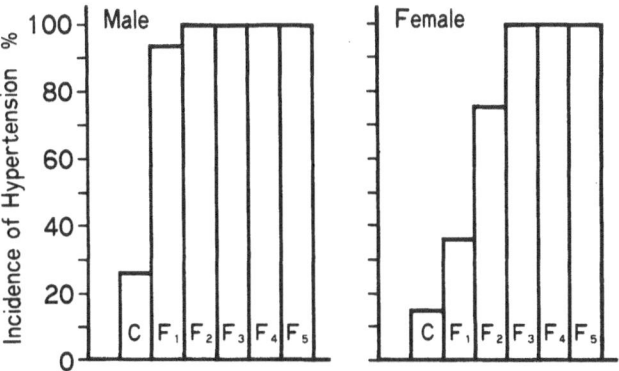

Fig. 3. Percentage incidence of hypertension in control rats and first to fifth generations of SHR
at age of 25 weeks. *C* control rats (34 males and 32 females). Generations of SHR: F_1 15 males and
19 females, F_2 22 males and 37 females, F_3 40 males and 49 females, F_4 31 males and 21 females,
F_5 25 males and 30 females. After Okamoto and Aoki [2]

   The third generation, which consisted of 56 males and 64 females, was obtained
by inbreeding the rats with the highest blood pressure from the second generation.
The blood pressure was 133 ± 14 and 192 ± 18 mmHg in males and 133 ± 14 and
179 ± 17 mmHg in females at the age of 5 and 25 weeks, respectively. The
incidence of hypertension in the third generation was 100% in both male and
female rats. All the offspring developed hypertension (Fig. 3). Thus, the develop-

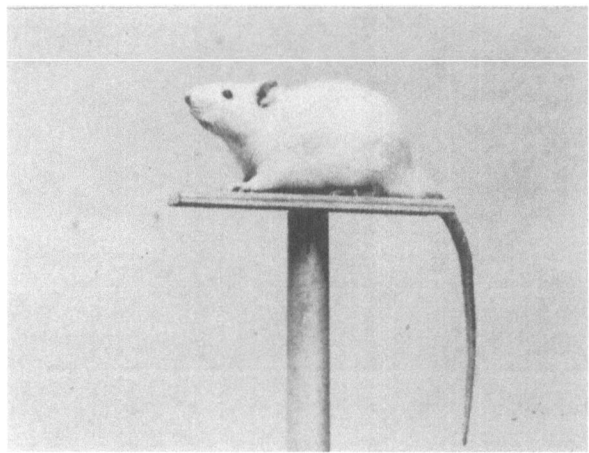

Fig. 4. An SHR

ment and establishment of a strain of spontaneously hypertensive rats were complete. These rats were called spontaneously hypertensive rats (SHR; Fig. 4).

By the selection of severe hypertension, its incidence was increased with successive generations. Severe hypertension was defined as blood pressure over 200 mmHg. The incidence was 35% in males and 16% in females at 25 weeks of age in the third generation.

For a study "Development of a strain of spontaneously hypertensive rats," 66 young rats were supplied from the Animal Center of Kyoto University as controls for the strain of SHR. There were some SHR in the control group. The blood pressure of the normotensive rats in the control group was 114 ± 12 and 135 ± 8 mmHg in males and 115 ± 11 and 133 ± 7 mmHg in females at the age of 5 and 25 weeks, respectively. The blood pressure of the hypertensive rats was 115 ± 6 and 160 ± 9 mmHg in males and 120 ± 7 and 158 ± 3 mmHg in females at the age of 5 and 25 weeks, respectively (Fig. 3). The incidence of hypertension in the control group was 26% in males and 16% in females [2–5].

The development of a strain of SHR was reported to Okamoto and an article was published in the Japanese Circulation Journal in 1963 [2–5].

Conclusion

A new apparatus for measuring rat blood pressure was made and an SHR was discovered while testing the accuracy of the apparatus. The original male SHR was bred with a female rat and the inbreeding of brothers and sisters selected from the offspring of SHR with the highest blood pressure was carried out; a strain of SHR was developed and established. I hope that the Aoki SHR will contribute to research on the mechanism and treatment of essential hypertension (major gene-induced hypertension) in humans.

Acknowledgments. I am very grateful to Professors Kozo Okamoto and Yasuaki Nishizuka for their interest in the establishment of a strain of SHR.

References

1. Okamoto K (1955) Experimental pathology of diabetes mellitus (Report II). III. Studies on rabbits from ancestors diabetic for several successive generations especially on spontaneous occurrence of diabetes in F_4 and F_5 rabbits. Tohoku J Exp Med 61 (Suppl, III): 62–112
2. Okamoto K and Aoki K (1963) Development of a strain of spontaneously hypertensive rats. Jpn Circ J 27: 282–293
3. Aoki K (1983) Hypertensiology, Essential and Secondary Hypertension, Concepts, Nature, Diagnosis, and Treatment (in Japanese). Shinkoh Igaku Shuppan, Tokyo, pp 144–169
4. Aoki K (1985) Memories of discovery and development of spontaneously hypertensive rats. The 25th anniversary of the discovery of spontaneously hypertensive rats (in Japanese). Coronary 2: 97–100
5. Aoki K (1985) Essential hypertension and secondary hypertension in humans and rats. Asian Med J 28: 529–548
6. William JR, Harrison TR, Grollman A (1939) A simple method for determining the systolic blood pressure of the unanesthetized rat. J Clin Invest 18: 373–376
7. Byrom FB, Wilson C (1938) A plethysmograhic method for measuring systolic blood pressure in the intact rat. J Physiol 93: 301–304
8. Sobin SS (1946) Accuracy of indirect determinations of blood pressure in the rat; Relation to temperature of plethysmograph and width of cuff. Am J Physiol 146: 179–186
9. Umezawa H (1952) An indirect method for measuring blood pressure of the unanesthetized rat (in Japanese). Tokyo Jikeikai Med J 66: 193–199

Classification of Hypertension

Etiological Classification of Hypertension

Essential Hypertension, Environment Hypertension, and Disease Hypertension

K. Aoki

Second Department of Internal Medicine, Nagoya City University
Medical School, Mizuho-ku, Nagoya, 467 Japan

Summary. In this paper, I shall present an overview of major studies on hypertension and propose a new etiological classification. Since the 1800s, investigators have questioned the concept, mechanism, and classification of hypertension in humans and animals. Bright reported hypertension as a renal disease. Gull and Sutton distinguished hypertension from renal disease. Albutt, Frank, and others assumed that subjects with essential hypertension differed qualitatively from subjects with normotension. Pickering rejected that essential hypertension was a specific disease entity and proposed that essential hypertension should be the name given to the syndrome of a group of subjects with high blood pressure caused by polygenic inheritance. Platt suggested that essential hypertension was the manifestation of a single gene inheritance. The values of the genetic parameters were calculated from the variance of crossbreedings of the spontaneously hypertensive rat (SHR), which demonstrated that the inheritance of hypertension in the SHR might be the incomplete dominant form transferred by three major genes and not completely polygenic. There are three qualitatively different kinds of hypertension animal models, including Aoki SHR of major gene hypertension, Dahl salt-sensitive rats of environment (accessory gene) hypertension, and Goldblatt renal hypertension animals of disease-induced (nongene) hypertension. On the basis of animal models and investigations of human hypertension, we have proposed an etiological classification in humans and animals as follows: Type 1, essential (major gene) hypertension; type 2, environment (accessory gene) hypertension; and type 3, disease (nongene) hypertension. This classification may be useful in the research on mechanisms, treatment, and prevention of hypertension.

Key words: Pickering's theory—Platt's hypothesis—Essential hypertension—Environment hypertension—Disease hypertension

Bright in 1827 recognized hypertension as a disease entity [1]. He described the cases of patients in which protein urine was associated with edema and hypertrophy of the heart without valvular disease. This evidence suggested that hypertrophy of the heart was induced by systemic disease of renal disturbance. In 1872, Gull and Sutton distinguished between hypertensive disease and nephritis [2]. They named the hypertensive disease arteriocapillary fibrosis, which was characterized by hypertrophy of the heart and alterations of the small arteries and arterioles not associated with kidney disease. Von Bash in 1893 confirmed patients with raised arterial pressure without evidence of kidney disease and termed the hypertensive disease latent arteriosclerosis [3]. Huchard in 1889 [4] used the term presclerosis and Allbutt in 1895 [5, 6] used the term senile hyperpiesis. In patients with hyperpiesis, blood pressure rose at around the age of 40 years and arterial changes accompanied the high blood pressure. In 1911, Frank termed raised arterial pressure "essentielle Hypertonie," which has been translated into English as essential hypertension [7]. The term essential hypertension has been widely used as the diagnostic name of a type of hypertension since 1911.

Pickering proposed in 1955 a new classification which was a two-way classification according to the kind and degree of hypertension: He attempted to differentiate hypertension qualitatively and quantitatively [8, 9]. High blood pressure with its consequences of cardiovascular hypertrophy constituted a disease of essential hypertension, which was a clinical entity [7]. He proposed that essential hypertension was dependent on inheritance and environment and defined secondary hypertension as hypertension occurring as a prominent symptom of a known disease.

In this chapter, I shall give an overview of the major studies on hypertension and present a new etiological classification.

Inheritance of Hypertension in Humans

Pickering's polygenic theory

The mode of hypertension inheritance in human was investigated in normotensive and hypertensive populations. Pickering reported that the frequency distribution curve of arterial blood pressure in population samples did not demonstrate a bimodality curve and thus concluded that separation of a disease of essential hypertension from the population was an artifact [8, 9]. He believed that

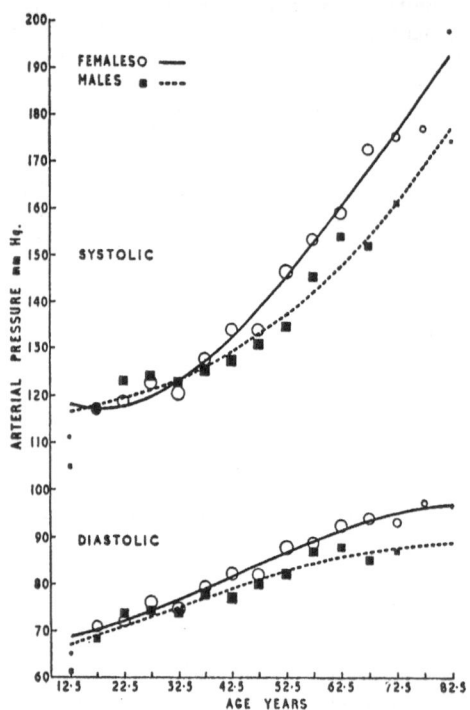

Fig. 1. Systolic and diastolic pressures for females (o) and males (■) for 5-year age-groups of a population sample. Blood pressure increases with age. From Hamilton et al. [10]

there was no unique cause of raised arterial blood pressure in essential hypertension. In 1964, Hamilton et al. pointed out that the differences between subjects
with essential hypertension were quantitative, not qualitative [10–12]. They
rejected that essential hypertension was a specific disease entity and proposed that
essential hypertension should be the name given to the syndrome of a group of
subjects with high blood pressure. Pickering suggested that the cause of essential
hypertension was polygenic and that the high blood pressure was the result of a
number of factors [9]. The three major factors were: first, age (Fig. 1); second,
inheritance; and third, environment. These factors operate to elevate arterial
blood pressure in essential hypertension.

    Albutt [5] and Frank [7] assumed that subjects with essential hypertension
differed qualitatively from subjects with normotension, that a sharp line could be
drawn between essential hypertension and normotension, and that essential
hypertension was a disease entity. Conversely, according to Pickering's concept
of essential hypertension, the difference between patients with essential hypertension and subjects with normotension is quantitative, not qualitative, and essential
hypertension is not a disease entity [13, 14]. Pickering concluded that blood
pressure was inherited by multifactorial or polygenic inheritance as a graded
character over the whole range from normotension to hypertension.

Platt's single gene hypothesis

The subjects (45–60 years of age) were selected from Pickering's subject [10]. The
frequency distribution curves of arterial pressure for their siblings showed a dip
at 150 mmHg systolic and 90 mmHg diastolic pressure (Fig. 2). The curves demonstrated a dividing line between normotension and hypertension [15, 16]. Platt
postulated that there were two populations. The blood pressure of the first group
rose steeply, but in the other group it was little affected by increasing age [15–18].

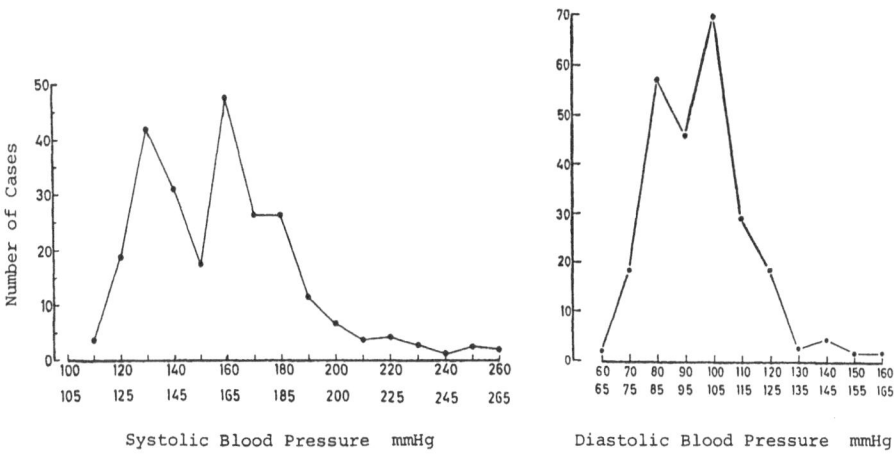

Fig. 2. The frequency distribution of systolic and diastolic blood pressures of siblings aged 45–60
years and of propositi aged 45–60 years with essential hypertension. The distribution curve is a
bimodality. From Platt [16]

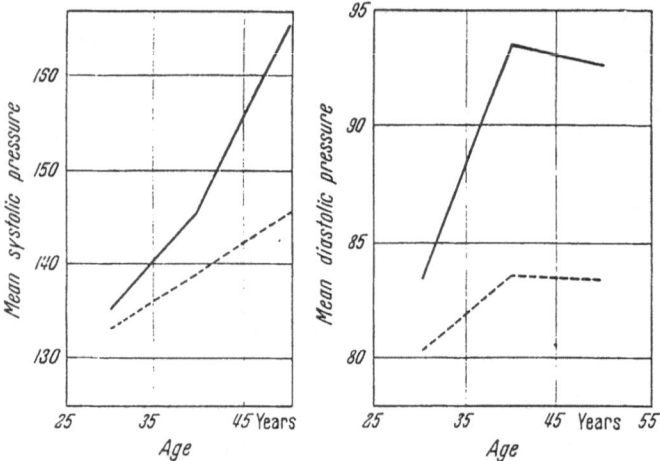

Fig. 3. The rise of blood pressure with age in the relatives of hypertensives (—) and normotensives (---). The increase is greater in relatives of hypertensives than in relatives of normotensives. From Platt [18]

From the blood pressures of employees of the Metropolitan Life Insurance Company of New York, Thomson in 1950 noted that the age of onset of diastolic hypertension was usually between 45 and 54 years and less common after that age, when hypertension was defined as a diastolic blood pressure of 90 mmHg or over [19]. Cruz-Coke in 1959 demonstrated that the rise in diastolic blood pressure per year was nearly 6 mmHg in those who developed hypertension between the ages of 30 and 49 and 3.5 mmHg after the age of 50, but in subjects with normotension the rise was less than 1 mmHg between the ages of 30 and 69 [20]. In 1959, Morrison and Morris showed from Pickering's data that the rise of pressure with age in the relatives of hypertensives was greater than that in the relatives of normotensives (Fig. 3) [21]. They suggested that the different rates of rise in blood pressure depended on genetic rather than environmental factors.

Evidence that there were two populations, normotensive and hypertensive, was very strong indeed and suggested that essential hypertension was the manifestation of a single gene inherited as a Mendelian dominant [15–21]. Platt suggested that there was single-gene inheritance in essential hypertension.

Genetic Hypertension in Rats

Dahl salt-hypertensive rats

Dahl et al. observed in 1962 that some rats remained normotensive despite the fact that they were fed chronically large amounts of salt (containing 11% salt in the diet) [22]. They pointed out that some animals never developed hypertension after the high-salt diet whereas a few became hypertensive. Dahl et al. reasoned that if the sensitivity to salt as a cause of hypertension was genetically controlled, it should be possible to separate two strains consisting of a group which developed hypertension from excess salt intake and the other which did not. A salt-hypertensive strain was obtained by the selective inbreeding of salt-hypertension rats; the salt-normotensive strain was developed by selective inbreeding of salt-normotension rats. The animals derived from the parents with salt hypertension and subsequent two generations were labeled S_1, S_2, and S_3, respectively. The animals derived from parents with normotension despite excess salt ingestion and subsequent two generations were labeled R_1, R_2, and R_3. The blood pressure response to salt intake differed between salt-sensitive S_3 and salt-resistance R_3 rats. None of the 39 R_3 rats showed hypertension with high-salt feeding. Neither the presence nor absence of excess dietary salt affected the blood pressure of the R_3 rats. Whereas 49 of the 60 S_3 rats were hypertensive with the high-salt diet. The mean systolic blood pressure of salt-fed S_3 males was 180 mmHg. When the S_3 rats were maintained on the control diet, hypertension did not develop. These S strain rats might have the gene to develop hypertension under environmental conditions of high-salt intake. A high-salt diet unmasked the hypertension gene and caused hypertension to develop in Dahl S rats.

By demonstrating two strains of rats, S and R, differing from one another in their susceptibility to excess salt ingestion, Dahl et al. concluded that the sensitivity of pressor response to excess salt intake was genetically transmitted in S and R rats (Fig. 4) [22].

Smirk genetically hypertensive rats
Smirk and Hall [23] and Phelan and Smirk [24] developed a colony of genetic hypertensive (GH) rats by breeding rats with above-average blood pressure. The average blood pressure of the rats, which consisted of some hypertensive and some normotensive rats, was 132 mmHg. In 1958, the rats of the Otago hypertensive colony had average systolic blood pressures of approximately 140 mmHg, and the incidence of hypertension was 30%.

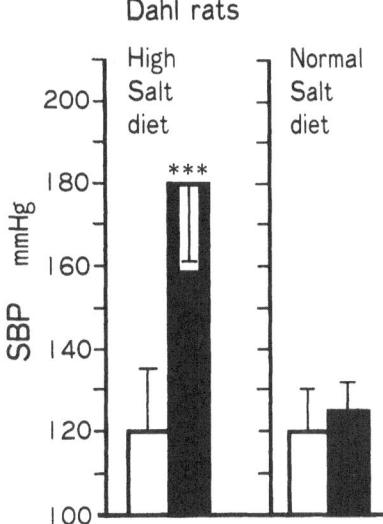

Fig. 4. Blood pressure of Dahl salt-sensitive (S) (■) and salt-resistant (R) (□) rats with high-salt feeding (*left*) and control-diet feeding (*right*). The high salt-fed S_3 rats developed hypertension, but the high salt-fed R_3 rats did not. The control diet-fed S_3 rats and R_3 rats did not develop hypertension. From Dahl et al. [22]

In 1983, the GH rats were in their 59th generation of selective inbreeding at the Wellcome Medical Research Institute, Department of Medicine, University of Otago [25, 26]. The blood pressure increased with age in both normotensive and GH rats, but the rate of increase was greater in GH than in normotensive rats [25]. The blood pressure of GH rats was in the range of 152–220 mmHg with an average of 170 mmHg; that of the normotensive rats was in the range of 115–137 mmHg with an average of 130 mmHg. A number of modified diets, e.g., low-salt and high-salt diets, did not affect the blood pressure in GH rats [26]. It was concluded that GH rats develop hypertension without any special dietary requirements [26].

Hypertension in the GH rats was inherited from parents to offspring. The inheritance mode of high blood pressure could be revealed by crossbreeding. GH rats were reciprocally mated with rats from another pure line. The gene analysis for blood pressure in the offspring showed that the inheritance of hypertension was additive. The number of effective genetic factors was at least five. Simpson and Phelan concluded that blood pressure in GH rats was under the control of a large number of genes possesing individual small effects [26].

Aoki spontaneously hypertensive rats
Now, there are three well-known hypertension strains of rats—Smirk GH, Dahl salt hypertension, and Aoki spontaneously hypertensive rats (SHR). Aoki bred a type of SHR by mating a male SHR with a normotensive female rat. All rats obtained from offspring of SHR developed hypertension after the F_3 generation (see Aoki, Discovery of the spontaneously hypertensive rat, this volume). The average blood pressure of F_4 SHR was 136, 188, and 197 mmHg at 5, 15, and 25 weeks of age in males, and 133, 178, and 189 mmHg in females, respectively (Fig. 5) [27].

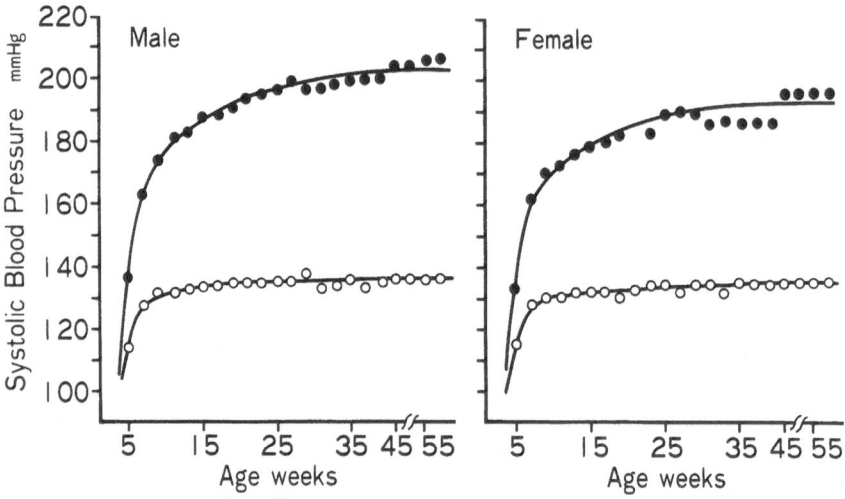

Fig. 5. The rise in blood pressure with age in F_4 of SHR (-•-) ($n = 30$ males and $n = 19$ females at 30 weeks of age) and normotensive rats (-o-) ($n = 24$ males and $n = 27$ females). The rise in SHR is greater than in normotensive rats. After Okamoto and Aoki [27]

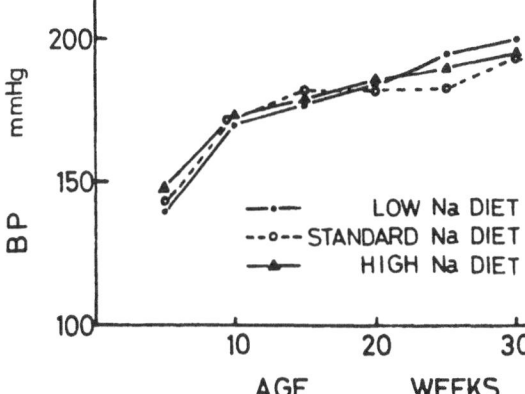

Fig. 6. Effects of salt intake on blood pressure. The low-salt (0.079% sodium) (-•-), standard-salt (0.276%) (--o--), and high-salt (2.76%) (-▲-) diet-fed SHR developed hypertension. From Aoki et al. [28]

SHR showed a striking increase in blood pressure at the age of 5–15 weeks. The rate of the rise in blood pressure was greater in SHR which showed a similar increase to GH rats, than in normotensive Wistar rats.

The effects of low-sodium (0.079% sodium), standard-sodium (0.0276%), and high-sodium (2.76%) diets on blood pressure were investigated in F_4 SHR. The blood pressure was 200, 192, and 193 mmHg in low-, standard-, and high-sodium diets in SHR, respectively, at the 25th week of the diet experiment. There was no difference in blood pressure with the different sodium diets. These results indicated that hypertension in SHR was independent of sodium intake (Fig. 6) [28].

Random brother-sister inbreeding resulted in a uniform population of SHR, and there was no significant difference in average blood pressure between F_2, F_3, F_4 SHR in NIH [29]. The result of F_1 hybrid crosses between normotensive and hypertensive rats showed that there was no significant difference between the blood pressures of the progeny of the two reciprocal crosses. The average blood pressure of the groups of F_1 hybrids was significantly lower than that of SHR, being intermediate between the values of normotensive and hypertensive rats [29]. The failure to obtain a uniform population of either hypertensive or normotensive rats in the F_1 hybrid group does not fit with a simple (dominant or recessive) form of Mendelian inheritance. The possibility of an incomplete dominant form of hypertension inheritance in SHR has been demonstrated. Louis et al. [29] concluded that the general decrease in the severity of hypertension in the hybrid progeny of SHR and normotensive rats favors a polygenic inheritance similar to the mode of inheritance suggested by Pickering for essential hypertension in man, and hypertension was inherited by both males and females.

The genetic determination of blood pressure was analyzed by the method of breeding three normotensive strains of rats with SHR [30]. The average blood pressure in F_1 hybrids was intermediate between those of the two parents, SHR and Wistar-Imamichi (WI) rats. The F_2 hybrids showed an intermediate blood pressure level between those of the parent strains. The means of the F_2 and backcross generations were lower than the expected values on an assumption of completely additive inheritance. There was no evidence either for bimodality of blood pressure distribution or backcross generations for the $1:2:1$ ratio in normotension, the intermediate level of blood pressure between WI rats and SHR, and hypertension in the F_2 generation. The degrees of genetic determination were calculated from the variance of the F_1 and F_2 generations. The values showed that this trait had a heritable character. The genetic determination of blood pressure in SHR was approximately 70% [30].

By cross-analysis between SHR and normotensive Wistar-Kyoto (WKY) rats, the F_1 hybrids showed an intermediate blood pressure level between SHR and WKY rats [30]. The degree of genetic determination derived from the variances of the F_1 and F_2 was 90%. These data indicated that hypertension was highly heritable and that the blood pressure was determined mostly by genetic factors. The calculated dominant ratio was higher than 90%. Tanase et al. suggested from these results that there was the possibility of dominant inheritance of major hypertension genes [30].

The value of the dominant ratio from the genetic parameters was calculated form the variances of their crosses. The value showed that dominance existed but was incomplete. If the inheritance was unconformable, the minimum number of the major hypertension genes would be three [30].

The blood pressure of Nagaoka stroke-prone SHR (Nagaoka SHRSP) (A_3) was significantly higher than that of stroke-resistant SHR (Nagaoka SHRSR) (C), which was suggestive of the positive correlation between high blood pressure and the incidence of cerebrovascular lesions [31]. The average blood pressure of the F_1 breeding with A_3 and C was roughly intermediate between both parental SHR. In addition, the blood pressure in the F_2 obtained by F_1 mated with F_1 showed a continuous distribution within the range of blood pressure in A_3 and C. The same kind of genetic data were demonstrated in the hybrid groups between A_3 and WKY rats. The F_1 was intermediate in blood pressure level between the levels of the parents, and the F_2 ranged from a blood pressure as high as that of A_3 to that of WKY rats (Figs. 7, 8). These results seem to be compatible with the findings by Tanase et al. [30], who indicated that three major genes transmit the hypertension in SHR [31].

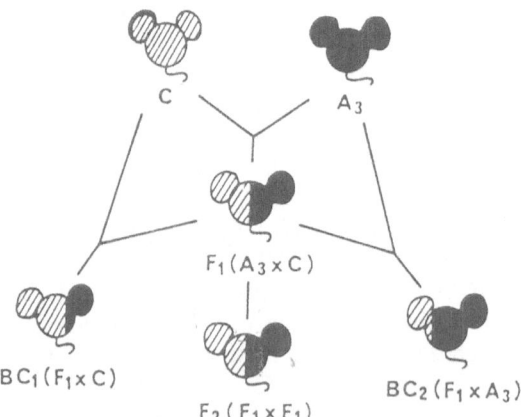

Fig. 7. Mating procedure between Nagaoka stroke-prone SHR (A_3) and stroke-resistant SHR (C). Theoretical gene constitution in each groups is represented. From Nagaoka et al. [31]

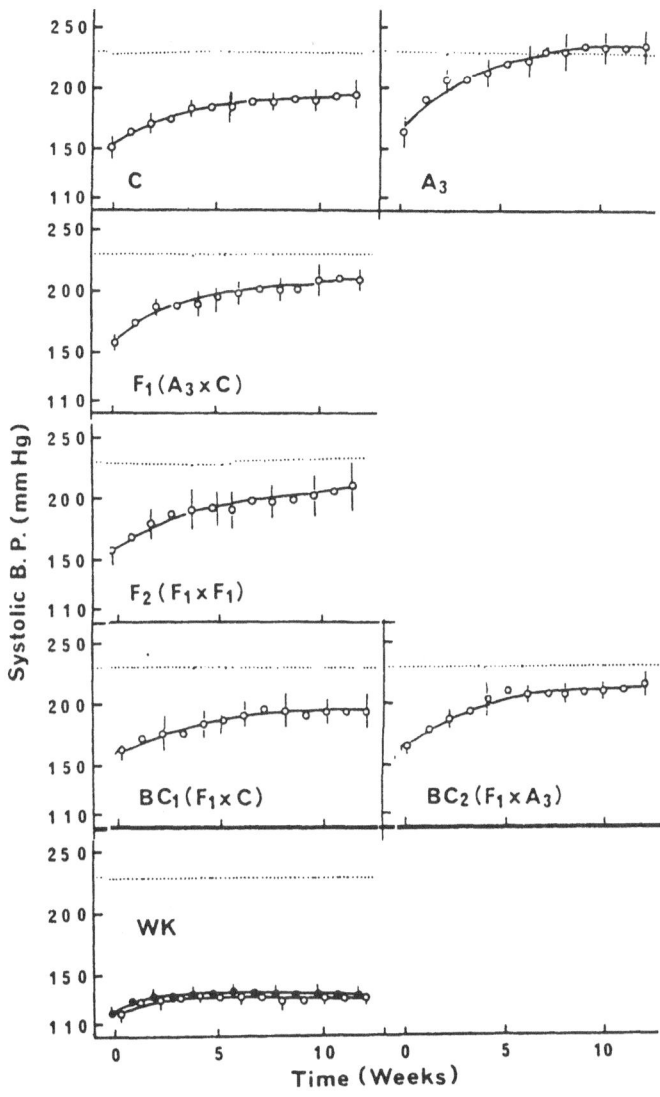

Fig. 8. Systolic blood pressure in Nagaoka stroke-prone SHR (A_3), stroke-resistant SHR (C), F_1, F_2, BC_1, BC_2, and Wistar-Kyoto normotensive rats (WK). The average blood pressure of the F_1 from A_3 bred with C was roughly intermediate between both parent SHR. From Nagaoka et al. [31]

Etiological Classification of Hypertension

The blood pressure in the general population including subjects both with nor-motension and hypertension is distributed in a normal Gaussian fashion. From this distribution, Pickering suggested that a division into hypertension and nor-motension was artificial and that there was qualitative difference between the two groups [8, 9]. If there is a lack of qualitative difference, there will be a practical and therapeutic need to distinguish hypertension from normotension.

Hypertension is divided into two major types—essential (primary, arterial) hypertension and secondary [7, 8]. We consider "essential hypertension" to be a disease entity in which hypertension is inherited and caused by abnormal contraction of the vascular smooth muscle of the arteries [32–34]. The abnormal contraction leads to an increase in blood pressure (see Aoki, Calcium membrane theory of essential hypertension, this volume) [32–34]. The term "secondary hypertension" is used when hypertension is associated with a disease or a factor which is known to increase blood pressure, such as renal disease or excessive salt intake. Thus, "secondary" does not imply that the cause or the exact mechanism of the elevation of blood pressure is known [8, 9, 14, 32–34].

The success of therapy and prevention of hypertension depends on a clear understanding of the etiological mechanisms, clinical manifestations, and a simple classification. We now have three qualitative and genetically different hypertension models in animals: Major gene hypertension of Aoki SHR [27–35], environment hypertension with accessory (satellite) gene of Dahl salt-sensitive rats [22], and disease hypertension of Goldblatt renal hypertension [36]. From genetic or nongenetic and environment or nonenvironment hypertension in animals, and Pickering's polygenic theory or Platt's single-gene hypothesis in human hypertension, I have proposed an etiological classification of hypertension as follows [34]. Systemic arterial hypertension is divided into three types: (1) Type 1, essential (major gene) hypertension; (2) type 2, environment (accessory gene) hypertension; and (3) type 3, disease (underlying disease, nongene) hypertension.

Essential (major gene) hypertension

Essential (major gene, arterial) hypertension is inherited, whereby the blood pressure is raised without any specific environmental factors. The blood pressure in essential hypertension increases strikingly over the age of 20–50 years, and hypertensive cardiovascular diseases are associated as a consequence of the hypertension. Essential hypertension can be divided into three groups with one, two, and three major hypertension genes, corresponding to mild, moderate, and severe hypertension. I shall present a theoretical natural history of increasing blood pressure in the three groups of essential hypertension (Fig. 9).

For the mechanism of development, an increase in calcium concentration in the cytosol of arterial smooth muscle may be caused in this type of hypertension. The increase in calcium concentration may be induced by abnormal proteins which are located in both the cell membrane and sarcoplasmic reticulum membrane. The proteins are located in the arterial smooth muscle. The proteins may have a causal relationship to the abnormalities of the calcium channels, calcium uptake sites, and calcium binding sites and may induce abnormal depolarization in the cell membrane and Ca^{2+} release from the sarcoplasmic reticulum, resulting in an excess increase in the concentration of cytosol calcium. The increase in intracellular calcium leads to an enhanced contraction, known as "overcoupling", and "incomplete relaxation" of the arterial smooth muscle, which reduces the lumen of the arterial vessel [32–35]. The reduction of the lumen results in an elevation of the total peripheral vascular resistance, which causes a rise in

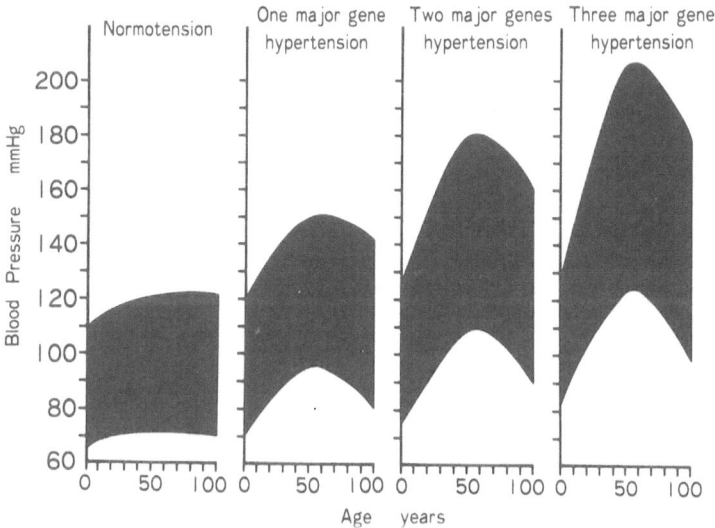

Fig. 9. Theoretical blood pressure is represented in nonhypertension gene normotension (*normotension*) and essential hypertension with one to three major hypertension genes. The rate of increase in blood pressure with age in subjects with essential hypertension is greater than that in subjects with normotension. The blood pressure of the three genes hypertension is higher than that of the two genes hypertension. The blood pressure of two genes hypertension is higher than that of the one gene hypertension

systemic arterial blood pressure and hypertension develops and persists. The molecular and cellular mechanism of high blood pressure in hypertension is dealt with elsewhere in this volume (Aoki, Calcium membrane theory of essential hypertension).

Environment (accessory gene) hypertension
In this type, environmental factors interacting with an accessory hypertension gene cause hypertension to develop. This hypertension is defined as environment (accessory gene) hypertension and is inherited (Table 1) [34]. There are many kinds of environment hypertension, such as salt, obesity, low-exercise, excessive exercise, mental stress, physical stress, anxiety, and doctor-induced hypertension [34]. Of these types, salt hypertension is well defined [22].

Salt hypertension develops in subjects with an accessory hypertension gene who are susceptible to the hypertensive effect of excess salt intake but not in subjects lacking the accessory gene. In salt hypertension, diminution of salt intake to the appropriate level decreases blood pressure [34]. Obesity hypertension is induced by overweight in subjects with an accessory hypertension gene who are susceptible to the pressor effect of obesity but not in subjects without the accessory gene [34]. In obesity hypertension, reduction to a desirable weight with the loss of body fat decreases the blood pressure to a normal level. The reduction of fat tissue in the wall of arterial vessel may widen the lumen of the arterial vessel, which reduces the total peripheral vascular resistance and decreases blood pressure.

Table 1. Etiological classification of hypertension (after Aoki [34])

Disease	Cause	Origin	Clinical diagnosis and abnormalities	Animal models
Type 1	Essential (primary) hypertension	Major gene inheritance	Arterial vessel	Arterial or essential hypertension, abnormality of arterial vessel, arterial smooth muscle, membrane calcium transport	Smirk GH rat, Aoki SHR
Type 2	Environmental (secondary) hypertension	Environment with accessory gene inheritance	Environment	Salt (excess intake) hypertension, obesity hypertension, low-exercise hypertension, excess-exercise hypertension, excess mental stress hypertension, excess physical stress hypertension, anxiety hypertension, doctor-induced hypertension	Dahl salt-hypertensive rat
Type 3	Underlying disease (secondary) hypertension	Underlying disease	Underlying disease		
			Endocrine	Primary aldosteronism, pheochromocytoma, Cushing's syndrome, hyperthyroidism, iatrogenic hypertension	
			Renal	Renal parenchymal disease, renovascular hypertension, primary reninism	Goldblatt hypertension
			Nervous	Sympathetic nerve hypertension, para-sympathetic nerve hypertension, cerebral nerve hypertension, neurogenic hypertension	
			Connective tissue	Arteriosclerotic hypertension	
			Drug	Liquorice hypertension, contraceptive hypertension, steroid hypertension	DOCA-salt hypertension
			Other	Hematological hypertension, immunological hypertension	

GH genetically hypertensive, *SHR* spontaneously hypertensive rats, *DOCA* deoxycorticosterone acetate.

Disease (nongene) hypertension

Disease (nongene, disease-induced) hypertension is defined as high blood pressure resulting from some known or unknown disease (Table 1). This type of hypertension is independent of any hypertension genes [34]. Disease hypertension is caused by different types of disease including renal, endocrine, nervous, and aortic valve diseases [36]. Renal parenchymal, renin-secreting tumor, primary aldosteronism, pheochromocytoma hypertension, etc. are classified in disease hypertension (Table 1). The causes and mechanisms of the blood pressure increase completely differ from one kind of disease hypertension to an other. For example, the clinical features of pheochromocytoma are due to an excessive production of catecholamines. Norepinephrine, which is secreted from the tumor, acts on the cell membrane of arterial smooth muscle to promote calcium influx and release. The excessive influx of calcium and its release increase the concentration of calcium in the cytosol, leading to "over-coupling" and an excessive contraction of the arterial smooth muscle and then narrowing of the lumen. The narrowing of the arterial lumen elevates the total peripheral vascular resistance, which causes hypertension [34]. The hypertension mechanism of primary aldosteronism is most likely related to sodium retention and volume expansion, although the mechanism remains unexplained [37].

Conclusion

An etiological classification of three types of hypertension—essential (major gene), environment (accessory gene), and disease (nongene) hypertension— is presented (Table 1). This classification will be applied in clinical cases of hypertension and may help in practical and theorteical research on the mechamism, therapy, and prevention of hypertension.

References

1. Bright R (1827) Reports of Medical Cases, Selected with a View of Illustrating the Symptoms and Cure of Diseases by a Reference to Morbid Anatomy. Longman, London
2. Gull WW, Sutton HG (1872) On the pathology of the morbid state commonly called chronic Bright's disease with contracted kidny; "Arterio-capillary fibrosis". Med-chir Trans 55:273
3. Bash S von (1893) Ueber latente Arteriosclerose und deren Beziehung zu Fettleibigkeit, Herzerkrankungen und anderen Begleiterscheinungen. Urban & Schwartzenberg, Viena
4. Huchard H (1889) Maladies du Coeur et des Vaisseaux. Doin, Paris
5. Allbutt TC (1895) Senile plethora or high arterial pressure in elderly persons. Trans Hunter Soc 77:38
6. Albutt TC (1915) Diseases of the Arteries, Including Angina Pectoris. Macmillian, London
7. Frank E (1911) Bestehen Beziehungen zwischen chromaffinem System und der chronischen Hypertonie des Menschen? Ein kritischer Beitrag zu der Lehre von der physio-pathologischen Bedeutung des Adrenalines. Dtsch Arch klin Med 103:397
8. Pickering GW (1955) The classification of hypertension. In: High Blood Pressure. Grune & Stratton, New York/J & A Churchill, London, pp 122–130
9. Pickering GW (1961) The aetiology of essential hypertension, the genetic factor. In: The nature of essential hypertension. J & A Churchill, London, pp 22–57

10. Hamilton M, Pickering GW, Roberts JAF, Sowry GSC (1954) The aetiology of essential hypertension. 1. The arterial pressure in the general population. Clin Sci 13:11–35
11. Hamilton M, Pickering GW, Roberts JAF, Sowry GSC (1954) The aetiology of essential hypertension. 2. Scores for arterial blood pressures adjusted for differences in age and sex. Clin Sci 13:37–49
12. Hamilton M, Pickering GW, Roberts JAF, Sowry GSC (1954) The aetiology of essential hypertension. 4. The role of inheritance. Clin Sci 13:273–304
13. Oldham PD, Pickering GW, Roberts JAF, Sowry GSC (1960) The nature of essential hypertension. Lancet I:1085
14. Pickering GW (1960) Inheritance of high blood pressure. In: Bock KD, Cottier PT (eds) Essential Hypertension. Springer-Verlag, Berlin, pp 30–38
15. Platt R (1947) Heredity in hypertension. Quart J Med NS 16:111
16. Platt R (1959) The nature of essential hypertension. Lancet II:55–57
17. Platt R (1959) The nature of essential hypertension. Lancet I:1189–1190
18. Platt R (1960) The nature of essential hypertension. In: Bock KD, Cottier PT (eds) Essential Hypertension. Springer-Verlag, Berlin, pp 39–44
19. Thomson KJ (1950) Proceedings of the 38th Annual Meeting of the Medical Section of the American Life Convention
20. Curz-Coke R (1959) The nature of essential hypertension. Lancet II:853
21. Morrison SL, Morris JN (1959) Epidemiological observations on high blood-pressure without evident cause. Lancet II:864–870
22. Dahl LK, Heine M, Tassinari L (1962) Effects of chronic excess salt ingestion. Evidence that genetic factors play an important role in susceptibility of experimental hypertension. J Exper Med 115:1173–1190
23. Smirk FH, Hall WH (1958) Inherited hypertension in rats. Nature 182:727–728
24. Phelan EL, Smirk FH (1960) Cardiac hypertrophy in genetically hypertensive rats. J Path Bact 80:445–448
25. Jones DR, Dowd DA (1970) Development of elevated blood pressure in young genetically hypertensive rats. Life Sciences 9 (I):247–250
26. Simpson FO, Phelan EL (1984) Hypertension in the genetically hypertensive strain. In: De Jong W (ed) Experimental and genetic models of hypertension. Handbook of Hypertension, vol 4. Elesevire, Amsterdam, pp 200–223
27. Okamoto K. Aoki K (1963) Development of a strain of spontaneously hypertensive rats. Jpn Circ J 27:282–293
28. Aoki K, Yamori Y, Ooshima A, Okamoto K (1972) Effects of high or low sodium intake in spontaneously hypertensive rats. Jpn Circ J 36:539–545
29. Louis WJ, Tabei R, Sjoerdsma A, Spector S (1969) Inheritance of high blood-pressure in the spontaneously hypertensive rat. Lancet I:1035–1036
30. Tanase H, Suzuki Y, Ooshima A, Yamori Y, Okamoto K (1970) Genetic analysis of blood pressure in spontaneously hypertensive rats. Jpn Circ J 34:1197–1212
31. Nagaoka A, Iwatsuka H, Suzuki Z, Okamoto K (1976) Genetic predisposition to stroke in spontaneously hypertensive rats. Am J Physiol 230:1354–1359
32. Aoki K (1982) Hypertensiology, Essential and Secondary Hypertension, Concepts, Nature, Diagnosis, and Treatment (in Japanese). Shinkoh Igaku Shuppan, Tokyo, pp 4–51
33. Aoki K, Kondo S, Mochizumi A, Sato K, Yoshida T, Kato S, Kato K (1978) Ca^{2+}-antagonist therapy for hypertension in combination with beta-blockade: A new concept of essential hypertension. In: Yamori Y, Lovenberg W, Freis ED (eds) Prophylactic Approach to Hypertensive Diseases. Raven Press, New York, pp 377–386
34. Aoki K (1985) Essential hypertension and secondary hypertension in humans and rats. Asian Med J 28:529–548
35. Aoki K, Ikeda N, Yamashita K, Tazumi K, Sato I, Hotta K (1974) Cardiovascular contraction in spontaneously hypertensive rat: Ca^{2+} interaction of myofibrils and subcellular membrane of heart and arterial smooth muscle. Jpn Circ J 38:1115–1121
36. Goldblatt H, Lynch J, Hanzal RF, Summercille WW (1934) Studies on experimental hypertension. J Exp Med 59:347–379
37. Conn JW (1955) Primary aldosteronism. J Lab Clin Med 45:661–664

Calcium Mechanism
in the Spontaneously Hypertensive Rat

Membrane Ca^{2+} Permeability and Calcium Antagonistic Effects in Resistance Vessels of Spontaneously Hypertensive Rats

C. Cauvin and C. van Breemen

Department of Pharmacology, University of Miami, Shool of Medicine, Miami, FL 33101, USA

Summary. This study compares resting and stimulated ^{45}Ca entry in vitro in mesenteric resistance vessels (MRV) of Wistar-Kyoto (WKY) rats and spontaneously hypertensive rats (SHR). The stimulating agent used was norepinephrine (NE). The results show clearly that Ca^{2+} influx into smooth muscle cells from resistance vessels was much higher in the SHR than in the WKY rats. Potential sensitive Ca^{2+} channels (PSC) and receptor-operated Ca^{2+} channels (ROC) may possibly be involved, although there is as yet no evidence for the existence of ROC in MRV in the rat. Further investigations are now needed to establish whether the enhanced stimulated Ca^{2+} entry is related causally to increased peripheral resistance, i.e., whether it occurs in vivo and what temporal relation it has to the onset of hypertension. Mechanistically, it remains to be established which aspect of channel function is involved in the enhanced Ca^{2+} entry, and how this is connected with cation stabilization of smooth muscle plasmalemmae in hypertensive individuals.

Key words: Arterial hypertension––Ca entry into smooth muscle—Peripheral resistance—Norepinephrine—Spontaneously hypertensive rat

Ca antagonists have proven to be effective in the treatment of essential hypertension [1, 2]. The mechanism of this antihypertensive effect is related to dilation of resistance vessels due to inhibition of stimulated Ca entry into smooth muscle cells [3]. These observations lead to the postulate that the excessive peripheral resistance in hypertensive patients results in part from increased Ca^{2+} entry into the smooth muscle cells of resistance vessels [4]. On the other hand, the excessively high peripheral resistance might be due to other causes, such as structural changes [5], in which case the beneficial effects of the Ca antagonists would be due to inhibition of the physiological component of tension, thereby relieving the extra resistance contributed by the physiological component of arterial resistance to flow.

Bohr and Webb have postulated that the Ca binding to smooth muscle cell membranes is deficient in hypertension, resulting in decreased membrane stabilization with increased permeability to cations and increased sensitivity to vasoactive agents [4]. If this theory is correct, we might ask which of the Ca entry mechanisms is most affected in hypertension. Evidence has been presented for four different Ca^{2+} entry mechanisms: (1) The Ca^{2+} leak (observed in the absence of stimulation and independent of intracellular Na^+), an inherent property of all biological membranes composed of phospholipids, cholesterol, and proteins. (2) Potential-sensitive Ca^{2+} channels (PSC), which are primarily activated by membrane depolarization [6, 7]. Recent results from patch clamp current measurements indicate that smooth muscle membranes contain several types of PSC characterized by different inactivation rates [8, 9]. (3) Receptor-operated Ca^{2+} channels (ROC), which are activated by agonists like norepinephrine (NE), histamine, angiotensin, etc., combining with their respective receptor proteins embedded in the plasmalemma [6, 7]. Recent evidence has indicated that ROC may, in addition, allow permeation of other cations and thus have a low selectivity for Ca^{2+} [10]. (4) Stretch-activated Ca^{2+} channels, which are thought to be activated by intraluminal pressure. Although little direct evidence for these channels exists, it is clear that myogenic tone is dependent on extracellular Ca^{2+} and appears to have a pattern of sensitivity to Ca entry blockers which seems to be different from that observed for the leak, PSC, or ROC [11].

The activating and relaxing mechanisms are far from being homogeneous throughout the arterial tree. Marked regional differences have been observed in receptor densities, nervous innervation, intracellular Ca^{2+} sources for activation, myogenic tone, and nearly every other parameter that has been studied. For this reason, we thought it necessary to study Ca entry and sensitivity to Ca antagonists in the resistance vessels. Furthermore, since the Aoki spontaneously hypertensive rat (SHR) is considered to be a good model for human essential hypertension [12], we compared resting and stimulated ^{45}Ca entry in mesenteric resistance vessels in SHR with that in WKY rats.

Materials and Methods

Contraction measurements

Rats were stunned, exsanguinated, and the entire mesentery removed and placed in a warmed, oxygenated (100% O_2) solution (PSS) of the following composition (in mM): NaCl, 140; MgCl, 1; $CaCl_2$, 1.5; KCl, 4.6; dextrose, 10; Hepes buffer, 5; the pH was 7.4. The dissection bath and tissue bath were maintained at 37°C and oxygenated.

The dissection and mounting of the vessels (as adapted from Mulvany and Halpern [13]) has been described previously [14]. Briefly, segments (2 mm long) of fourth or fifth generation vessels of the mesenteric artery were threaded onto two 40-μm parallel wires, which were attached under tension to two support arms in a tissue bath. One of the arms was mounted on a displacement device, and the other to an isometric force transducer (U-gage; Shinkoh, Inc.) The optimum passive tension for NE activation of the vessels was determined in preliminary studies to be 20 mg/mm vessel length. The internal diameter of the vessel that corresponded to this passive tension was determined by using a calibrated micrometer eye-piece attached to the dissecting microscope.

Concentration-response curves for NE were obtained by cumulative addition of the agent to the bathing medium. The effects of NE on phasic and tonic contractions were determined. All contractions are expressed as percentage of maximum steady state NE contraction for the individual vessel, and EC_{50} were obtained graphically. Concentration-response curves for NE were compared using analysis of variance. When significant differences were indicated, Student's t-tests were performed to compare responses to individual concentrations ($P <$ 0.05 was considered significant). Alterations that were found in contractions with NE in the SHR vessels were further examined for mechanisms of alteration using ^{45}Ca fluxes. These measurements were normalized for tissue wet weight and cell volume; therefore, any changes in ^{45}Ca fluxes in SHR vessels should be independent of changes in the vascular geometry. For contraction and ^{45}Ca flux studies (see below), NE activation was induced in the presence of propranolol (3×10^{-6} M to eliminate β-receptor effects by NE). In one set of experiments, cocaine (3×10^{-6} M) was used to inhibit the neuronal uptake of NE, and in another set 3×10^{-7} M desipramine was used.

Concentration—response curves were also obtained for the inhibitory effects of the dihydropyridine Ca^{2+} antagonists nisoldipine and PN200–110. These were obtained by first preincubating the vessels in the desired concentration of Ca^{2+} antagonist, then reexposing them to the activating agent. For these studies, 10^{-4} M NE and 80 mM K^{+} were used to activate the tissues under control conditions (i.e., in PSS alone) and then in the presence of increasing Ca^{2+} antagonist concentrations.

^{45}Ca fluxes

Net Ca content. In order to determine the net content of tissue Ca, tissues were labeled for 2.5 in ^{45}Ca^{2+}-PSS ($2–5 \times 10^{-6}$ cpm/ml), and then the efflux of the ^{45}Ca from the tissues in ice-cold, vigorously bubbled O Ca^{2+} 2 mM EGTA was monitored every 5 min for 50 min. The tissues were then blotted gently, weighed to 0.001 mg (Metler microbalance), and placed in 5 mM ethylenediamine tetraacetic acid (EDTA) overnight prior to addition of scintillation fluid and counting (Tracor analytical model 43). Samples of ^{45}Ca loading media and blanks were also counted, so that cell Ca^{2+} could be calculated as: [(CPM sample − background)/tissue weight] × [medium [Ca]/(medium cpm-background)]. When the decay in Ca content became monoexponential, the curve was extrapolated back to time zero to determine the orginal cellular Ca content. In SHR and WKY vessels, the decay of tissue Ca content in Ca^{2+}-free solution became monoexponential in 20 min. This time was, therefore, used as a quench or wash time to remove extracellular ^{45}Ca in subsequent ^{45}Ca-uptake experiments.

Undirectional influx. The initial ^{45}Ca uptake in SHR and WKY mesenteric resistance vessels (MRV) was found to be linear up to to 3 min, suggesting that measurement of the initial rate of ^{45}Ca uptake provides an estimate of the unidirectional ^{45}Ca influx rate into these vascular smooth muscles. Therefore, unidirectional ^{45}Ca influx rate in MRV (two to three tissue samples from each of four to five rats per group) was studied by exposing them to control (PSS) and experimental media containing ^{45}Ca for 90 sec, then washing them for 20 min in ice-cold, vigorously bubbled Ca-free PSS containing 2 mM EGTA in order to remove extracellular ^{45}Ca^{2+}. The tissues were then processed as described above for determination of Ca content.

Efflux. Tissue samples (three to four per rat) were labeled in ^{45}Ca PSS for 2.5 h. The washout of ^{45}Ca was then monitored by passing the tissue samples through a

Table 1. Compartmental parameters of Ca exchange in MRV

No. of compartments		r	Size of compartment (μmol/l cells)	Rate constant (min^{-1})	$t_{1/2}$ (min)
^{45}Ca efflux					
WKY	2	0.822	2717 + 1130	0.74 + 0.34	0.94 + 0.43
			731 + 205	0.066 + 0.032	10.5 + 5.1
SHR	2	0.742	1460 + 686	1.41 + 0.30[a]	0.50 + 0.11
			493 + 90	0.059 + 0.024	11.7 + 4.76
^{45}Ca uptake					
WKY	1	0.888	451 + 30	0.11 + 0.029	6.3 + 1.7
SHR	1	0.723	333 + 39	0.083 + 0.033	8.3 + 3.3

Values given as means are indicated + 2 SEM
[a] Significant difference between SHR and WKY rats

series of tubes containing 1.5 ml O Ca^{2+} 2 mM EGTA at 37°C, moving the tissues from tube to tube at 1-min intervals for 10 min. Following washout, the tissues were blotted, weighed, and processed to measure residual label. The amount of ^{45}Ca in the tissue at any point during washout was calculated by adding in reverse fashion the label in the tissue and the ^{45}Ca in the series of washout tubes. The apparent rate constant of efflux (fraction of ^{45}Ca lost/min) during each efflux interval was calculated by dividing the amount of label lost during 1 min by the average tissue ^{45}Ca during that minute. To study intracellular Ca^{2+} release, NE (10^{-4} M) was added to the efflux media after 3 min. When an agonist induces release of intracellular Ca^{2+}, an increase in the ^{45}Ca efflux rate occurs [14].

Extracellular space. This was measured by the uptake of ^{14}C sorbitol during 15-min exposure, assuming that sorbitol is distributed only in the extracellular water. The extracellular space (ECS) was used to compute the Ca fluxes per liter of cells.

Drugs. The following drugs were used in this study: 1-norepinephrine bitartrate (Sigma), propranolol hydrochloride (Sigma), desipramine hydrochloride Sigma), and phentolamine hydrochloride (Ciba-Geigy).

Results

Table 1 shows the characteristics of ^{45}Ca exchange in MRV from SHR and WKY rats obtained from ^{45}Ca uptake and ^{45}Ca efflux under control steady state conditions. ^{45}Ca efflux exhibited two components—the fast one presumably due to loss of extracellular ^{45}Ca and the slow one due to cellular ^{45}Ca loss. The ^{45}Ca uptake was best fitted with one cellular Ca compartment, since the extracellular ^{45}Ca is removed during the cold quench. The cellular Ca compartment in SHR was somewhat smaller than that in WKY; both exchanged at 37°C with a rate constant of about 0.06 min^{-1} from efflux or 0.09 min^{-1} calculated from ^{45}Ca uptake. Considering the different methods of analysis used, the agreement between the values is quite good.

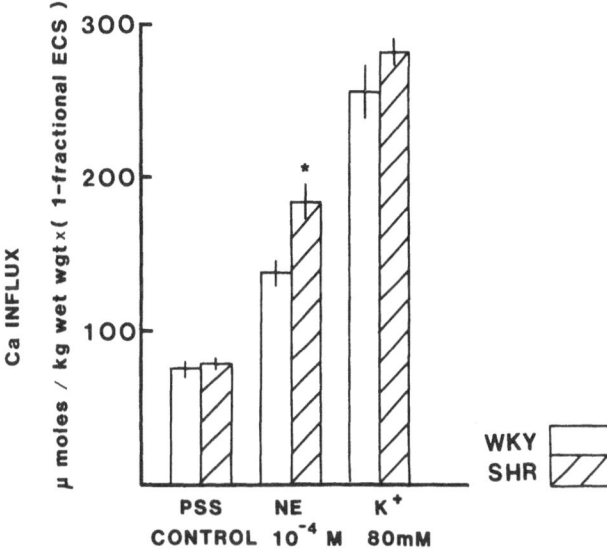

Fig. 1. ^{45}Ca influx was measured during 90-s incubation in the labeling solutions. Tissues were then washed in ice-cold Ca-free PSS containing $2mM$ EGTA for 20 min; the values for Ca content were then extrapolated to time zero using the rate constants obtained from previous washout curves. ^{45}Ca fluxes are normalized for wet weight corrected for differences in the extracellular space in the two strains as measured using ^{14}C = sorbital (WKR rats, 0.42 ± 0.04; SHR, 0.27 ± 0.02). *Asterisk* indicates significant difference between SHR and WKY rats ($P < 0.05$)

In order to measure Ca influx, we used a 90-exposure to ^{45}Ca since this provided a highly reproducible measurement at a time when ^{45}Ca uptake was only 10% equilibrated. To ensure further that comparisons of 90-s ^{45}Ca uptakes reflected differences in inward Ca permeability rather than differences in Ca extrusion, we also measured ^{45}Ca efflux rates under parallel conditions. The results of these experiments are illustrated in Fig. 1. It is clear that a maximal dose of NE stimulated a much greater Ca^{2+} influx in the MRV of SHR than it did in WKY rats. Both forms of activation (i.e., NE and 80 mM K$^+$) can also stimulate a transient increase in the rate of ^{45}Ca efflux, but no differences between SHR and WKY rats could be discerned in these latter measurements. The inhibitory effects of two dihydropyridine Ca antagonists, nisoldipine and PN 200–110, on high K$^+$ and NE-induced contractions are shown in Table 2. An interesting aspect of these results is that a tenfold higher dose of nisoldipine was required to cause 50% blockage of the MRV in the SHR than was needed for the same inhibition in the WKY rats. No difference in sensitivity was apparent for the high K$^+$-induced contractions.

Discussion

Arterial hypertension is a disease of complex etiology and it is unlikely that a defect in a single molecular mechanism can be identified as the cause of the

Table 2. Ca^{2+} antagonist sensitivities

	WKY rats	SHR
IC_{50} PN200-110		
vs. 10^{-4} M NE	3×10^{-9} molar	3×10^{-8} molar
vs. 80 mM K^+	2×10^{-8} molar	3×10^{-8} molar
IC_{50} nisoldipine		
vs. 10^{-4} M NE	2×10^{-10} molar	2×10^{-9} molar
vs. 80 mM K^+	1×10^{-8} molar	1×10^{-8} molar

IC_{50} concentration of Ca^{2+} antagonist which inhibited the tonic NE-induced or the phasic K^+-induced contraction by 50%

disease. However, since the arterial smooth muscle in the resistance vessels from hypertensive patients and rats can be relaxed, it is clear that defects must be present within the feedback systems which link systemic blood pressure and smooth muscle myofilaments. Bohr and Webb have postulated that a major defect in hypertensive patients is related directly to Ca^{2+} stabilization of arterial smooth muscle membranes [4]. One of several pieces of evidence cited to support this concept is that high concentrations of Ca^{2+} are effective in relaxing depolarization-induced contractions in arteries from normotensive rats but are much less effective in arteries obtained from hypertensive animals [15]. Mulvany and Nyborg [16] showed that tonic NE-induced contractions of mrvs in SHR occur at lower Ca^{2+} concentrations than in WKY rats, again suggesting that stimulated Ca entry may be enhanced.

Our data show conclusively that the NE-stimulated Ca^{2+} influx into smooth muscle cells from resistance vessels is much greater in hypertensive than in normotensive rats. We have recently presented evidence that rabbit MRV possess ROC and PSC [17]. No such evidence is as yet available for the rat; however, it would not be unreasonable to suggest that both ROC and PSC are involved in the increased Ca^{2+} influx. The questions which are now open to further research are: Is the enhanced stimulated Ca^{2+} entry causally related to increased peripheral resistance? In other words, does it occur in vivo and what is its temporal relation to the onset of hypertension? On a mechanistic level, we are left with the questions: Which aspect of channel function, i.e., number of channels, single-channel conductance or open probability, is involved in the enhanced Ca^{2+} entry and how are these related to different cation stabilization of the smooth muscle plasmalemmae in the hypertensive subject?

References

1. Klein W, Brandt D, Vrecko K, Harringer M (1983) Role of calcium antagonists in the treatment of essential hypertension. Circ Res 52 (Suppl I): 174–181
2. Buhler FR, Bolli P, Kiowski W, Muller FB, Erne P (1985) Calcium antagonists for identification of mechanisms and treatment in patients with essential hypertension. In: Fleckenstein A, van Breemen C, Gross R, Hoffmeister F (eds) Cardiovascular effects of dihydropyridine-type calcium antagonist and agonists. Springer-Verlag, Berlin

3. Von Witzleben H, Frey M, Keidel A, Fleckenstein A (1980) Normalization of blood pressure in spontaneously hypertensive rats by long term treatment with verapamil and nifedipine. Pflugers Arch Ges. (Suppl 384)
4. Bohr DR, Webb RC (1984) Vascular smooth muscle function and its changes in hypertension. Am J Med 77:3–17
5. Folkow B (1982) Physiological aspects of primary hypertension. Physiol Res 62:347–428
6. van Breemen C, Aaronson P, Loutzenhiser R (1979) Sodium-calcium interactions in mammalian smooth muscle. Pharmacol Rev 30:167–208
7. Bolton TB (1979) Mechanisms of action of transmitters and other substance on smooth muscle. Physiol Rev 1979 (3) 606–718
8. Bean BP, Sturek M, Pugo A, Hermsmeyer K (1985) Ca^{2+} channels in smooth muscle cells from mesenteric arteries. J Gen Physiol 86, 23a (abstract)
9. Friedman M, Kaczorowski C, Wandlen K, Katz G, Reuben JP (1985) Ca^{2+} and Ca^{2+} activated K$^+$ currents in cultured smooth muscle cells. Feb Proc (abstract)
10. Benham CD, Bolton TB, Lang RJ (1985) Acetylcholine activates an inward current in single mammalian smooth muscle cells. Nature 316:345–347
11. Bevan JA, JJ Laher I, Owen MP (1985) Calcium, dihydropyridines and resistance vessel tone in cardiovascular ATPase of dihydropyridine-type calcium antagonists and agonists. In: Fleckenstein A, van Breemen C, Gross R, Hoffmeister F (eds) Cardiovascular effects of dihydropyridine-type calcium antagonists and agonists. Springer-Verlag, Berlin
12 Trippodo NL, Frolich ED (1981) Similarities of genetic (spontaneous) hypertension in man and rat. Circ Res 48:309–319
13. Mulvany MJ, Halpern W (1977) Contractile properties of small arterial resistance vessels in spontaneously hypertensive and normotensive rats. Circ Res 41:19–26, 1977
14. Cauvin CA, Malik S (1984) Induction of Ca^{2+} influx and intracellular Ca^{2+} release in isolated rat aorta and mesenteric resistance vessels by activation of alpha-1 receptors. J Pharm Exp Ther 230:413–418
15. Hansen TR, Bohr DF (1975) Hypertension transmural pressure and vascular smooth muscle response in rats. Circ Res 36:590–598
16. Mulvany MJ, Nyborg N (1980) An increased calcium sensitivity of mesenteric resistance vessels in young and adult spontaneously hypertensive rats. Br J Pharmacol 71:585–596
17. Cauvin C, Lukeman S, Cameron J, Hwang O, van Breemen C (1985) Differences in norepinephrine activation and diltiazem inhibition of Ca^{2+} channels in isolated rabbit aorta and mesenteric resistance vessels. Circ Res 56:822–828

Actions of Calcium Agonists and Antagonists on Femoral Arteries of Spontaneously Hypertensive Rats

M. Asano[1], K. Aoki[2], and T. Matsuda[1]

Department of Pharmacology[1] and Second Department of Internal Medicine[2], Nagoya City University Medical School, Nagoya, 467 Japan

Summary. The Ca^{2+} agonist actions of Bay k 8644, a Ca^{2+} agonist, on femoral arteries from 6-week-old spontaneously hypertensive rats (SHR) were investigated and the data compared with findings in normotensive Wistar-Kyoto rats (WKY). The addition of Bay k 8644 produced a dose-dependent contraction in the SHR femoral artery with a pD_2 value of 8.55. The maximum contraction induced by this Ca^{2+} agonist ($1 \times 10^{-7} M$) was comparable with the maximum developed by either K^+ depolarization or alpha adrenoceptor stimulation. The SHR femoral artery was more sensitive to the contractile response to Bay k 8644 than to that to alpha adrenoceptor stimulation. Bay k 8644 was much less effective in eliciting the contractile effects on the WKY femoral artery. Two other Ca^{2+} agonists, CGP 28392 and YC-170, also exhibited greater contractions in SHR than in WKY arteries. Increased responsiveness to exogenously added K^+ was also observed in the SHR femoral artery. Contractions induced by alpha adrenoceptor stimulation were not different between SHR and WKY. Contractile responses of the SHR femoral artery to Bay k 8644 were antagonized competitively by both nifedipine ($pA_2 = 8.36$) and verapamil ($pA_2 = 6.77$), but noncompetitively by diltiazem. Nifedipine showed a typical competitive antagonism toward Ca^{2+}-induced contractions in K^+-depolarized strips of SHR femoral arteries with a pA_2 value of 9.42. These results suggest that: (1) The SHR femoral artery possesses increased Ca^{2+}-handling properties; (2) Bay k 8644 acts primarily on the same site, presumably the voltage-dependent Ca^{2+} channels at which both nifedipine and verapamil act; and (3) the state of the channel may differ between the stimulation of Bay k 8644 and K^+ depolarization.

Key words: Calcium agonist—Calcium antagonist—Femoral artery—Vasoconstriction—Spontaneously hypertensive rats—Voltage-dependent calcium channel

Differences from normotensive animals in responsiveness to a variety of vaso-constrictor and vasodilator agents exist in arterial smooth muscle isolated from hypertensive animals [reviews—1-5]. In particular, a number of studies have demonstrated that there may be an abnormality in the Ca^{2+}-handling property of arterial smooth muscle from spontaneously hypertensive rats (SHR). Holloway and Bohr [6] have demonstrated that femoral arterial strips isolated from various types of hypertension, including SHR, renal, and deoxycorticosterone acetate-hypertensive rats, are more sensitive to KCl (K^+) than normotensive rats. Since the response of vascular smooth muscle to K^+ is known to depend on the influx of extracellular Ca^+ [review—7], the increase in K^+ sensitivity may reflect the increased permeability of the plasma membrane to Ca^+. Several investigators have demonstrated the evidence for the plasma membrane of vascular smooth muscle from hypertensive animals including SHR being more sensitive to changes in extracellular Ca^{2+} concentration than normotensive animals [7–10]. Such abnormalities have been related to the initiation and maintenance of the elevated peripheral resistance associated with hypertension in the SHR.

Dihydropyridine Ca^{2+} antagonists, such as nifedipine, are useful pharmacological tools for investigating the role of Ca^{2+} influx in intact smooth and cardiac muscles, since these antagonists have been shown to block Ca^{2+} influx through the voltage-dependent Ca^{2+} channels [11–13]. Recently, a new dihydropyridine derivative, Bay k 8644 (Bay k) (methyl-1,4-dihydro-2,6-dimethyl-3-nitro-4-(2-trifluoromethylphenyl)-pyridine-5-carboxylate, Bayer AG, Wuppertal, Federal Republic of Germany) (Fig. 1), has been reported to have the opposite effects to those of nifedipine. Bay k 8644 has positive inotropic and vasoconstrictor effects [14, 15]. Recent studies have confirmed agonist actions of Bay k on the voltage-dependent Ca^{2+} influx in vascular smooth muscles [16–23]. Therefore, Bay k appears to serve as a Ca^{2+} agonist suitable for evaluating the Ca^{2+} sensitivity and Ca^{2+} reactivity of the tissue. A combination study of the dihydropyridine Ca^{2+} agonist (Bay k 8644) and antagonist (nifedipine) is needed to gain more insight into the nature of the regulatory mechanisms of Ca^{2+} influx in intact smooth muscles.

In the present study, we have examined the agonist actions of Bay k on the femoral arteries isolated from 6-week-old SHR, which is an early stage of hypertension, and age-matched WKY. Evidence is presented that Bay k 8644 itself caused a dose-dependent contraction that was much greater in the SHR femoral artery than in the WKY artery. We propose that the state of voltage-dependent Ca^{2+} channels in SHR femoral artery may differ between stimulation by Bay k and K^+ depolarization.

Methods

Male SHR, 6 week old, and age-matched male WKY were used in the study. The rats were inbred in our laboratory. Systolic blood pressure was measured in conscious rats by the tail-cuff method [24]. The number of rats, their body weights, systolic blood pressures, and strip weights are shown in Table 1.

Table 1. Characteristics of the 6-week-old SHR and WKY

Characteristics	SHR	WKY
Number	20	20
Age (days)	43 ± 1	43 ± 1
Animal weight (g)	111 ± 4	115 ± 5
Blood pressure (mmHg)[a]	134 ± 8*	114 ± 3
Strip weight (mg)[b]	0.52 ± 0.02	0.50 ± 0.02

[a] Systolic blood pressure was measured by the tail-cuff method as described under "Methods"
[b] Weight of femoral arterial strips was measured in 40 strips/group
* Significantly different when compared with WKY ($P < 0.05$). Values are expressed as mean $\pm$S.E.

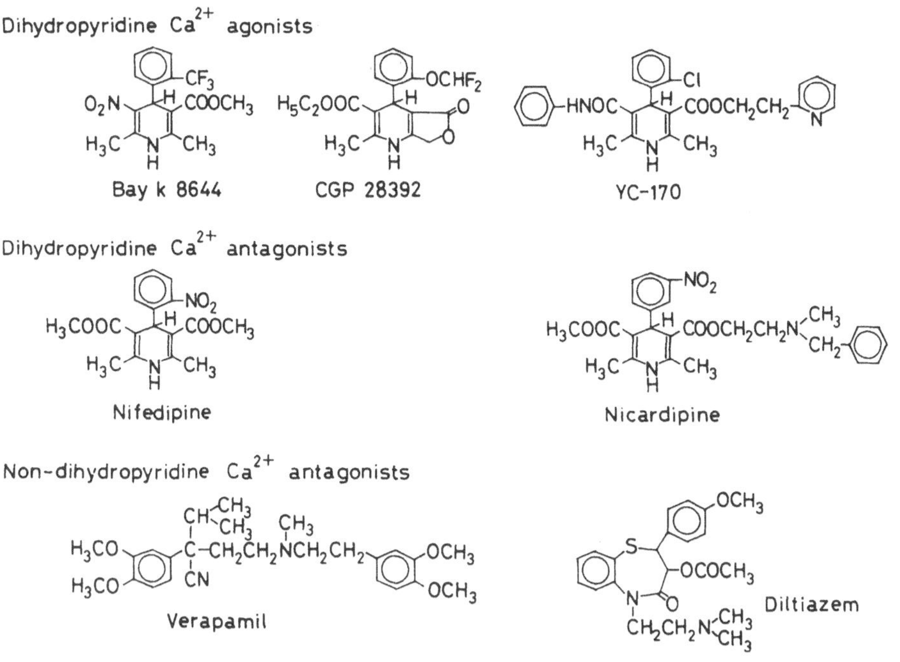

Dihydropyridine Ca^{2+} agonists

Bay k 8644   CGP 28392   YC-170

Dihydropyridine Ca^{2+} antagonists

Nifedipine   Nicardipine

Non-dihydropyridine Ca^{2+} antagonists

Verapamil   Diltiazem

Fig. 1. Chemical structures of Ca^{2+} agonists and antagonists

Preparation of femoral arterial strips for recording mechanical activity

The rats were stunned and exsanguinated. The femoral arteries (0.5–0.7 mm outside diameter) were quickly dissected. After removal of adhering fat and connective tissue, the arteries were helically cut into strips, 0.8 mm wide and 7 mm long, according to the method of Furchgott and Bhadrakom [25]. The strips were mounted vertically between hooks in a water-jacketed ($37° \pm 0.5°C$) muscle bath containing 20 ml modified Krebs' bicarbonate solution of the following composition (in mM): NaCl, 115.0; KCl, 4.7; $CaCl_2$, 2.5; $MgCl_2$, 1.2; $NaHCO_3$, 25.0; KH_2PO_4, 1.2; and dextrose, 10.0. The muscle bath solutions were maintained at $37° \pm 0.5°C$ and continuously bubbled with a gas mixture of 95% O_2 and 5% CO_2. The upper end of the strip was connected to the lever of a force-displacement transducer (TB-612T, Nihonkohden Kogyo Co., Tokyo, Japan). The strips were stretched passively by imposing a resting tension of 0.4 g. The degree of passive stretch of strips from both SHR and WKY is nearly optimal for active tension development. Length-passive tension studies failed to demonstrate differences in passive stiffness between strips from SHR and WKY. This tension was maintained throughout the experiments. After application of passive tension, arterial strips were equilibrated for 90 min in aerated Krebs' bicarbonate solution, and during this period, the solutions were replaced every 15 min.

Contractile responses of the strips to KCl, Bay k 8644, and norepinephrine

After the 90-min equilibration period, the maximally effective concentration (10^{-5} M) of norepinephrine (NE) (l-NE bitratrate, Signa Chemical Co., MO,

USA) was administered two or three times at 40-min intervals until the successive response remained constant. Throughout the NE response, Krebs' bicarbonate solution contained 3×10^{-7} M timolol to block beta adrenoceptor responses, since the beta adrenoceptor activities in the femoral arteries were significantly different between the SHR and WKY [26]. Isometric contractions were recorded on an ink-writing oscillograph (RJG-4006, Nihonkohden Kogyo Co.).

A cumulative dose-response curve for the contractile effects of KCl(K^+) was determined by a stepwise increase in the concentration of K^+ as soon as a steady response to the preceding dose had been obtained. Following the determination of the response to K^+, a dose-response curve for the contractile effects of Bay k was determined in the same strip. Therefore, the responses to Bay k can be expressed as a ratio to the maximum contraction induced by K^+ [27]. Osmotic adjustment was not made when K^+ was added. Contractile responses of the strips to other Ca^{2+} agonists, 4-[2-(difluoromethoxy) phenyl]-1,4,5,7-tetrahydro-2-methyl-5-oxofuro [3, 4–b] pyridine-3-carboxylic acid ethylester (CGP 28392, CGP, Ciba-Geigy Ltd, Basel, Switzerland) and 2-(2-pyrididyl) ethyl 4-(o-chlorophenyl-)-2, 6-dimethyl-5-phenylcarbamoyl-1,4-dihydropyridine-3-carboxylate ethanol (YC-170, YC, Yamànouchi Phàrma, Co., Ltd, Tokyo, Japan) (Fig. 1), were determined in a similar fashion.

Dose-response curves for NE were determined in another series of experiments. After the 90-min equilibration period, K^+ in a concentration of 60 mM was added two or three times until the successive response remained constant. A dose-response curve for NE was then determined in the presence of 3×10^{-7} M timolol to eliminate the possible beta adrenoceptor responses as described above.

A dose-response curve for Ca^{2+} in K^+-depolarized strips was determined. In this experiment, strips were washed several times over a period of 60 min with (nominally) Ca^{2+}-free K^+-depolarizing solutions (80 mM K^+ substitution for Na^+) [28, 29] and a cumulative dose-response curve for Ca^{2+} was determined. Dose-response curves for Ca^{2+} were also determined after the strips had been washed with Ca^{2+}-free Krebs' bicarbonate solutions containing either 10^{-7} M Bay k or 10^{-5} M NE (plus 3×10^{-7} M timolol and 100 μg/ml asorbic acid).

Effects of Ca^{2+} antagonists on the contractile response of the SHR femoral artery to Bay k 8644

The effect of nifedipine, a dihydropyridine Ca^{2+} antagonist, on the dose-response curve of the SHR femoral artery for Bay k was determined in the following way. The reproducibility of the contractile responses to Bay k was first determined in strips from the SHR femoral artery. In this experiment, following the determination of the dose-response curve for K^+, five dose-response curves for Bay k were obtained from a single strip with an interval of 80 min between each determination. Following the determination of the first dose-response curve for Bay k, the responses of SHR femoral arteries to this agonist were fast, such that it took a relatively short time to complete a dose-response curve. The maximum contractions induced by Bay k were fairly constant throughout the five sequential dose-response curves. As the pD_2 values obtained from the second and subsequent dose-response curves were found to be identical, the second curve was taken as a control and the effects of three concentrations of Ca^{2+} antagonists were determined at the third, fourth, and fifth curves.

The pA_2 value of nifedipine against Bay k 8644 was determined from the regression analysis of log (dose-ratio-l) against log [B]. Dose-ratio refers to the concentration of Bay k required to produce 50% of the maximum response (ED_{50}) in the presence of a concentration [B] of nifedipine, divided by the ED_{50} in the absence of nifedipine [30].

The effects of nifedipine on the dose-response curves for either Ca^{2+} (in K^+-depolarized solution) or NE in strips of SHR femoral arteries were determined according to the method as described previously [28, 29].

The effects of verapamil and diltiazem, structurally different Ca^{2+} antagonists, were also determined as in the nifedipine experiments.

Statistical analysis

When assessing the ED_{50} value, responses to agonists were calculated as a percentage of the maximum response obtained with that agonist. The ED_{50} value was obtained visually from a plot of percentage response versus log concentration of the agonist and was expressed as the negative logarithm (pD_2 value) with the exception of K^+.

Unless otherwise specified, the results shown in the text, table, and figures were expressed as mean values $\pm$ SE. For statistical evaluation, data were analyzed by Student's t-test, paired t-test, or analysis of variance. Statistical significance was assumed when $P < 0.05$.

Drugs and chemicals

Bay k 8644 or nifedipine was dissolved in ethanol to make a stock solution of 10^{-3} M. CGP 28392 (10^{-2} M) was dissolved in ethanol. YC-170 (2×10^{-3} M) was dissolved in 0.05 N HCl and the pH was adjusted to 4.0 with 0.1 N NaOH. These dihydropyridine derivatives were stored under refrigeration and protected from light. Phenoxybenzamine (10^{-3} M) was prepared in 50% ethanol. Other drugs were daily prepared in Kreb's bicarbonate solution and kept on ice during the course of the experiment. The chemical structures of the dihydropyridine Ca^{2+} agonists, antagonists and the structures of nondihydropyridine Ca^{2+} antagonists, verapamil and diltiazem are shown in Fig. 1.

Results

Contractile responses of femoral arteries to K^+, Bay k 8644, and NE

Contractile responses to exogenously added K^+ (5–90 mM) were first determined in strips of femoral arteries from SHR and WKY. Following the determination of the dose-response curve for K^+, the addition of Bay k in concentrations ranging from 1×10^{-10} to 3×10^{-7} M caused a dose-dependent contraction in strips of the SHR femoral artery (Fig. 2). The maximum contraction was observed when 1×10^{-7} M Bay k was added, and higher concentrations of this agonist (1×10^{-6} M) produced significant relaxation. The maximum contractile tension developed by Bay k in the SHR femoral artery was 198 ± 16 mg

($n = 28$) and was much the same as the maximum tension induced by K^+ depolarization. As shown clearly in Fig. 2, spontaneous rhythmic contractions were observed far more frequently in femoral arterial strips from SHR (23 of 28) than in strips from WKY (7 of 28). Comparison of the dose-response curve for the contractile effect of either K^+ or Bay k is made between the femoral arteries from SHR and WKY (Fig. 3). As shown in Fig. 3A, strips from the SHR femoral artery had a lower threshold to K^+ than did strips from the WKY femoral artery. The ED_{50} value of the response to K^+ in strips from the SHR femoral artery (8.2 ± 0.6 mM, $n = 28$) was significantly ($P < 0.001$) lower than the value in strips from the WKY artery (11.8 ± 0.5 mM, $n = 28$). The differences between the contractile responses of femoral arteries from SHR and WKY were more evident in the case of Bay k than in the case of K^+ (Fig. 3B). The threshold concentration of Bay k was significantly lower in the SHR artery than in the WKY artery. The pD_2 value of the response to Bay k in the SHR femoral artery (8.55 ± 0.05, $n = 28$) was significantly ($P < 0.001$) larger than the value obtained in the WKY artery (7.54 ± 0.06, $n = 28$). Mean values of the ratio of maximum contraction induced by Bay k to that by K^+ depolarization were 0.956 ± 0.039 (SHR, $n = 28$, significantly different from WKY, $P < 0.001$) and 0.263 ± 0.057

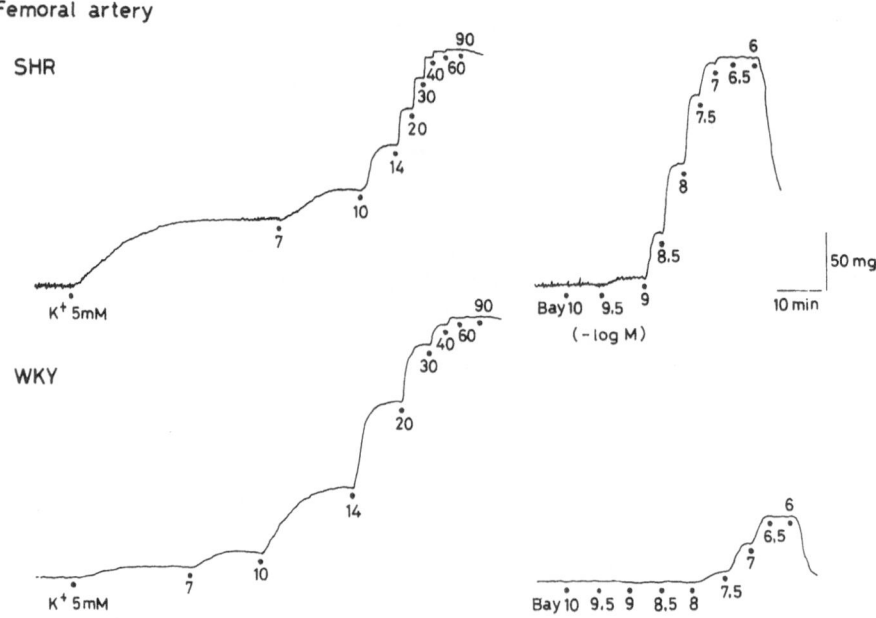

Fig. 2. Typical recording of the responses of a strip of femoral artery from either 6-week-old SHR (*top panel*) or age-matched WKY (*bottom panel*) to KCl (K^+) and Bay k 8644 (*Bay*). Following the 90-min equilibration, repeated administration of 10^{-5} M NE (in the presence of 3×10^{-7} M timolol, a beta-adrenoceptor antagonist) and subsequent 40-min washing, the dose-response curve for K^+ was determined. The dose-response curve for Bay k 8644 was then determined in the same strip after 80-min washing. The concentrations of Bay k 8644 are expressed as a negative logarithm of the molar concentration

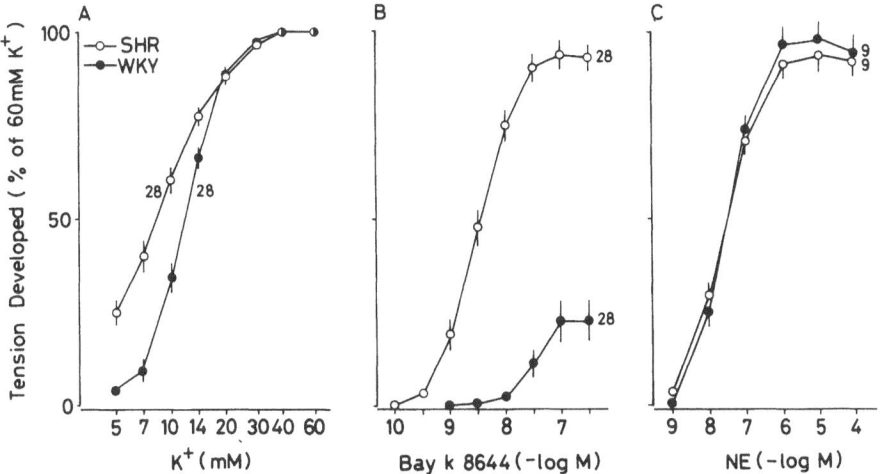

Fig. 3A–C. Dose-response curves for the contractile effects of **A** KCl (K$^+$), **B** Bay k 8644, and **C** norepinephrine (NE) in strips of femoral arteries isolated from SHR and WKY. Experimental conditions were the same as in Fig. 1. Maximum contraction was obtained when 60 mM K$^+$ was added and was taken as 100%. Mean values of the maximum contractile tensions developed by 60 mM K$^+$ were 214 $\pm$ 20 mg (SHR, n = 28, not significantly different from WKY) and 233 $\pm$ 9 mg (WKY, n = 28), respectively. Contractile responses to Bay k 8644 are expressed as a percentage of the maximum contraction induced by 60 mM K$^+$. Contractile responses to NE were determined in the presence of 3 $\times$ 10^{-7} M timolol to eliminate the possible beta-adrenoceptor responses and expressed as a percentage of the contraction induced by 60 mM K$^+$. *Vertical bars* represent SE. *Numbers* beside the dose-response curves indicate the number of preparations used [34]

(WKY, n = 28), respectively. However, the contractile responses to NE via alpha adrenoceptors were not significantly different between the femoral arteries from SHR and WKY (Fig. 3C). It is noteworthy that the SHR femoral artery was more sensitive to the contractile effect of Bay k than to that of NE.

When the femoral arterial strips were fully depolarized by replacing the normal solution with a Ca^{2+}-free 80 mM K$^+$ solution, contractile responses to Ca^{2+} were not significantly different between SHR and WKY (Fig. 4A). Contractile responses to Ca^{2+}, determined after the incubation of the strips with a Ca^{2+}-free solution containing 10^{-7} M Bay k, were significantly different between SHR and WKY (Fig. 4B). Ca^{2+} influx through the receptor-operated channels determined after the incubation of the strips with a Ca^{2+}-free solution containing 10^{-5} M NE was not significantly different between SHR and WKY (Fig. 4C). Thus, the difference in the contractile response to Ca^{2+} between SHR and WKY can be obtained only in the presence of Bay k. These results strongly suggest that femoral arteries possess increased Ca^{2+}-handling properties at this age. This abnormality appears to be dependent on Ca^{2+} influx through the voltage-dependent channels.

Dose-response curves of femoral arteries for CGP and YC are shown in Fig. 5. CGP acts as a partial agonist, since the maximum contraction induced by this compound is significantly smaller than the maximum induced by Bay k. On the other hand, responses to YC were somewhat different from those to Bay k and

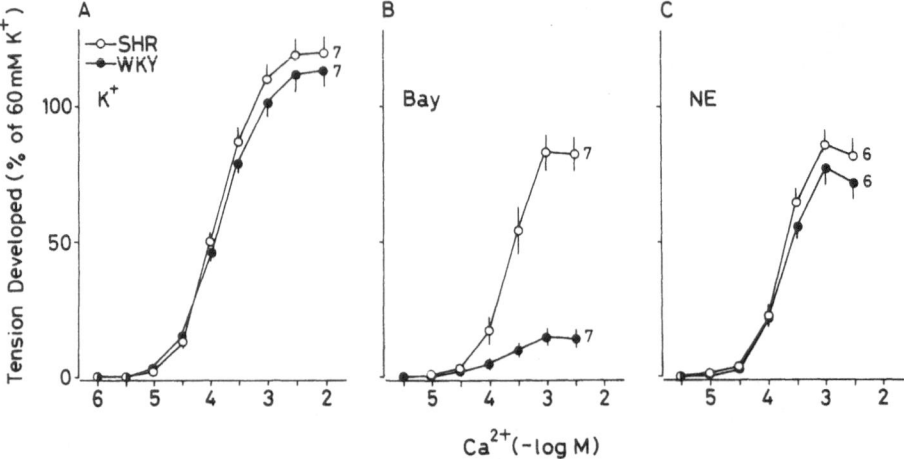

Fig. 4A–C. Dose-response curves of femoral arterial strips for Ca^{2+} determined in various Ca^{2+}-free Krebs' bicarbonate solutions. **A** Dose-response curves for Ca^{2+} in K^+-depolarized strips. Following the determination of 60 mM K^+ response, the strip was incubated with a Ca^{2+}-free, K^+-rich solution (80 mM K^+ substitution for Na^+) for 60 min. **B** Dose-response curves for Ca^{2+} determined after the incubation of the strip with a Ca^{2+}-free solution containing 10^{-7} M Bay k 8644. Following the determination of the dose-response curve for Bay k 8644 in normal Krebs' bicarbonate solution (as in Fig. 3B), the solution was replaced with the Ca^{2+}-free solution containing 10^{-7} M Bay k 8644. **C** Dose-response curves for Ca^{2+} determined after the incubation of the strip with a Ca^{2+}-free solution containing 10^{-5} M NE (plus 3×10^{-7} M timolol and 100µg/ml ascorbic acid). Following the determination of the dose-response curve for NE in normal Krebs' bicarbonate solution (as in Fig. 3C), the solution was replaced with the Ca^{2+}-free solution containing NE. In all the panels, the response to 60 mM K^+ determined in the same strip was taken as 100%. *Vertical bars* represent SE. *Numbers* beside the dose-response curves indicate the number of preparations used [34]

CGP. Maximum contractions induced by YC were not significantly different between the femoral arteries from SHR and WKY, whereas the pD_2 value of this compound in SHR was larger than the value in WKY.

Contractile responses to K^+ and Bay k were also determined in distal portions of the superior mesenteric artery from both SHR and WKY (data not shown). In this artery, dose-response curves for K^+ and Bay k were not significantly different between SHR and WKY. Spontaneous rhythmic contractions were not observed in mesenteric arteries from SHR and WKY.

Effects of Ca^{2+} antagonists in the contractile responses of femoral arteries to Bay k 8644

The effects of nifedipine on the dose-response curves of the SHR femoral artery for Ca^{2+} (K^+ depolarization), Bay k, and NE are shown in Fig. 6. Nifedipine showed a competitive antagonism against both Ca^{2+} (K^+ depolarization) and Bay k, producing a rightward displacement of the dose-response curve for each agonist (Fig. 6A, B). These results support the view proposed by Schramm et al.

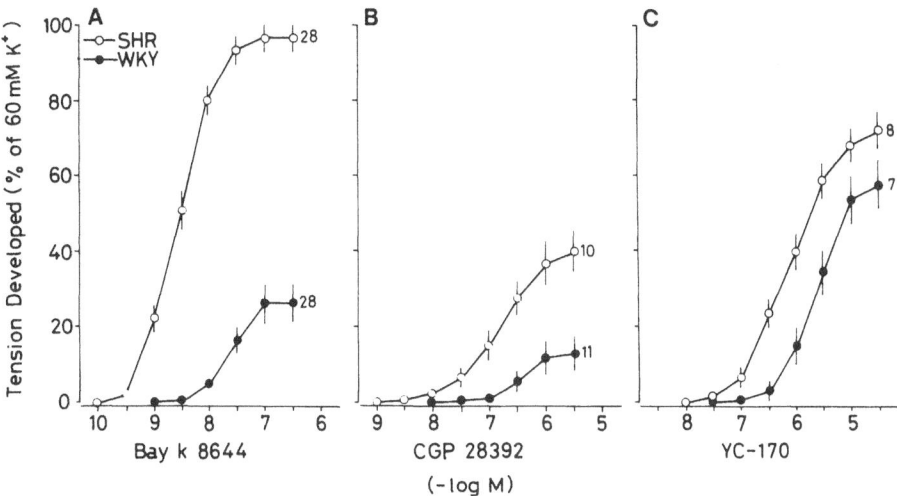

Fig. 5A–C. Dose-response curves for the contractile effects of **A** Bay k 8644, **B** CGP 28392, **C** YC-170 in strips of femoral arteries isolated from SHR and WKY. Experimental conditions were the same as in Figs. 2 and 3. Contractile responses to these Ca^{2+} agonists are expressed as a percentage of the contraction induced by 60 mM K$^+$. *Vertical bars* represent SE. *Numbers* beside the dose-response curves indicate the number of preparations used

[14, 15] that Bay k and nifedipine may act on a common site of the voltage-dependent Ca^{2+} channels. In contrast, the antagonism by nifedipine of the response to NE was of a noncompetitive type (Fig. 6C). The Schild plot for nifedipine against Ca^{2+} (K$^+$ depolarization) gave a regression line with a slope of 1.06 and a pA_2 value of 9.42. The pA_2 value and slope of nifedipine antagonism of the responses to Bay k were 8.36 and 1.09, respectively (Fig. 6D). Thus, the pA_2 value of nifedipine is much smaller in the antagonism of Bay k 8644 than in the antagonism of K$^+$ depolarization.

Antagonism by verapamil of the contractile responses to Bay k in the SHR femoral artery was competitive, with a pA_2 value and slope of 6.77 and 1.09, respectively (Fig. 7, left). In contrast, the addition of diltiazem in concentrations ranging from 3×10^{-7} to 3×10^{-6} M produced a reduction of the maximum response of the SHR femoral artery to Bay k, suggesting a noncompetitive antagonism (Fig. 7, right).

The addition of 1×10^{-6} M phentolamine and treatment of the strip with 2×10^{-6} M phenoxybenzamine [26] did not affect the dose-response curve of the SHR femoral artery for Bay k. Contractile responses of this artery to Bay k were not altered by 3×10^{-7} M timolol. These results suggest that arterial contractile responses to Bay k are not mediated by the release of endogenous NE or the direct stimulation of alpha adrenoceptors. Bay k failed to produce the contraction after the 60-min incubation of the strips in Ca^{2+}-free Krebs' bicarbonate solution containing 10^{-4} M ethylene glycol-bis (β-aminoethyl ether) N,N,N',N'-tetra-acetic acid (EGTA).

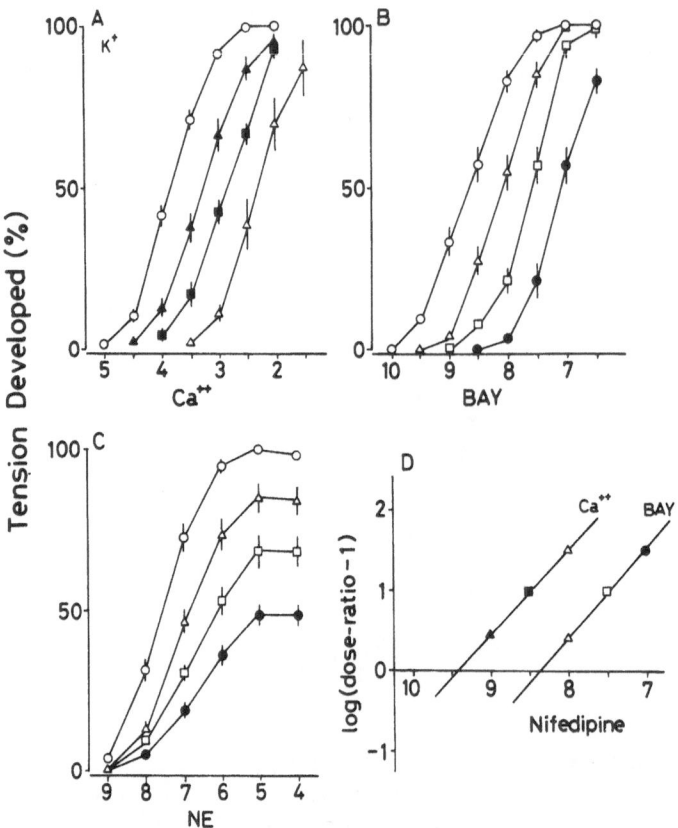

Fig. 6A–D. Effects of nifedipine on the dose-response curves for Ca^{2+} in **A** K^+ depolarized strips and for **B** Bay k 8644 or **C** NE in strips of femoral arteries isolated from SHR. Effects of nifedipine were determined as described in "Methods." The concentrations of each agonist were expressed as a negative logarithm of the molar concentration. In each *panel*, maximum contractile tension developed by each agonist in the absence of nifedipine (○) was taken as 100%. The concentrations of nifedipine used were 1×10^{-9} M (▲), 3×10^{-9} M (■), 1×10^{-8} M (△), 3×10^{-8} M (□), and 1×10^{-7} M (●). Note the competitive antagonism by nifedipine of the contractile responses to both Ca^{2+} (K^+-depolarized strip) and Bay k 8644. In contrast, nifedipine showed a typical noncompetitive antagonism of the contractile response to NE. **D** Schild plot of the data. the pA_2 value of nifedipine was determined from the regression analysis of log (dose-ratio − 1) against log [B]. Dose-ratio refers to the ED_{50} of Bay k 8644 in the presence of a concentration of [B] of nifedipine, divided by the ED_{50} in the absence of nifedipine. Dose-response curves shown represent the mean ± SE for six to seven preparations [34]

Discussion

The major finding in this study is a difference between the contractile effects of three Ca^{2+} agonists, Bay k, CGP, and YC, on strips of the femoral arteries from SHR and WKY. Bay k alone elicited greater contractions in the SHR artery than in the WKY artety. Extremely low concentrations of Bay k (3×10^{-10} M) caused a contraction in the SHR artery and the maximum contraction incuded by

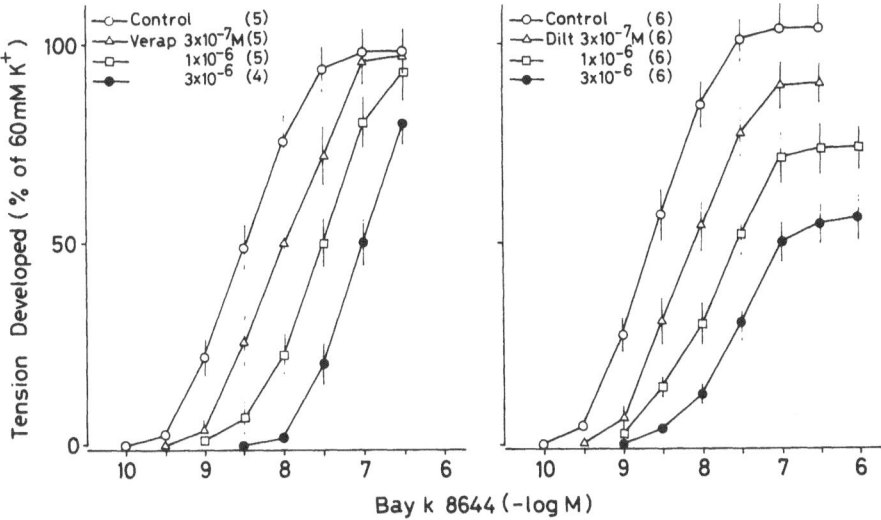

Fig. 7. Effects of verapamil and diltiazem on the dose-response curves for Bay k 8644 in strips of SHR femoral arteries. Experimental conditions were the same as in Fig. 6B except that the contraction induced by Bay k 8644 is expressed as a percentage of the contraction induced by 60 mM K$^+$. Note the competitive antagonism by verapamil, whereas the antagonism by diltiazem is of a noncompetitive type. *Vertical bars* represent SE. *Numbers in parentheses* indicate the number of preparations used

this agonist (1×10^{-7} M) was much the same as the maximum developed by K$^+$ depolarization. On the other hand, the WKY artery had a higher threshold concentration of Bay k (1×10^{-8} M) than the SHR artery, and the maximum contraction in the WKY was approximately one-fourth of the maximum in SHR. The affinity for the contractile effects of Bay k in the SHR artery was significantly higher than that in the WKY artery. The ED$_{50}$ value for the response to K$^+$ in this artery was also significantly greater in SHR than in WKY. These results strongly suggest the increased Ca^{2+}-handling properties in femoral arteries from 6-week-old SHR, which is the early stage of elevated blood pressure. It is noteworthy that the SHR femoral artery was more sensitive to Bay k than to NE.

Schramm et al. [14, 15] have demonstrated that Bay k alone did not induce a contraction of rabbit aortic strips incubated in Tyrode's solution (K$^+$ concentration, 2.6 mM), probably because this vessel is quiescent and therefore the voltage-dependent Ca^{2+} channels in this tissue under resting conditions are not activated. They demonstrated that this Ca^{2+} agonist lowered the threshold for the contractile response to elevated extracellular K$^+$. Recent investigations have also demonstrated that Bay k did not elicit mechanical responses unless the K$^+$ concentration in the bathing solution was elevated in strips of the rat tail artery [18], rabbit mesenteric artery [19], and cat femoral artery [23]. In strips of cat basilar arteries [20], Bay k inconsistently contracted the strips, and in the presence of 10 mM K$^+$, this agonist exhibited potent vasoconstriction with a pD$_2$ value of 8.68 and a maximum of 0.83 (expressed as a ratio to the 124 mM K$^+$-induced contraction). Similar results were obtained in cat middle cerebral arteries [23]. Bay k exhibited a potent vasoconstriction in the rat thoracic aorta [21] and human umbilical artery [22], with a pD_2 value of 6.66 and 7.89, respectively. The maximum response of the human umbilical artery to Bay k was the same as the maximum induced by K^+ depolarization [22]. In the present study of the SHR femoral artery, Bay k consistently exhibited potent vasoconstriction under resting conditions (K^+ concentration, 5.9 mM) with a pD_2 value of 8.55 and a maximum of 0.96 (expressed as a ratio to the maximum induced by K^+ depolarization). When the dose-response curve of this artery for Bay k was determined after the K^+ concentration in the bathing solution was elevated to 8.9 mM, the pD_2 value and maximum response were not significantly changed. On the other hand, responses of the WKY femoral artery to Bay k were significantly potentiated by the elevation of K^+ concentration in the bath. Therefore, the differences in the responses to Bay k 8644 were not evident between SHR and WKY under the conditions where the concentration of K^+ was elevated (data not shown). These results strongly suggest that in the SHR femoral artery the voltage-dependent Ca^{2+} channels might normally be activated or are directly activated by the Ca^{2+} agonists.

This assumption also comes from the observation that spontaneous rhythmic contractions were obtained more frequently in strips of the SHR femoral artery than in strips of the WKY artery. Moreover, these activities were not observed in mesenteric arteries from both SHR and WKY. In strips of the SHR mesenteric artery, Bay k was much less effective in producing the contractile effects than in the SHR femoral artery. The responses of the mesenteric artery to either Bay k or K^+ were not significantly different between SHR and WKY, suggesting that the Ca^{2+} sensitivity in this artery was not altered at this age.

The assumption that the contractile responses of the SHR femoral artery to Bay k are exerted at Ca^{2+} channels comes from the observation that the responses to this agonist are antagonized by Ca^{2+} antagonists, nifedipine, verapamil, and diltiazem. The antagonisms by nifedipine and verapamil were competitive, producing a rightward displacement of the dose-response curve of the SHR femoral artery for Bay k. In contrast, diltiazem exhibited a noncompetitive antagonism. This supports the view proposed by Schramm et al. [14, 15] that Bay k and nifedipine, but not diltiazem, may act on a common dihydropyridine receptor regulating the Ca^{2+} influx through the Ca^{2+} channels. The differences between the antagonism by nifedipine and that by diltiazem are also consistent with other investigations [14, 15, 18].

The Schild plot for nifedipine against Bay k gave a regression line with a slope of 1.09 and a pA_2 value of 8.36. This pA_2 value is significantly smaller than the value (9.42) for nifedipine antagonism of Ca^{2+}-induced contractions in K^+-depolarized strips in the present study and other smooth muscle preparations, in which the values range from 9.4 to 9.7 [18, 31–33]. These results raise the question of whether the Ca^{2+} channels activated by Bay k are the same as those activated by K^+ depolarization. The difference in the pA_2 value may suggest two distinct populations of Ca^{2+} channels or the different state of the channels with a 10- to 20-fold difference in affinity for nifedipine.

Recent findings by Hess et al. [17] suggest that dihydropyridine Ca^{2+} antagonists promote a mode of Ca^{2+}-channel gating in which the channels are unavailable for opening, whereas dihydropyridine Ca^{2+} agonists promote a mode of gating where the channels exhibit long-lasting openings. The most likely explanation of the contractile activities of Bay k shown in the present study is that the mechanism of action of Bay k is to enhance the opening mode of the channels either by increasing the probability of openings or shortening the closed periods.

The contractile effects of Bay k on the SHR femoral artery were not affected by either alpha adrenoceptor antagonists or a beta adrenoceptor antagonist and thus are not due to the release of endogenous NE or the direct stimulation of alpha adrenoceptors. When a Ca^{2+}-free solution containing 10^{-4} M EGTA replaced the normal Krebs' bicarbonate solution in the bath, Bay k failed to elicit a contraction in this artery. Contractile responses of the SHR femoral artery to Bay k were highly reproducible. These results suggest that Bay k seems to be a useful pharmacological tool for investigating the voltage-dependent Ca^{2+} influx in intact vascular smooth muscles. It has been suggested that Bay k is a partial Ca^{2+} agonist with Ca^{2+} antagonistic effects [17, 18]. These antagonistic effects of Bay k were observed at higher concentrations of this agonist (above 10^{-6} M). In this study, 10^{-6} M Bay k also produced arterial relaxation, which may indicate the Ca^{2+} antagonistic effects. Thus, the Ca^{2+} agonistic effects of Bay k could be observed only over a relatively limited concentration range (below 10^{-6} M) in vascular smooth muscles.

In conclusion, Bay k appears to be a potent Ca^{2+} agonist in strips of the SHR femoral artery and is thus a useful pharmacological tool for investigating the Ca^{2+} sensitivity of the vascular smooth muscle. Competitive antagonism observed between Bay k and nifedipine clearly suggests that this agonist may act primarily on the same site, presumably the voltage-dependent Ca^{2+} channel at which nifedipine acts. Whether or not the Ca^{2+} channels activated by Bay k are identical to or are in the same state as those activated by K^+ depolarization is the subject of ongoing investigations [34, 35].

Acknowledgments. The authors wish to thank Kazuko Misawa for skillful technical assistance. Gifts of Bay k 8644 (Bayer AG), CGP 28392 (Ciba-Geigy), YC-170 (Yamanouchi Pharmaceutical), nifedipine (Bayer Yakuhin), verapamil (Eisai), diltiazem (Tanabe Pharmaceutical), phentolamine (Ciba-Geigy), and timolol (Banyu Pharmaceutical) are gratefully acknowledged.

References

1. Webb RC, Bohr DF (1981) Recent advances in the pathogenesis of hypertension: Consideration of structural, functional, and metabolic vascular abnormalities resulting in elevated arterial resistance. Am Heart J 102:251–264
2. Webb RC, Vanhoutte PM, Bohr DF (1981) Adrenergic neurotransmission in vascular smooth muscle from spontaneously hypertensive rats. Hypertension 3:93–103
3. Daniel EE, Kwan CY (1981) Control of contraction of vascular smooth muscle: Relation to hypertension. Trends Pharmacol Sci 2:220–223
4. Winquist RJ, Webb RC, Bohr DF (1982) Vascular smooth muscle in hypertension. Fed Proc 41:2387–2393
5. Mulvany MJ (1983) Do resistance vessel abnormalities contribute to the elevated blood pressure of spontaneously-hypertensive rats? A review of some of the evidence. Blood Vessels 20:1–22

6. Holloway ET, Bohr DF (1973) Reactivity of vascular smooth muscle in hypertensive rats. Circ Res 33:678–685

7. Bolton TB (1979) Mechanism of action of transmitters and other substances on smooth muscle. Physical Rev 59:606–718

8. Bohr DF, Sitrin M (1970) Regulation of vascular smooth muscle contraction. Changes in experimental hypertension. Circ Res 26 and 27 (Suppl II):83–90

9. Shibata S, Kurahashi K, Kuchii M (1973) A possible etiology of contractility impairment of vascular smooth muscle from spontaneously hypertensive rats. J Pharmacol Exp Ther 185:406–417

10. Noon JP, Rice PJ, Baldessarini RJ (1978) Calcium leakage as a cause of the high resting tension in vascular smooth muscle from the spontaneously hypertensive rats. Proc Natl Acad Sci USA 75:1605–1607

11. Fleckenstein A (1977) Specific pharmacology of calcium in myocardium, cardiac pacemakers and vascular smooth muscle. Ann Rev Pharmacol Toxicol 17:149–166

12. Fleckenstein A (1983) History of calcium antagonists. Circ Res 52 (Suppl I):3–16

13. Janis RA, Triggle DJ (1983) New development in Ca^{2+} channel antagonists. J Med Chem 26:775–785

14. Schramm M, Thomas G, Towart R, Franckowiak G (1983) New dihydropyridines with positive inotropic action through activation of Ca^{2+} channels. Nature (Lond) 303:536–538

15. Schramm M, Thomas G, Towart R, Franckowiak G (1983) Activation of calcium channels by novel 1,4-dihydropyridines. A new mechanism for positive inotropics or smooth muscle stimulants. Arzneim-Forsch 33:1268–1272

16. Yamamoto H, Hwang O, van Breemen C (1984) Bay k 8644 differentiates between potential and receptor operated Ca^{2+} channels. Eur J Pharmacol 102:555–557

17. Hess P, Lansman JB, Tsien RW (1984) Different modes of Ca channel gating behavior favoured by dihydropyridine Ca agonists and antagonists. Nature (Lond) 311:538–544

18. Su CM, Swamy VC, Triggle DJ (1984) Calcium channel activation in vascular smooth muscle by BAY K 8644. Can J Physiol Pharmacol 62:1401–1410

19. Kanmura Y, Itoh T, Kuriyama H (1984) Agonist actions of Bay k 8644, a dihydropyridine derivative, on the voltage-dependent calcium influx in smooth muscle cells of the rabbit mesentric artery. J Pharmacol Exp Ther 231:717–723

20. Uski TK, Andersson K-E (1985) Some effects of the calcium promotor BAY K 8644 on feline cerebral arteries. Acta Physiol Scand 123:49–53

21. Mikkelsen E, Nyborg NCB, Kazda S (1985) A novel 1, 4 dihydropyridine, BAY K 8644, with contractile effects on vascular smooth muscle. Acta Pharmacol Toxicol 56:44–49

22. Gopalakrishnan V, Park LE, Triggle CR (1985) The effect of the calcium channel agonist, Bay K-8644 on human vascular smooth muscle. Eur J Pharmacol 113:447–451

23. Salaices M, Marin J, Sanchez-Ferrer CF, Reviriego J (1985) The effects of BAY-K-8644 on the contraction of cat middle cerebral and femoral arteries. Biochem Pharmacol 34:3131–3135

24. Okamoto K, Aoki K (1963) Development of a strain of spontaneously hypertensive rats. Jpn Circ J 27:282–293

25. Furchgott RF, Bhadrakom S (1953) Relations of strips of rabbit aorta to epinephrine, isopropylarterenol, sodium nitrite and other drugs. J Pharmacol Exp Ther 108:129–143

26. Asano M, Aoki K, Matsuda T (1982) Reduced *beta* adrenoceptor interactions of norepinephrine enhance contraction in the femoral artery from spontaneously hypertensive rats. J Pharmacol Exp Ther 223:207–214

27. Asano M, Aoki K, Matsuda T (1984) Quantitative changes of maximum contractile response to norepinephrine in mesenteric arteries from spontaneously hypertensive rats during the development of hypertension. J Cardiovasc Pharmacol 6:727–731

28. Kanamori M, Naka M, Asano M, Hidaka H (1981) Effects of N-(6-aminohexyl)-5-chloro-1-naphthalenesulfonamide and other calmodulin antagonists (calmodulin interacting agents) on calcium induced contraction of rabbit aortic strips. J Pharmacol Exp Ther 217:494–499

29. Asano M, Hidaka H (1985) Pharmacological properties of N-(6-aminohexyl)-5-chloro-1-naphthalesulenesulfonamide (W-7), a calmodulin antagonist in arterial strips from rats and rabbits. J Pharmacol Exp Ther 234:476–484

30. Arunlakshana O, Schild HO (1959) Some quantitative uses of drug antagonists. Br J Pharmacol 14:48–58
31. Rosenberger LB, Ticku MK, Triggle DJ (1979) The effects of Ca^{2+} antagonists on mechanical responses and Ca^{2+} movements in guinea pig ileal longitudinal smooth muscle. Can J Physiol Pharmacol 57:333–347
32. Hashimoto K, Takeda K, Katano Y, Nakagawa Y, Tsukada T, Hashimoto T, Shimamoto N, Sakai K, Otorii K, Imai S (1979) Effects of niludipine (Bay a 7168) on the cardiovascular system. With a note on its calcium-antagonistic effects. Arzneim Forsch 29:1368–1373
33. Spedding M (1982) Assessment of "Ca^{2+}-antagonists" effects of drugs in K^+-depolarized smooth muscle. Differentiation of antagonist subgroups. Naunyn-Schmiedeberg's Arch Pharmacol 318:234–240
34. Aoki K, Asano M (1986) Effects of Bay k 8644 and nifedipine on femoral arteries of spontaneously hypertensive rats. Br J Pharmacol 88:221–230
35. Aoki K, Mochizuki A, Hotta K (1981) Noradrendline and calcium induced tension in aortic strips of normotensive and spontaneously hypertensive rats. Jpn Circ J 45:547–551

Altered Vascular Calcium Metabolism
As a Possible Cause of Increased Blood Pressure
in Essential Hypertension

M. J. Mulvany

Biophysics Institute, Aarhus University, 8000 Aarhus C, Denmark

Summary. In human essential hypertension, there is some limited evidence for vascular EC coupling abnormalities, and abnormalities are also found in the SHR. There is little information from human studies as to whether such abnormalities play a role in the development of hypertension, but from rat studies the available evidence does not support a direct connection between EC coupling abnormalities and increased blood pressure, although the possibility cannot be excluded that the increased sensitivity is a substrate upon which other factors may act. Further work is required, particularly using human isolated vascular preparations, to delineate more precisely the role of vascular abnormalities in the pathogenesis of essential hypertension.

Key words: Calcium —Resistance vessels—Excitation-contraction coupling—Hypertension—Therapy---Hybrids

There is little doubt that the vasculature plays an important role in the pathogenesis of human essential (primary) hypertension. Numerous studies have demonstrated that in established essential hypertension, the total peripheral resistance is elevated [1], and this increased resistance appears to be equally divided between the various systemic circuits [2]. It is, therefore, clear that hypertension is associated with a generalized narrowing of the vasculature. It is likely that this narrowing is in part due to increased levels of activation: Increased sympathetic drive is widely reported [3]. Raised levels of blood-borne pressor agents, such as the currently canvassed natriuretic hormone [4], could also be causes of the increased vascular resistance. However, there is also substantial evidence that at least part of the increased vascular resistance is due to alterations within the vasculature itself.

Since the aim of hypertension research is not so much to identify differences between hypertensives and normotensives as to determine which factors represent the primary defects in the pathogenesis of the disease, it is necessary to consider whether the vasculature plays a primary role in the development of high blood pressure. In a sense, the complexity of the cardiovascular system, where each part not only acts on, but is also acted on by the system, makes the question one of semantics—we should perhaps consider hypertension a *system* defect. Nevertheless, one can envisage a situation where some defect in the vasculature causes this to constrict in a manner which none of the cardiovascular feedback systems is able to counteract, so that we could indeed consider a vascular defect as a prime cause of hypertension.

The vascular abnormalities which can be associated with hypertension can be broadly divided into two types—alterations in vascular structure and alterations in the excitation-contraction coupling (EC coupling) properties of the vasculature (i.e., the sensitivity of the vasculature to agonists). The question of the importance of abnormal vascular structure as a prime cause of hypertension has recently been discussed elsewhere [5], where it was concluded that the available evidence supports the possibility that abnormal vascular structure may be among the causes of increased blood pressure. The present contribution aims to discuss whether alterations in EC coupling, in particular as regards calcium metabolism, could also be a cause of the increased peripheral resistance associated with hypertension.

Evidence for Altered Vascular EC Coupling in Hypertension

Evidence for hypertension being associated with altered EC coupling in the vasculature has been obtained both from human and animal studies; in the latter, particular use has been made of the spontaneously hypertensive rat (SHR) [6], a model which has a number of features in common with human primary or essential hypertension [7].

Human studies
The main evidence for altered EC coupling properties in the vasculature of patients with essential hypertension comes from studies where it is found that the threshold dose which would give rise to a response was lower. Thus, Ljungman et al. [8] have shown that the threshold dose to angiotensin II for the renal vasculature was lower in essential hypertension. Other clinical evidence for a difference in the EC coupling properties of the hypertensive vasculature comes from the finding that calcium antagonists such as verapamil have a greater vasodilating effect in the forearm of hypertensives [9]. In contrast, the threshold dose for noradrenaline vasoconstriction in the hand vasculature is unaltered in hypertensives [10].

Evidence obtained from isolated human vessels is sparse. Moulds [11] reported a reduced noradrenaline response in digital arteries from hypertensives, while Wyse [12] found little difference in the noradrenaline responsiveness of cystic arteries from borderline hypertensives and normotensives. In preeclampsia, we [13] found unaltered noradrenaline sensitivity but an increased sensitivity to angiotensin II in isolated omental resistance vessels.

The available evidence suggests, therefore, that there may be some alterations in the EC coupling properties of the hypertensive vasculature but that the differences are related specifically to the drug used to investigate it.

Animal studies
Although the sensitivity of vascular preparations from SHR has been extensively studied, the overall picture is far from clear. One problem, as discussed earlier [14], is that "sensitivity" is sometimes confused with "reactivity." The latter term refers only to the magnitude of the response for a given agonist, and may,

therefore, be influenced by structural factors [15]. The former term refers to the concentration giving a threshold (or sometimes half-maximal) contraction, such that if these concentrations are low this indicates a high sensitivity. Thus "sensitivity" refers solely to EC coupling properties. Another problem, as Bohr [16] pointed out earlier, is that many different techniques, preparations, and control animals have been used. Nevertheless, in the past few years, the situation has improved; in particular, it is generally agreed now that the control animal for the SHR of most interest is the genetically related Wistar-Kyoto rat (WKY). Presumably, the genetic differences between the SHR and WKY must include those factors responsible for the increased blood pressure. On this basis, it seems that although in many investigations no difference in the sensitivity of SHR and WKY vascular preparations has been detected, where differences have been seen it is almost always the SHR preparation which is the most sensitive.

As regards noradrenaline sensitivity, it would appear from perfusion experiments both in the hindquarter [17] and in the kidney [18] that the noradrenaline sensitivity is greater in SHR than in WKY. Similar observations have been made in comparisons of these vascular beds in stroke-prone SHR (SHRSP) and WKY [19, 20]. The results of experiments with isolated preparations suggest, however, that it is only part of the SHR vasculature which shows increased sensitivity. An increased noradrenaline sensitivity of helical strips from SHR tail arteries has been reported [21, 22], although later experiments using ring preparations could not confirm this [23]. Likewise, femoral small arteries (lumen ca. 200 μm) from SHR did not have an increased noradrenaline sensitivity [23]. By contrast, mesenteric small arteries were found to have an increased noradrenaline sensitivity [24–26], provided that the increased uptake of noradrenaline by the nerve terminals in the SHR vessels was inhibited [25, 27]. Under in vivo, but anesthetized conditions, Wiegman et al. [28] found no difference in the sensitivity of ca. 100-μm arteries in the exposed cremaster muscle of SHR to topically applied noradrenaline, while Bohlen [29] found that vessels with a diameter less than ca. 70 μm in this preparation were hypersensitive to noradrenaline.

These differences in sensitivity to noradrenaline suggest either that there are differences in the various receptors or that there are differences in the manner in which the final trigger for contraction, the intracellular free calcium concentration, is controlled. The available evidence [30] suggests, however, that at least as regards alpha receptors the affinity of these for noradrenaline is normal is SHR (similar results are reported for alpha receptors in hypertensive and normotensive humans [31]). Therefore, differences in calcium handling may be expected, and there is much evidence to suggest that this is the case although, as for agonist sensitivity, different parts of the vasculature appear to react differently to calcium.

In the aorta, the presence of a calcium-dependent tone [32, 33] and an increased labeled calcium efflux [34] has been taken as evidence that the SHR aortic plasma membrane has an increased calcium permeability. In support of this, Pedersen et al. [35] found that the noradrenaline response of the SHR aorta had an increased sensitivity to the calcium antagonist nifedipine. On the other hand, Pedersen et al. [35] also found that the calcium sensitivity of the SHR aorta was *reduced.* That is, at low extracellular calcium concentrations, the noradrenaline response of the SHR aorta was more depressed than in control preparations, and we have made similar observations [36]. The calcium sensitivity of the SHR basilar artery [37] and of the superior mesenteric artery [38] is also decreased. In more distal vessels, where the functional role of intracellular calcium stores may be less [39], it seems that increased plasma membrane permeability plays a dominant role. Although in the SHR tail artery, calcium sensitivity is normal [23], in SHR mesenteric small arteries (Figs. 1, 2; Table 1) [40], SHR femoral small

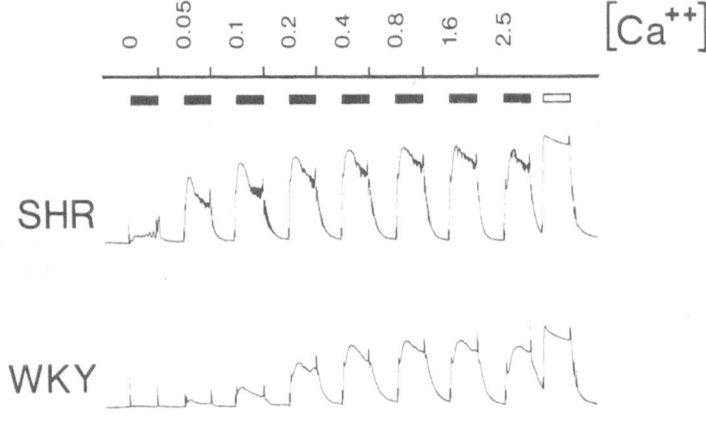

Fig. 1. Records showing how calcium dose-response curves were obtained. Double myograph used allows comparison of mesenteric resistance vessel from SHR (*upper record*) and WKY (*lower record*). Vessels stimulated repetitively with noradrenaline (10 μmol/l), first in calcium-free solution and then in solutions containing increasing concentrations of calcium as indicated (in mmol/l). After Nilsson and Mulvany [41]

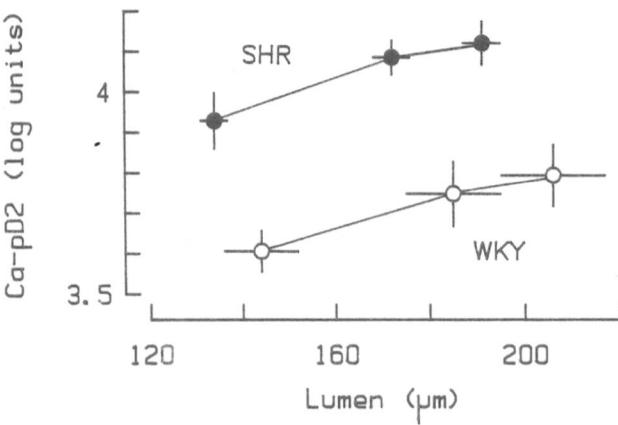

Fig. 2. Calcium sensitivity ($Ca\text{-}pD_2$) of SHR and WKY mesenteric resistance vessels determined at different internal lumen diameters (= internal circumference/π). *Points* show mean ± SE. Data obtained from six SHR and six WKY. Since lumen diameters of SHR vessels are for a given transmural pressure less than those of WKY vessels [40], the increased SHR vessel calcium sensitivity cannot be ascribed to the normalization procedure

Table 1. Calcium sensitivity of SHR and WKY resistance vessels

Activator	Vessel	Animal Age (weeks)	Therapy	Ca-pD$_2$ SHR	Ca-pD$_2$ WKY	Reference
Noradrenaline	Mesenteric	4	None	**3.96 ± 0.07 (10)	3.66 ± 0.06 (10)	40
		16	None	**4.07 ± 0.07 (9)	3.76 ± 0.06 (9)	40
		60	None	***4.19 ± 0.03 (8)	3.71 ± 0.01 (10)	a
		14	Hydralazine	***4.17 ± 0.07 (5)	3.83 ± 0.01 (12)	66
		27	Hydralazine	*4.06 ± 0.05 (11)	3.89 ± 0.04 (8)	66
		14	Felodipine	***4.42 ± 0.08 (9)	4.01 ± 0.03 (9)	65
	Femoral	14	None	[b]4.07 ± 0.08 (9)	3.91 ± 0.06 (9)	41
	Renal	16	None	4.16 ± 0.02 (10)	4.15 ± 0.02 (10)	a
K	Mesenteric	4	None	[c]3.16 ± 0.02 (10)	3.10 ± 0.04 (10)	40
		16	None	[c]3.12 ± 0.03 (9)	3.07 ± 0.03 (9)	40

Calcium sensitivity of resistance vessels from vascular bed expressed as Ca-pD$_2$ = −log concentration (mol/l) of calcium giving half maximal response for vessels activated with 10 μmol/l noradrenaline or 125 mmol/l K$^+$. Hydralazine and felodipine treatments instituted at age 4–6 wk. Values given as mean ± SE (number of animals in parentheses) *** $P < 0.01$, ** $P < 0.01$, * $P < 0.05$ student's t-test [a]Mulvany, unpublished results [b] $P < 0.05$: dose-response-ANOVA [c] $P < 0.05$, age-strain ANOVA

arteries [41], and the SHR portal vein [42], calcium sensitivity is increased. Also in the SHR perfused hindquarter, the calcium sensitivity of the noradrenaline response is enhanced [43]. However, increased calcium sensitivity is not found in renal resistance vessels (Table 1). This suggests that increased vascular calcium sensitivity may not be a general feature of the SHR resistance vasculature and thus not an expression of a general membrane defect [14]. One possibility is that it is related to an increased innervation, which appears to be particularly prevalent in the SHR mesenteric bed [23], as denervation has been found to reduce calcium sensitivity (Nyborg, Korsgaard, and Mulvany, J. Hypertension, in press).

The available evidence thus suggests that the vasculature of the SHR has different EC coupling properties to those of the WKY. In the larger vessels, this is expressed as a reduced sensitivity to a number of agonists, while in the more peripheral vessels the sensitivity is increased. Since it is the latter which are responsible for the increased peripheral resistance of the SHR, it is presumably these which are of most interest when considering whether abnormal EC coupling is a cause of the increased blood pressure. We may, therefore, consider the mechanisms which may be responsible for the abnormalities.

EC Coupling in Peripheral Vascular Smooth Muscle

Cellular mechanisms

The interaction of the contractile proteins in smooth muscle is, as in other muscle types, dependent in part on the cytoplasmic calcium concentration and in part on the level of other second messengers, such as cyclic AMP. The level of the cytoplasmic calcium is the result of the balance between the influx of extracellular calcium, the release or uptake of calcium into the intracellular stores (mainly the sarcoplasmic reticulum), and the extrusion of calcium across the plasma membrane. The influx of calcium is mediated by potential-dependent channels (PDC) [44] and, possibly, by receptor-operated channels (ROC). The release of calcium from intracellular stores may be mediated through some interaction between the membrane caveoli and the sarcoplasmic reticulum. Uptake of calcium into the sarcoplasmic reticulum is mediated by a Ca-ATPase, a mechanism which is also responsible for extrusion of calcium across the plasma membrane [45, 46]. Another extrusion mechanism which may be of importance in some vessels is a Na-Ca exchange mechanism, whereby calcium is extruded using the energy of the inwardly directed sodium gradient [47]. The importance of this mechanism in peripheral vessels has, however, been questioned [48–50]. In any event, increases in cytoplasmic calcium may be expected to increase the interaction of the contractile proteins through binding to calmodulin and hence affecting the phosphorylation level of myosin light chain kinase.

Receptor activation

Activation of receptors through neural stimulation causes, in most blood vessels, a release of calcium from intracellular stores and a depolarization (either an action potential or a graded decrease in potential), and this is accompanied by a vasoconstriction. The action potential is probably due to the influx of calcium ions, not sodium as in other muscle types [51]. The effect of neural stimulation on rat mesenteric resistance vessels has been recently investigated [52]. In this study, it was found that with a constant rate of stimulation, frequencies of up to 10 to 15 Hz were required to obtain a maximal response. These frequencies are suprisingly high considering that the mean firing rate in autonomic nerves is probably much lower [53]. However, Nilsson and colleagues also found that the pattern of stimuli played an important role in the response of these small vessels [52]. Thus, if vessels were stimulated at the normal (slow) firing rate but with the usual irregular pattern of neural firing the vessels did respond, even though there was no response if the same rate of stimulation was given at a constant rate. This difference is presumably related to the mechanisms which reduce cytoplasmic calcium being slower than those which increase it.

Receptor activation with exogenous stimuli may or may not be accompanied by alterations in membrane potential. In some vessels, such as for example the rabbit ear artery, the vasoconstrictor response to exogenous noradrenaline produces no change in membrane potential [54]. In others, for example rat mesenteric resistance vessels, noradrenaline activation does produce depolarization [55]. Moreover, in these vessels, at least, it appears that the depolarization is a potentiating factor as regards the vasoconstrictor response, for the oscillatory mechanical response caused by noradrenaline stimulation is accompanied by similar changes in the membrane potential which *precede* the mechanical changes by about 1 s. This, therefore, suggests that the electrical changes are responsible for the mechanical changes and that they are probably mediated through the PDC. The PDC thus appear to play an important role in the determination of peripheral vascular smooth muscle tone.

Mechanism of Altered Calcium Sensitivity in SHR Mesenteric Resistance Vessels

The molecular basis for altered calcium metabolism is unknown. A number of authors have found that the ability of intracellular fractions of SHR vascular smooth muscle to bind calcium is reduced [56–58, 59], such that for a given total intracellular calcium level the cytoplasmic calcium concentration could be enhanced. Furthermore, there is some evidence that the rate of calcium extrusion by the calcium pump is reduced in SHR plasma membrane preparations [59], an abnormality which could again account for increased cytoplasmic calcium. Recent experiments which we have performed, however, suggest that the increased calcium sensitivity may also be due to alterations in the plasma membrane, since the increased calcium sensitivity of SHR mesenteric small arteries is eliminated by the calcium antagonist felodipine (Fig. 3) [60]. Since it has been shown [61] that felodipine acts primarily on the PDC (see above), this suggests that the enhanced calcium sensitivity of noradrenaline-activated SHR mesenteric resistance vessels may be due either to increased permeability of these channels or to noradrenaline causing a greater depolarization of the vessels. The latter possibility does not seem to be the case since we have found by direct intracellular measurements (Table 2) that the membrane potential of SHR and WKY vessels is the same, both under

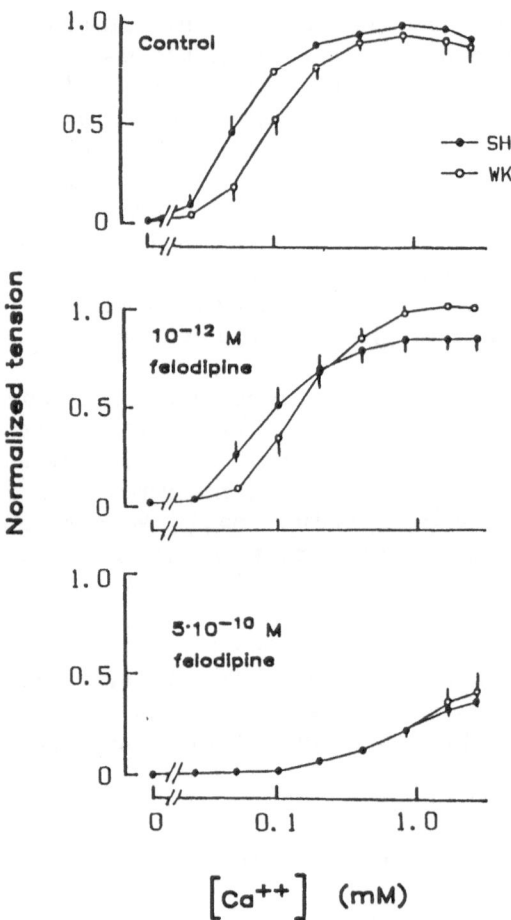

Fig. 3. Effect of felodipine on calcium sensitivity of noradrenaline-activated mesenteric resistance vessels from five SHR (*filled circles*) and five WKY (*open circles*). Points show mean ± SE. Note that increased calcium sensitivity was eliminated by 10^{-12} M felodipine. After Nyborg et al. [60]

Table 2. Membrane potential of SHR and WKY mesenteric resistance vessels

	SHR	WKY
Control	-55.6 ± 1.4 (12)	-55.9 ± 1.9 (10)
Activated	-28.9 ± 1.2 (12)	-29.9 ± 0.2 (10)

Vessels had internal diameter of ca. 150 μm. Membrane potential (mV) measured with intracellular electrodes [55]. Vessels held either in normal saline (*Control*) [40] or normal saline plus ca. 7 μmol/l noradrenaline (*Activated*). Values show mean ± SE (number of rats in parentheses). No significant differences between SHR and WKY values. (Nilsson and Mulvany unpublished data)

resting conditions and when activated with exogenous noradrenaline. Thus, it seems more likely that the increased calcium sensitivity is due to an increased permeability of the PDC (either because the individual channels are more permeable or because there are more of them), support for which is obtained from our

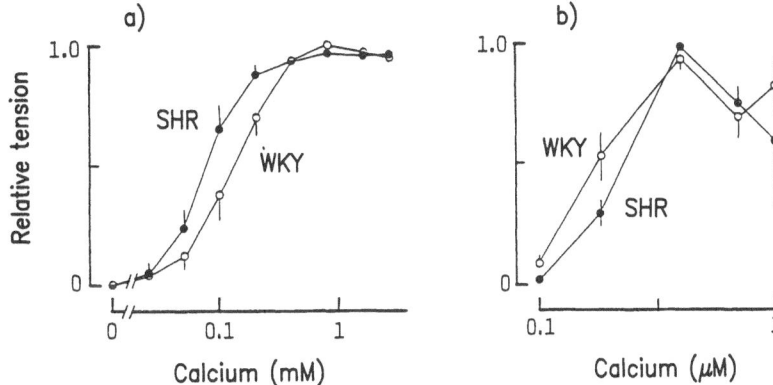

Fig. 4a, b. Calcium sensitivity of mesenteric resistance vessels from five SHR (*filled circles*) and five WKY (open circles) **a** before and **b** after "skinning" with Triton X. *Points* show mean ± SE. Note lack of difference in sensitivity after "skinning." After Byg Hansen [70]

previous findings (Table 1) [40] that the calcium sensitivity of SHR vessels which have been depolarized with potassium is also slightly increased. However, more direct support for this concept must await measurements of calcium uptake in these vessels [62]. Further evidence that the difference in calcium sensitivity is due to a defect in the plasma membrane has been provided by recent experiments in my laboratory which indicate that the calcium sensitivity of SHR "skinned" mesenteric resistance vessels is not different to that of WKY vessels (Fig. 4).

Are Vascular Abnormalities a Cause of Hypertension?

Experimental approaches

Although it is clear from the above discussion that, in the SHR at least, there appear to be certain vascular abnormalities associated with hypertension, it still needs to be determined whether the abnormalities are a cause of, a consequence of, or just incidental to the increased blood pressure. To investigate this, five approaches may be considered. First, the abnormality must be such that there are theoretical grounds for believing that the defect could cause increased blood pressure [e.g., 63]. Second, examination of how the defect develops with age may provide clues: Since the elevation of blood pressure in hypertension develops gradually, it may be possible to exclude the possibility that defects are consequences of the high blood pressure if the defects are already present at a very early age. Third, the effects of antihypertensive treatment may be determined; again, if the defect is a consequence of high blood pressure, it may be expected to regress with reduction of blood pressure. Fourth, in the case of animal models, genetic investigations may be made in the progeny obtained in controlled cross-breeding experiments between hypertensive and normotensive hybrids. Fifth, the abnormality can be investigated in a variety of hypertensive models to determine to what extent the abnormality might be a general determinant of hypertension.

With respect to an abnormality giving increased vascular sensitivity, it is clear that such a defect, all else being equal, would tend to cause an increased peripheral resistance and hence increased pressure. The theoretical basis for supposing that such an abnormality could be a cause of hypertension is thus sound, but there are other approaches to the problem as outlined below.

Age and therapy studies
Regarding effects of age and antihypertensive treatment on vascular EC coupling properties, this has not been studied in essential hypertensives in any detail. In the SHR, where vascular sensitivity differences have been seen, these do not seem to change greatly with age [24, 40, 64]. On the other hand, the available evidence suggests that the effect of antihypertensive treatment of SHR on the EC coupling properties of the vasculature is to increase its sensitivity. Pang and Sutter [65] found that treatment of SHR with D600 caused an increase in the sensitivity of the aorta and portal vein to calcium. Treatment of SHR with felodipine caused an increase in the calcium sensitivity of mesenteric small arteries but not in the noradrenaline sensitivity (Table 1) [66]. Conversely, hydralazine treatment of SHR increased the noradrenaline sensitivity of mesenteric small arteries but not the calcium sensitivity (Table 1) [67]. Whether the changes seen are compensatory mechanisms or effects of the reduced pressure remains to be determined.

Cross-breeding experiments
In an extensive study, Rapp [68] found that in the F_2 generation of SHR/Dahl-salt-insensitive rats, there was a correlation between blood pressure and the sensitivity of the aorta to cobalt (a marker of EC coupling properties). Some support for this was provided by an earlier limited investigation of ours, in which we saw a weak correlation between the blood pressure of F_2-hybrid SHR/WKY and the calcium sensitivity of their mesenteric resistance vessels when activated with noradrenaline [69]. However, in an extended study (Table 3) in which we looked at both SHR/WKY hybrids ($n = 54$) and SHRSP/WKY hybrids ($n = 42$) and where we took multiple vessels per animal, we were unable to confirm this. Clearly, therefore, any

Table 3. Calcium sensitivity of mesenteric resistance vessels in hybrid hypertensive/normotensive rats

	Blood pressure quartile	SHR/WKY	SHRSP/WKY
Systolic blood pressure (mmHg)	Highest	173 ± 1 (11)	182 ± 2 (11)
	Lowest	135 ± 2 (11)	139 ± 3 (9)
Ca-pD$_2$ (log units)	Highest	3.96 ± 0.04 (11)	4.04 ± 0.10 (11)
	Lowest	3.89 ± 0.04 (11)	3.94 ± 0.05 (9)

From measurements of systolic blood pressure (tail cuff method, average of three to six daily measurements), SHR/WKY ($n = 54$) and SHRSP/WKY ($n = 42$) were ranked. The table shows the blood pressures and Ca-pD$_2$ values for the highest and lowest blood pressure quartiles for each type of hybrid. Values show mean $\pm$ SE (number of rats in parentheses). No significant difference in Ca-pD$_2$ values for highest and lowest quartiles in either hybrid type

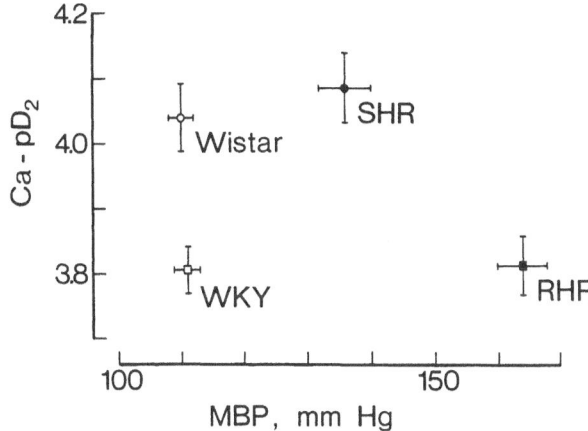

Fig. 5. Calcium sensitivity of mesenteric resistance vessels from ten SHR, ten WKY, ten 2-kidney, 1-clip Goldblatt hypertensive WKY (RHR), and ten outbred Wistar rats plotted against mean blood pressure, measured intraarterially. *Points* show mean $\pm$ SE. Note lack of correlation. After Mulvarny and Korsgaard [69]

correlation must be very weak and it must be concluded that the calcium sensitivity of noradrenaline-activated mesenteric resistance vessels is not a parameter which is closely associated with the factor causing high blood pressure in SHR and SHRSP.

Other models
Further evidence that altered vascular EC coupling is not an overriding factor in the determination of blood pressure comes from investigations where different strains of hypertensive and normotensive rats were investigated. Regarding aortic cobalt sensitivity, for example, although this was greater in SHR than in WKY, Dahl salt-sensitive and -resistant rats had even lower aortic cobalt sensitivities [68]. Likewise, we have found (Fig. 5) that although SHR mesenteric resistance vessels have an increased calcium sensitivity compared with WKY vessels, there is no difference in the calcium sensitivity of SHR and outbred normotensive Wistar rats [69].

Interpretations
On the basis of these findings, certain deductions may be made as to whether the EC coupling abnormalities are causes or consequences of the increased blood pressure associated with hypertension.

As indicated above, abnormalities of vascular EC coupling properties are in general rather small and difficult to demonstrate. Furthermore, since the age studies indicate that any such vascular EC coupling abnormalities are present at a very early age and do not increase with the development of hypertension, it is unlikely that they are consequences of hypertension. The lack of effect of antihypertensive treatment on vascular EC coupling abnormalities also supports this conclusion. Whether they could be associated with the causes of hypertension is not, however, clear. The reports referred to above indicating that in aortic vascular preparations there is a correlation between vascular EC coupling abnormalities and blood pressure suggest that the genetic abnormality causing abnormal vascular EC coupling properties could be associated with the genetic abnormality which causes high blood pressure. It is also clear from the effectiveness of vasodilators as antihypertensive drugs that alterations in vascular sensitivity can cause changes in blood pressure. However, our recent experiments in which we failed to find any correlation between the calcium sensitivity of mesenteric resistance vessels and blood pressure do not support this view; nor does the finding that the calcium sensitivity of normotensive Wistar vessels is the same in the SHR vessels. Therefore, in our view, much further work needs to be done before it can be established whether altered vascular EC coupling properties could be one of the factors which initiate the onset of hypertension.

Acknowledgments. This paper was prepared while the author was receiving support from the Danish Medical Research Council.

References

1. Lund-Johansson P (1980) Haemodynamics in essential hypertension. State of the art review. Clin Sci 59:343s–354s
2. Ferrone RA, Walsh GM, Tsuchiya M, Frohlich ED (1979) Comparison of hemodynamics in conscious spontaneous and renal hypertensive rats. Am J Physiol 236:H403–H408
3. Julius S, Esler M (eds) (1976) The Nervous System in Arterial Hypertension. Thomas, Springfield
4. Sakamaki T, Johnson JA, Zielgler DW, Koivunen DG, Siripaisarnpipat S, Fowler WL, Payne CG (1984) Pressor hyperresponsiveness in saline-infused rabbits. Hypertension 6:503–510
5. Mulvany MJ (1985) Role of vascular structure in blood pressure development of the SHR. J Hypertens (in press)
6. Okamoto K, Aoki K (1963) Development of a strain of spontaneously hypertensive rats. Jpn Circ J 27:283–293
7. Trippodo NC, Frohlich ED (1981) Similarities of genetic (spontaneous) hypertension. Man and rat. Circ Res 48:309–319
8. Ljungman S, Aurell M, Hartford M, Wikstrand J, Berglund G (1983) Effects of subpressor doses of angiotensin II on renal hemo-dynamics in relation to blood pressure. Hypertension 5:368–374
9. Robinson BF, Dobbs RJ, Bayley S (1982) Response of forearm resistance vessels to verapamil and sodium nitroprusside in normotensive and hypertensive men: evidence for a functional abnormality of vascular smooth muscle in primary hypertension. Clin Sci 63:33–42
10. Sivertsson R (1970) The hemodynamic importance of structural vascular changes in essential hypertension. Acta Physiol Scand Suppl 343
11. Moulds RFW (1980) Reduced responses to noradrenaline of isolated digital arteries from hypertensives. Clin Expt Pharmacol Physiol 7:505–508
12. Wyse DG (1984) Relationship of blood pressure to the responsiveness of an isolated human artery to selected agonists and to electrical stimulation. J Cardiovasc Pharmacol 6:1083–1091
13. Aalkjær C, Danielsen H, Johannesen P, Pedersen EB, Rasmussen A, Mulvany MJ (1985) Abnormal vascular function and morphology in preeclampsia: a study of isolated resistance vessels. Clin Sci 69:477–482
14. Mulvany MJ (1983) Do resistance vessel abnormalities contribute to the elevated blood pressure of spontaneously-hypertensive rats? A review of some of the evidence. Blood Vessels 20:1–22
15. Folkow B, Hallback M, Lundgren Y, Weiss L (1970) Background of increased flow resistance and vascular reactivity of spontaneously hypertensive rats. Acta Physiol Scand 80:93–106

16. Bohr DF (1974) Reactivity of vascular smooth muscle from normal and hypertensive rats: effect of several cations. Fed Proc 33:127–129
17. Lais LT, Shaffer RA, Brody MJ (1974) Neurogenic and humoral factors controlling vascular resistance in the spontaneously hypertensive rat. Circ Res 35:764–774
18. Collis MG, Vanhoutte PM (1977) Vascular reactivity of isolated perfused kidneys from male and female spontaneously hypertensive rats. Circ Res 41:759–767
19. Schömig A, Dietz R, Rascher W, Luth JB, Mann JFE, Schmidt M, Weber J (1978) Sympathetic vascular tone in spontaneous hypertension in rats. Klin Wochenschr 56 (Suppl I):131–138
20. Berecek KH, Stocker M, Gross F (1980) Changes in renal vascular reactivity at various stages of deoxycorticosterone hypertension in rats. Circ Res 46:619–624
21. Hermsmeyer K (1976) Electrogenesis of increased norepinephrine sensitivity of arterial vascular muscle in hypertension. Circ Res 38:362–267
22. Webb RC, Vanhoutte PM, Bohr DF (1981) Adrenergic neurotransmission in vascular smooth muscle from spontaneously hypertensive rats. Hypertension 3:93–103
23. Mulvany MJ, Nilsson H, Nyborg N, Mikkelsen E (1982) Are isolated femoral resistance vessels or tail arteries good models for the hindquarter vasculature of spontaneously hypertensive rats. Acta Physiol Scand 116:275–283
24. Mulvany MJ, Aalkjær C, Christensen J (1980) Changes in noradrenaline sensitivity and morphology of arterial resistance vessels during development of high blood pressure in spontaneously hypertensive rats. Hypertension 2:664–671
25. Whall CW, Myers MM, Halpern W (1980) Norepinephrine sensitivity, tension development and neuronal uptake in resistance arteries from spontaneously hypertensive and normotensive rats. Blood Vessels 17:1–15
26. Gray SD, Demey JG (1985) Vascular reactivity in neonatal spontaneously hypertensive rats. Prog Appl Microcirc 8:173–180
27. Zsoter TT, Sirko S, Wolchinsky C, Kadar D, Endrenyi L (1981) Adrenergic activity in arteries of spontaneously hypertensive rats. Can J Physiol Pharmacol 59:1104–1107
28. Wiegman DL, Joshua IG, Morff RJ, Harris PD, Miller FN (1979) Microvascular responses to norepinephrine in renovascular and spontaneously hypertensive rats. Am J Physiol 236:H545–H548
29. Bohlen HG (1979) Arteriolar closure mediated by hyperresponsiveness to norepinephrine in hypertensive rats. Am J Physiol 236:H157–H164
30. Strecker RB, Hubbard WC, Michelakis AM (1975) Dissociation constant of the norepinephrine-receptor complex in normotensive and hypertensive rats. Circ Res 37:658–663
31. Horwitz D, Clineschmidt BV, van Buren JM, Ommaya AK (1974) Temporal arteries from hypertensive and normotensive man. Circ Res 34–35 (Suppl I):115–109
32. Noon JP, Rice PJ, Baldessanne RJ (1978) Calcium leakage as a cause of high resting tension in vascular smooth muscle from SHR. Proc Nat Acad Sci 75:1605
33. Fitzpatrick DF, Szentivanyi A (1980) The relationship between increased myogenic tone and hyporesponsiveness in vascular smooth muscle of spontaneously hypertensive rats. Clin Exp Hypertens 2:1023–1037
34. Zsoter TT, Wolchinsky C, Henein NF, Ho LC (1977) Calcium kinetics in the aorta of SHR. Cardiovasc Res 11:353–357
35. Pedersen OL, Mikkelsen E, Andersson KE (1978) Effects of extracellular calcium on potassium and noradrenaline induced contractions in the aorta of spontaneously hypertensive rats—increased sensitivity to nifedipine. Acta Pharmacol Toxicol 43:137–144
36. Mulvany MJ (1983) Arterial abnormalities in spontaneously hypertensive rats (abstract). Proceedings of the International Union of Physiological Sciences 15:14
37. Winquist RJ, Bohr DF (1983) Structural and functional changes in cerebral arteries from spontaneously hypertensive rats. Hypertension 5:292–297
38. Kawaguchi Y, Aoki K, Yamamoto M, Hotta K (1982) Calcium-induced tension development and effect of calcium antagonist in mesenteric arteries from spontaneously hypertensive rats. In: Rascher W, Clough D, Ganten D (eds) Hypertensive mechanisms. Schattauer, Stuttgart, pp 264–267
39. Devine CE, Somlyo AV, Somlyo AP (1972) Sarcoplasmic reticulum and excitation-contraction coupling in mammalian smooth muscle. J Cell Biol 52:690–718

40. Mulvany MJ, Nyborg N (1980) An increased calcium sensitivity of mesenteric resistance vessels in young and adult spontaneously hypertensive rats. Br J Pharmacol 71:585–596
41. Nilsson H, Mulvany MJ (1981) Prolonged exposure to ouabain eliminates the greater noradrenaline-dependent calcium sensitivity of resistance vessels in spontaneously hypertensive rats. Hypertension 3:691–697
42. Pegram BL, Ljung B (1981) Neuroeffector function of isolated portal vein from spontaneously hypertensive and Wistar-Kyoto rats: dependence on external calcium concentration. Blood Vessels 18:89–99
43. Folkow B, Hallback M, Jones JV, Sutter M (1977) Dependence of external calcium for noradrenaline contractility of resistance vessels in spontaneously hypertensive and renal hypertensive rats, as compared with normotensive controls. Acta Physiol Scand 101:84–97
44. Bolton TB (1979) Mechanisms of action of transmitters and other substances on smooth muscle. Physiol Rev 59:606–718
45. Wuytack F, Raeymakers L, de Schutter G, Casteels R (1982) Demonstration of the phosphorylated intermediates of the Ca^+-transport ATPase in a microsomal fraction and in a $(Ca^{2+} + Mg^{2+})$-ATPase purified from smooth muscle by means of a calmodulin affinity chromatography. Biochim Biophys Acta 693:45–52
46. Kwan CY, Triggle CR, Grover AK, Lee RMKW, Daniel EE (1983) An analytical approach to the preparation and characterization of subcellular membranes from canine mesenteric arteries. Preparative Biochem 13:275–314
47. Blaustein MP (1977) Sodium ions, calcium ions, blood pressure regulation and hypertension: a reassessment and a hypothesis. Am J Physiol 232:C165–C173
48. Droogmans G, Casteels R (1979) Sodium and calcium interactions in vascular smooth muscle cells of the rabbit ear artery. J Gen Physiol 74:57–70
49. Hermsmeyer K (1983) Sodium pump hyperpolarization-relaxation in rat caudal artery. Fedn Proc 42:246–252
50. Mulvany MJ, Aalkjær C, Petersen TT (1984) Intracellular sodium, membrane potential and contractility in rat mesenteric small arteries. Circ Res 54:740–749
51. Harder DR, Sperelakis N (1979) Action potentials induced in guinea pig arterial smooth muscle by tetraethylammonium. Am J Physiol 237:C75–C80
52. Nilsson H, Ljung B, Sjoblom N, Wallin BG (1985) The influence of the sympathetic impulse pattern on contractile responses of rat mesenteric arteries and veins. Acta Physiol Scand 123:303–309
53. Thoren P, Ricksten SE (1979) Recordings of renal and splanchnic sympathetic nervous activity in normotensive and spontaneously hypertensive rats. Clin Sci 57:197s–199s
54. Droogmans G, Raeymakers L, Casteels R (1977) Electro- and pharmacomechanical coupling in the smooth muscle cells of the rabbit ear artery. J Gen Physiol 70:129–148
55. Mulvany MJ, Nilsson H, Flatman JA (1982) Role of membrane potential in the response of rat small mesenteric arteries to exogenous noradrenaline stimulation. J Physiol 332:363–373
56. Aoki K, Ikeda N, Yamashita K, Tazumi K, Sato I, Hotta K (1974) Cardiovascular contraction in spontaneously hypertensive rat: Ca^{2+} interaction of myofibrils and subcellular membrane of heart and arterial smooth muscle. Jpn Circ J 38:1115–1121
57. Webb RC, Bhalla RC (1976) Altered calcium sequestration by sub-cellular fractions of vascular smooth muscle from spontaneously hypertensive rats. J Mol Cell Cardiol 8:651
58. Moore L, Hurwitz L, Davenport GR, Landon EJ (1975) Energy-dependent calcium uptake activity of microsomes from the aorta of normal and hypertensive rats. Biochim Biophys Acta 413:432–443
59. Kwan CY, Belbeck L, Daniel EE (1979) Abnormal biochemistry of vascular smooth muscle plasma membrane as an important factor in the initiation and maintenance of hypertension in rats. Blood Vessels 16:259–268
60. Nyborg N, Byg Hansen J, Mulvany MJ (1985) Effect of felodipine on resistance vessels from spontaneously hypertensive and normotensive rats. J Cardiovasc Pharmacol (in press)
61. Nyborg N, Mulvany MJ (1984) Effect of felodipine, a new dihydropyridine vasodilator on contractile responses to potassium, noradrenaline, and calcium in mesenteric resistance vessels of the rat. J Cardiovasc Pharmacol 6:499–505

62. Cauvin C, Saida K, van Breemen C (1982) Effects of calcium antagonists on calcium fluxes in resistance vessels. J Cardiovasc Pharmacol 4: S287–S290
63. Rapp JP (1983) A paradigm for identification of primary genetic causes of hypertension in rats. Hypertension 5 (Suppl 1): I-198–I-203
64. Lais LT, Brody MJ (1978) Vasoconstrictor hyper-responsiveness: an early pathogenic mechanism in the spontaneously hypertensive rat. Eur J Pharmacol 17: 177–189
65. Pang CCY, Sutter MC (1981) Effect of chronic treatment of spontaneously hypertensive rats with D600. Hypertension 3: 657–663
66. Nyborg NCB, Mulvany MJ (1985) Lack of effect of antihypertensive treatment with felodipine on cardiovascular structure of young spontaneously hypertensive rats. Cardiovasc Res 19: 528–536
67. Jespersen LT, Nyborg NCB, Pedersen OL, Mikkelsen EO, Mulvany MJ (1985) Cardiac mass and peripheral vascular structure in hydralazine-treated spontaneously hypertensive rats. Hypertension 7: 734–741
68. Rapp JP (1982) A genetic locus (*Hyp-2*) controlling vascular smooth muscle response in spontaneously hypertensive rats. Hypertension 4: 459–467
69. Mulvany MJ, Korsgaard N (1983) Correlations and otherwise between blood pressure, cardiac mass and resistance vessel characteristics in hypertensive, normotensive and hypertensive/normotensive hybrid rats. J Hypertension 1: 235–244
70. Byg Hansen J (1985) Calcium sensitivity in mesenteric resistance vessels from spontaneously hypertensive and control Wistar-Kyoto rats, demonstrated with mechanical experiments and the use of ouabain, felodipine, skinning and denervation. Research Prize, Aarhus University, Aarhus

Calcium-Membrane Interactions in Smooth Muscle in Relation to Hypertension

A Subcellular Membrane Approach

C. Y. Kwan

Smooth Muscle Research Program, Department of Neurosciences, McMaster University, Hamilton, Ontario, L8N 3Z5 Canada

Summary. This article provides an overview on the studies of calcium-membrane interactions in smooth muscle during the past decade using subcellular membrane fractionation technique with special reference to the relationship between the alterations of calcium ion handling in vascular smooth muscle and the pathogenesis of spontaneous hypertension in rats. The calcium-membrane interactions include ATP-dependent Ca-transport, Na-dependent Ca-transport (Na-Ca exchange) and Ca-binding. A collection of experimental evidence consistently suggest that the ATP-dependent Ca-transport is decreased in membrane vesicles isolated from the vascular smooth muscles of spontaneously hypertensive rats compared to those of normotensive control rats. This Ca-transport deficit occurs in large as well as small arteries, is an intrinsic change of the cell membranes and cannot be interpreted solely as the consequence of elevated blood pressure in hypertension. It also occurs in several forms of experimentally induced hypertension in rats. Such a Ca-transport deficit is present in nonvascular smooth muscles as well in spontaneous hypertension, but not in experimental hypertension. This suggests that the altered ATP-dependent Ca-transport may be genetically programmed and may represent a widespread membrane defect in tissues not confined to the cardiovascular system.

Key words: Hypertension—Calcium—Ion transport—Vascular smooth muscle—Cell membrane

The close association of altered body and tissue electrolytes and the development of hypertension has long been one of the most active areas of research into the etiological mechanisms of essential hypertension. It has long been accepted that sodium is an etiological factor in hypertension [1, 2]. Some considerable attention has recently been focussed upon the roles of calcium in the pathogenesis of hypertensive diseases [3–6]. This is consistent with the rapidly growing interest in the calcium antagonists as a group of effective therapeutic antihypertensives in the treatment of cardiovascular diseases, including hypertension [7–10]. Essential hypertension is associated with increased total peripheral resistance due to increased arteriolar tone. Therefore, a variety of hypotheses for the pathogenesis of hypertension have been based upon the proposed regulatory mechanisms that control the vascular muscle tone, e.g., myogenic, neurogenic, and humoral controls (Fig. 1).

The association between calcium metabolism and blood pressure regulation was implicated in early epidemiological studies relating the lower incidence of death from cardiovascular disease in some geographical areas to the hardness of drinking water [11]. More recent studies on the epidemiology of dietary calcium and blood pressure have identified low dietary calcium intake as a risk factor for

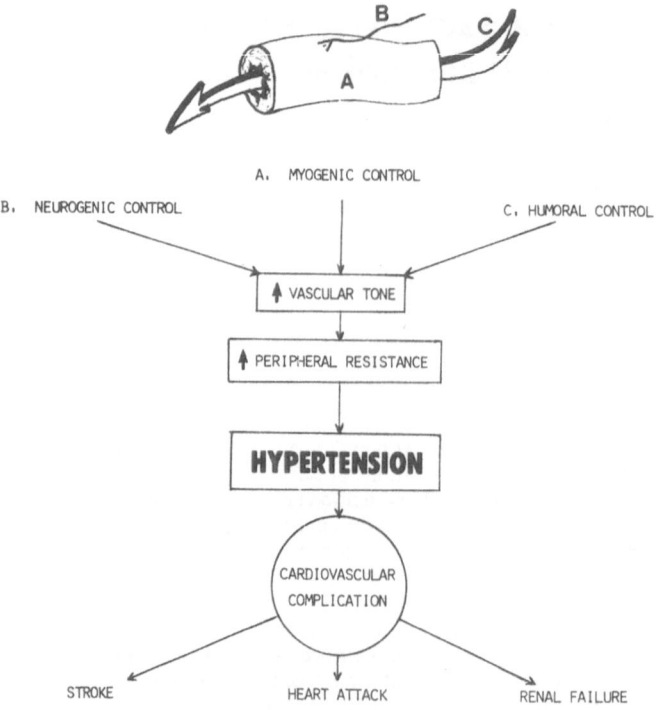

Fig. 1. Possible controls of vascular muscle tone in hypertension

the development of essential hypertension [12, 13], and this has also been observed in animal studies using spontaneously hypertensive rats (SHR) [14, 15].
Since the contractile apparatus in vascular muscle is activated by a rise in the
cytoplasmic concentration of ionized calcium, derangement of regulation of the
Ca^{2+} level in vascular muscle cells may conceivably provide a logical interpretation of some of the altered contractile properties of vascular muscles associated
with hypertension, including elevated vascular muscle tone, hyperreactivity to
vasoactive substances, and decreased rate of relaxation [16]. Extracellular Ca^{2+},
on the other hand, not only serves as the activator Ca^{2+} to support vascular
muscle contraction by crossing the cell membrane, but also acts as a membrane
stabilizer to prevent further influx of Ca^{2+}, thus inhibiting the vasoconstriction
and ultimately leading to relaxation [17]. Therefore, the activity of cytoplasmic
Ca^{2+} is the major determinant of the contractile state of the vascular muscle; the
level of extracellular Ca^{2+} provides modulation of the intracellular Ca^{2+} activity
via interactions with cell membranes as well as being a source of intracellular
Ca^{2+}.

Methods

Among the various methods used in studying the distribution and handling of
Ca^{2+} in vascular muscles [for a review, see 18, 19], the subcellular fractionation

technique circumvents some of the technical limitations inherently associated with intact tissue preparations, such as the anatomical complexity of blood vessel walls and the extremely low intracellular Ca^{2+} content of smooth muscle cells. The fractionation technique involves basically three major steps: (a) Trimming of blood vessels; (b) homogenization and separation of membranes, and (c) characterization of isolated subcellular fractions.

Trimming of blood vessels

In earlier studies, a large elastic artery such as the aorta was commonly used, presumably due to its size because the vascular muscle could be isolated and collected with reasonable ease and sufficient quantity. In this laboratory, smaller mesenteric arteries, which are more muscular and resemble the resistant vessel type, were employed for most studies. Handling the mesenteric vasculature to remove the large amounts of mesenteric connective tissue surrounding fat and the collateral veins requires special tissue-trimming procedures and was described previously in great detail [20, 21]. Failure to remove effectively the nonarterial tissues may complicate the interpretation of the results obtained [22, 23].

Homogenization and separation of membranes

Conventionally, a vigorous homogenization procedure is required to achieve effective disruption of the cellular membrane components to allow subsequent separation based upon physical properties of subcellular membranes such as size and density. It was generally assumed that the major subcellular membrane components such as nuclei, intact and broken mitochondria, endoplasmic reticulum, and plasma membranes sediment with different velocities in a given medium under a given centrifugal force. Microsomal membranes, usually quite heterogeneous, were frequently obtained by differential centrifugation and used without further purification [24–26; review—19]. To determine the subcellular site of vascular membrane lesions in hypertension, the heterogeneous microsomal fraction was further subfractionated on a sucrose density gradient to separate the light-density plasma membrane fraction and other denser fractions more enriched in internal membranes.

Characterization of subcellular membranes

Positive identification of the membranes in a given isolated fraction requires an analytical approach that utilizes the analysis of a group of membrane markers, usually some membrane-specific enzyme activities, sometimes in combination with the morphological examination, in all isolated subcellular fractions. Marker enzymes include: 5′-nucleotidase, phosphodiesterase I, Mg^{2+}-ATPase, adenylate cyclase and alkaline phosphatase for plasma membranes; NADPH cytochrome c reductase for endoplasmic reticulum; cytochrome c oxidase for mitochondria. The validity and limitation of the use of these and other enzymes as membrane markers in smooth muscle fractionation have recently been reviewed [19].

Study of Ca^{2+}-membrane interactions

Ca^{2+} interacts with the smooth muscle membranes (isolated primarily in the form of vesicles as examined electron microscopically) in a complex manner, depending upon the experimental conditions. This was studied as the accumulation or loss of

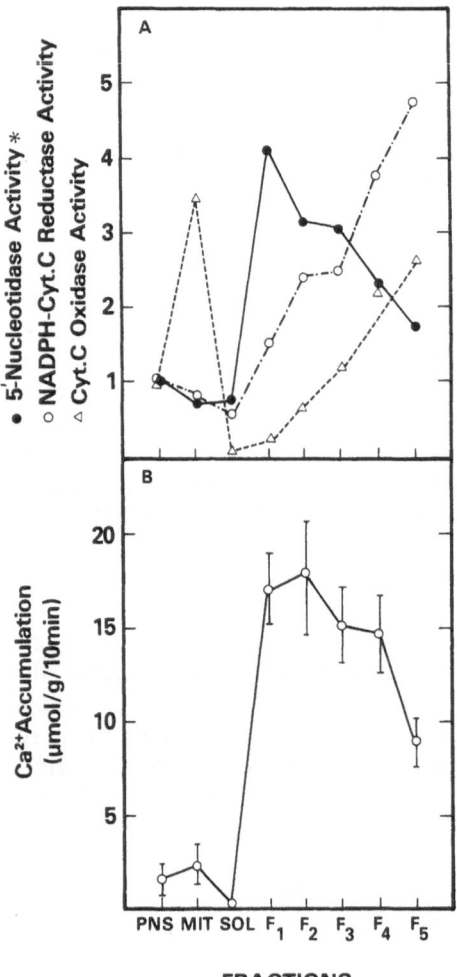

Fig. 2. Marker enzyme distribution and ATP-supported Ca^{2+} accumulation by subcellular fractions isolated from rat mesenteric arteries. *PNS* postnuclear supernatant after centrifugation of tissue homogenate at 1000 g for 10 min, *MIT* mitochondrial fraction after centrifugation of PNS at 10 000 g for 10 min, *SOL* soluble protein fraction after centrifugation of postmitochondrial supernatant. The resultant microsomal pellet was resuspended and subfractionated on a discontinuous sucrose density gradient to obtain *F1* (8/26.5% sucrose interphase), *F2* (26.5% sucrose layer), *F3* (26.5% sucrose interphase), *F4* (32.5% sucrose layer), and *F5* (26.5/32.5% sucrose interphase). Enzyme activities were expressed as relative activities with that of PNS set as unity. For details, see Kwan et al. [20]

$^{45}Ca^{2+}$ by the isolated membranes using a Millipore filtration technique; the method includes: (a) Ca^{2+} binding—Ca^{2+} accumulated in the absence of chemical energy from ATP or diffusion energy from the ionic gradient; (b) ATP-dependent Ca^{2+} transport—active transport of Ca^{2+} in the presence of ATP hydrolysis; and (c) Na^+-Ca^{2+} exchange—active transport of Ca^{2+} into or out of the membrane vesicles at the expense of an oppositely directed Na^+ gradient. The methodological details have previously been described in great detail using isolated smooth muscle plasma membrane vesicles [20, 27–29]. Figure 2 shows a typical profile of characterization of various subcellular fractions isolated from rat mesenteric arteries.

Results and discussion

Sites of Ca^{2+}-handling defects

A decreased rate of relaxation in vascular muscle strips isolated from hypertensive animals can conceivably be interpreted as the indication of a possible defect in the ability of the smooth muscle cells to lower their cytoplasmic free Ca^{2+} concentration. Therefore, a defective Ca^{2+} extrusion mechanism in the cell membranes or a derangement of the Ca^{2+} sequestration system in the internal organelles, such as the endoplasmic (or sarcoplasmic) reticulum, has been suspected. Aoki et al. [24] in 1974 reported that the ATP-supported Ca^{2+} transport was significantly lower in the aortic microsomes isolated from the SHR than in those from the corresponding Kyoto-Wistar normotensive control (WKY). This finding was later confirmed by Moore et al. [25] and Webb and Bhalla [26] in aortic microsomes isolated from SHR and rats with deoxycorticosterone (DOC)-salt induced hypertension. These studies also showed that such a vascular muscle membrane lesion was not due to the changes in the affinity of the transport system for the Ca^{2+}. They attributed this microsomal membrane defect in Ca^{2+} transport to an abnormality of the sarcoplasmic reticulum. However, Wei et al. [30] further subfractionated the aortic microsomes from SHR on a sucrose density gradient and showed that aortic microsomes prepared by differential centrifugation were highly heterogeneous and heavily contaminated by the plasma membranes and that it was the aortic plasma membranes that showed a prominent decrease in ATP-supported Ca^{2+} transport in SHR. Kwan et al. [23, 31] using rat mesenteric arteries of SHR also found a similar defect in the light-density plasma membrane fraction (Fig. 3). These studies strongly suggest that in hypertension

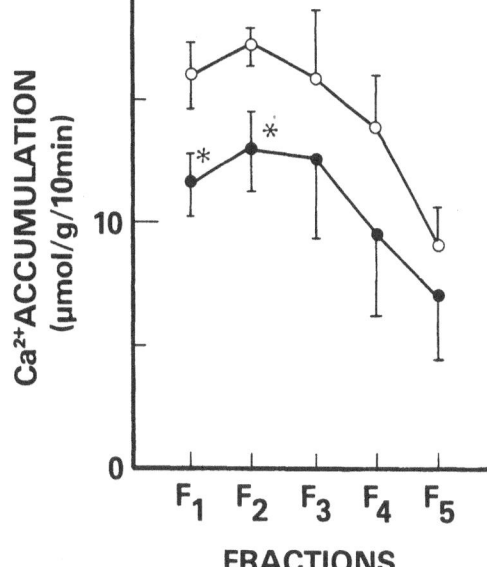

Fig. 3. Distribution of ATP-supported Ca^{2+} accumulation by submicrosomal fractions isolated from mesenteric arteries of spontaneously hypertensive (●) and normotensive (○) rats. *Significantly different from control values ($P < 0.05$). *Vertical bars* represent standard deviation for the mean of five separate experiments. Adapted from Kwan et al. [23]

decreased Ca^{2+} transport in the presence of ATP occurs at the level of plasma membranes in both large and small arteries.

Nature of Ca^{2+}-handling defects

Kwan et al. [31] and others [25, 26, 30] have shown that in the absence of ATP the binding of Ca^{2+} at 20 μM free Ca^{2+} to the plasma membrane-enriched fractions isolated from the vascular muscles of SHR was not different from that of WKY. They also demonstrated that the addition of the Ca^{2+}-specific ionophore A23187 prevented the ATP-supported Ca^{2+} transport and caused a rapid and substantial release of Ca^{2+}, and the residual Ca^{2+} binding (in the presence of A23187) was not different in fractions isolated from SHR and WKY. However, Wei et al. [30] reported a significant decrease of Ca^{2+} binding to the plasma membrane fraction of mesenteric arteries from SHR at millimolar concentrations of Ca^{2+}. This finding seems to be consistent with the hypothesis that reduced binding of Ca^{2+} to the vascular muscle cell membranes may be responsible for the decreased membrane stability that leads to increased influx of Ca^{2+} and reduced ability of the vascular muscle to relax in hypertension [32]. Thus, it is possible that stabilization of cell membranes requires millimolar, not micromolar, concentrations of Ca^{2+}. Kwan and Daniel [33] also reported that the plasma membrane fractions isolated from mesenteric veins, unlike those from the accompanying mesenteric arteries, showed increased Ca^{2+} binding but unaltered ATP-supported Ca^{2+} transport in spontaneous hypertension. This suggests that the Ca-handling defect present in SHR may take several forms in vascular muscles.

Another way in which Ca^{2+} distribution across the vascular muscle cell membrane may be affected is via Na^+-Ca^{2+} exchange, a process that utilizes the diffusion energy from the countercurrent of the Na^+ gradient to transport Ca^{2+}. It has been speculated that Na^+-Ca^{2+} exchange could be a working mechanism to relate the altered Na^+ distribution across the vascular muscle cell membrane to the altered contractile function of vascular muscle strips in hypertension [34]. The existence of such an Na^+-Ca^{2+} exchange system has been demonstrated using plasma membrane vesicles isolated from vascular [35, 36] as well as nonvascular muscles [27]. The physiological importance of such an exchange system in smooth muscle contractile function is still questionable [37]. The transport of Ca^{2+} via the Na^+ gradient, compared with that via ATP hydrolysis, by the smooth muscle plasma membrane vesicles showed an initial rate of transport and affinity for Ca^{2+} too low to be physiologically relevant. Recently, Matlib et al. [36] have reported that the plasma membrane-enriched fraction isolated from the mesenteric arteries of SHR under conditions similar to ours [20] showed slightly but not significantly higher Ca uptake in the presence of an outward Na^+ gradient than that obtained from WKY. The interpretation of these data was complicated by the possible changes in SHR of Ca^{2+} binding to the membranes and the competition for such Ca^{2+}-binding sites by Na^+. To date, optimal conditions for retaining Na^+-Ca^{2+} exchange in isolated plasma membrane vesicles from vascular smooth muscle may not have been achieved; so a final decision about this mechanism may await future studies.

It appears that the most consistent finding in Ca^{2+} deficit in vascular muscle membranes from SHR reported from various laboratories is the reduced amount of Ca^{2+} accumulated against its electrochemical gradient in the presence of ATP compared with that obtained from WKY. This change could result from: (a) the higher contamination by other membranes or proteins, (b) a lower proportion of inverted membrane vesicles, (c) an increased Ca^{2+} leak, and (d) a reduced Ca^{2+}-pump activity. We have ruled out the first possibility by showing that the vascular muscle plasma membrane fractions isolated from SHR and WKY were enriched in plasma membrane marker enzymes to a similar extent and did not differ in other membrane marker enzyme activities. The second possibility also seems unlikely because a similar latency of ouabain-sensitive K^+-activated p-nitrophenyl phosphatase activity (revealed by osmotic shock of the membrane vesicles) was obtained using the rat mesenteric artery plasma membranes from SHR and WKY [38]. To assess the Ca^{2+} leak, plasma membrane vesicles from mesenteric arteries of SHR and WKY were loaded with Ca^{2+} via the Ca^{2+} pump in the presence of ATP and then diluted by Ca^{2+}-free ethylene glycol-bis (β-aminoethyl ether) N,N,N',N'-tetraacetic acid (EGTA) containing medium. Figure 4 shows that the rates of loss of Ca^{2+} from the vesicles over a 3-h period at 37°C followed a complex profile. The SHR membranes showed a slightly but not significantly faster loss of Ca^{2+} than WKY membranes. This may be interpreted to mean that SHR membrane vesicles were no leakier than WKY membrane vesicles. This result is also consistent with the lack of change in Na^+-Ca^{2+} exchange as mentioned previously, since increased Ca^{2+} leak may in fact lead to

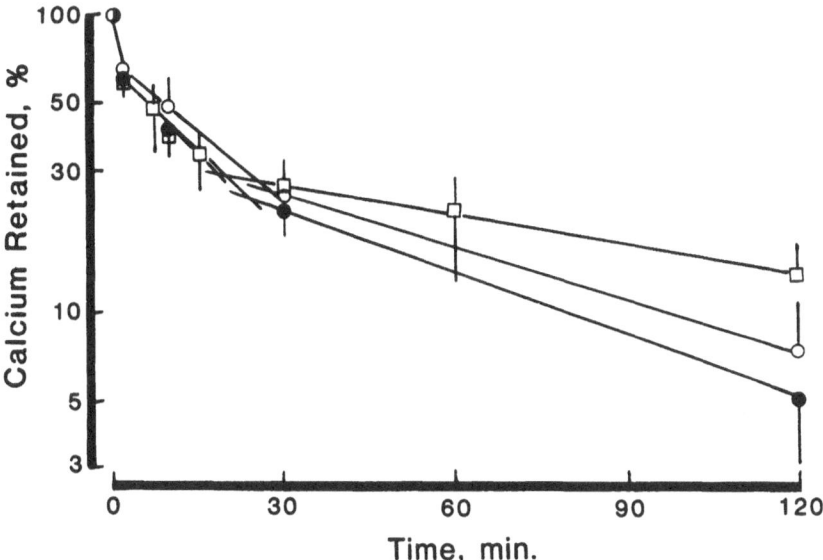

Fig. 4. Ca^{2+} leakage from the plasma membrane-enriched fractions isolated from mesenteric arteries of SHR (●), WKY (○), and normotensive Wistar rats (□). Each *value* for SHR and WKY represents mean ± SD of triplicates from a paired experiment. The $^{45}Ca^{2+}$ accumulation was first performed in the presence of ATP and then diluted ten fold into isotonic Ca^{2+}-free sucrose buffer containing 1 *mM* EGTA. Aliquots were removed at various time intervals and assayed for $^{45}Ca^{2+}$ retained by Millipore filtration (Kwan CY, Grover AK, Daniel EE, unpublished observation)

reduced Na^+-Ca^{2+} exchange. However, the complexity of the interpretation and the technical difficulties in providing sufficient data points for the analysis of the Ca^{2+} efflux curves caused us not to rule out increased leakage as an explanation of the altered Ca^{2+} handling. Very little is known about the change in Ca^{2+}-pump activities in vascular smooth muscle in hypertension. This aspect awaits future studies.

Relationship between Ca^{2+}-handling defects and hypertension

Several lines of evidence suggest that the deficit in ATP-supported Ca^{2+} transport in vascular muscle plasma membrane vesicles from hypertensive rats cannot be interpreted as a direct consequence of increased wall stress on the vessel walls due to elevated blood pressure.

First, this Ca^{2+}-handling defect was shown to precede the onset of detectable hypertension in our SHR colony [31]. This is shown in Fig. 5. In addition, the activities of two of the plasma membrane marker enzymes, alkaline phosphatase and 5'-nucleotidase, were also elevated in accordance with the development of blood pressure. However, the elevation of alkaline phosphatase activity closely paralleled the decrease in Ca^{2+} transport, whereas the elevation of 5'-nucleotidase activity closely paralleled the increase in arterial mass. It is possible that vascular muscle alkaline phosphatase may attenuate the Ca^{2+}-pump activity via

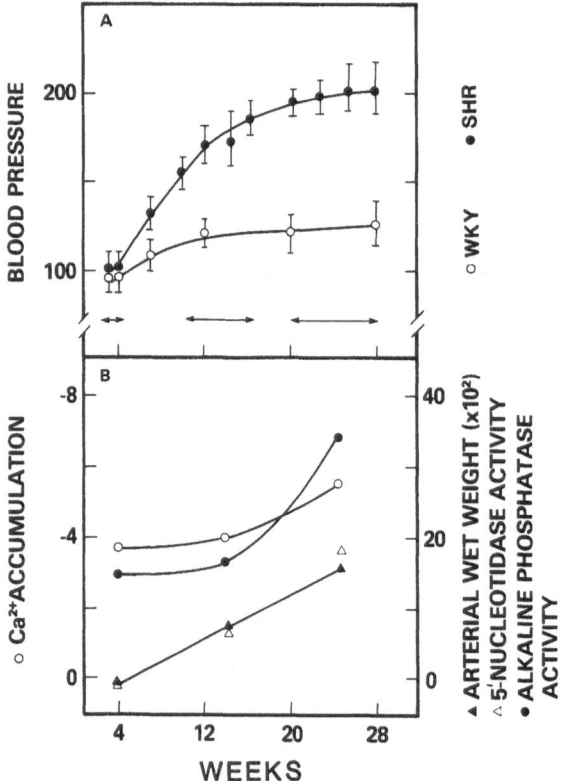

Fig. 5. A Development of systolic blood pressure (mmHg) of SHR and WKY. B Changes in wet weight of mesenteric arteries (g/kg body weight), 5'-nucleotidase activity (μmol-mg^{-1}/h), alkaline phosphatase activity (μmol-mg^{-1}/h), and ATP-supported Ca^{2+} accumulation (μmol-g^{-1}/ 10 min) of the plasma membrane fractions of mesenteric arteries in SHR. *Negative values* denote lower activity in SHR than in WKY. Adapted from Kwan et al. [31]

a dephosphorylation mechanism. Alternatively, alkaline phosphatase activity may be affected independently of the Ca^{2+}-pump activity via a common, but yet unknown, mechanism. These results also suggest that functional changes (Ca^{2+} transport) may precede the structural changes (arterial mass). Such a hypothesis obviously deserves more experimental exploration in the future.

Second, in DOC-salt hypertension, this Ca^{2+}-handling defect behaved in accordance with the blood pressure. In those animals with blood pressure returning to normal after the withdrawl of the cause of hypertension, i.e., the DOC treatment, this Ca^{2+}-handling defect was no longer present [23, 31], but the defect persisted in those animals in which hypertension persisted. On the other hand, normalization of the blood pressure in SHR by long-term hydralazine treatment, which does not correct the causal mechanism and "cure" hypertension, failed to correct this Ca^{2+}-handling defect [39].

Third, a similar decrease in ATP-supported Ca^{2+} transport was also observed using microsomes prepared from cultured aortic smooth muscle cells from adult SHR compared with those from age-matched WKY [40] under similar culture conditions.

Fourth, in spontaneous hypertension, a similar Ca^{2+}-transport defect also occurred in microsomes obtained from nonvascular smooth muscles [41]. If it is not unreasonable to assume that vascular and nonvascular smooth muscles elicit fundamentally similar membrane properties in regulating the Ca^{2+} distribution, this result can be interpreted to mean that the Ca^{2+}-handling defects in vascular smooth muscle, as in nonvascular smooth muscle, are not a consequence of hypertension. Such a Ca^{2+}-handling defect in nonvascular smooth muscle (vas deferens) membranes, however, was not found in DOC-salt hypertension [42]. This is in excellent agreement with the finding of altered contractile function of the vas deferens in spontaneous hypertension but not in DOC-salt hypertension [43, 44]. These results suggest that in spontaneous hypertension, the deficit in ATP-supported Ca^{2+} transport may be genetically programmed such that it occurs in smooth muscles not necessarily confined to the cardiovascular system.

Widespread phenomenon of Ca^{2+}-handling defects
Table 1 summarizes the deficits of Ca^{2+} handling in vascular and nonvascular smooth muscles in five different modes of hypertension in rat studies. It is

Table 1. Summary of changes in ATP-supported Ca^{2+} transport by membranes isolated from vascular and nonvascular smooth muscles of rats with different modes of hypertension

Mode of hypertension	Vascular	Nonvascular	Reference
Spontaneous	↓	↓, ↔	22, 23, 30, 31
Deoxycorticosterone-salt	↓	↔	23, 31
1-kidney, 1-clip	↓	ND	45
2-kidney, 2-clip	↓	ND	45
Dahl salt-sensitive	↔	↓	46

↓ decreased, ↔ unaltered compared with corresponding normotensive controls, *ND* not determined

interesting to note that although the Ca^{2+} handling defect was present in the vascular muscle plasma membranes in spontaneous hypertension [23, 31], DOC-salt hypertension [23, 31], and two types of renovascular hypertension [45], the salt-induced hypertension in the S strain of Dahl rats did not elicit such a membrane defect in the mesenteric artery, but it did in the vas deferens [46]. The results obtained using Dahl hypertensive rats were interpreted to mean that the vascular muscle membrane defect in Ca^{2+} handling should not be generalized to all types of hypertension and such a defect cannot be a direct consequence of hypertension. Furthermore, the presence of this Ca^{2+}-handling defect in the vas deferens in salt-induced hypertension, as in spontaneous hypertension, seems to suggest that a genetically programmed membrane defect may still be present but expressed in a nonvascular system. This also points to the possibility that salt-induced genetic hypertension may involve changes of Ca^{2+} membrane interac-

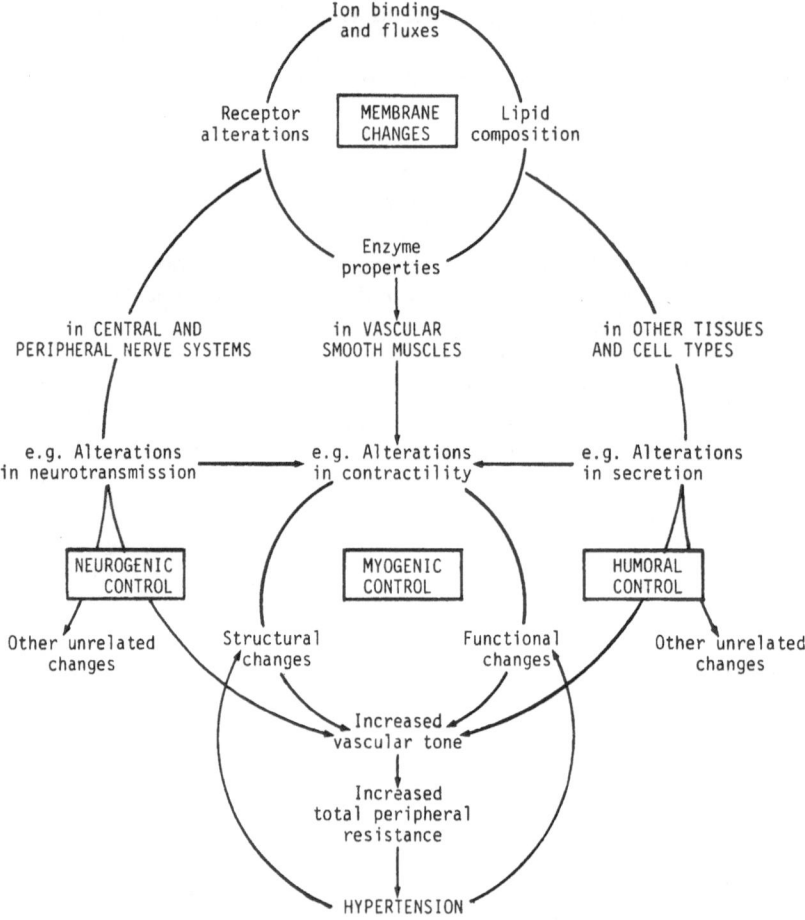

Fig. 6. Schematic representation of the membrane hypothesis of hypertension. See text and Kwan [40] for discussion

Table 2. Summary of Ca^{2+}-handling abnormalities in cell membranes of tissues from spontaneously hypertensive rats

	Reference	Ca^{2+} transport	Ca^{2+} binding
Brain (synaptosomes)	49	↓	↓
Heart (ventricle)	50, 51	↔ (ER↓)	↓
Aorta	30	↓	↔
Mesenteric artery	30, 31	↓	↔, ↓
Mesenteric vein	33	↔	↑
Vas deferens	41	↓	↔
Gastric fundus	41	↓	↔
Kidney	25, 51	↔	↓
Adipocyte	52	↔ (ER↓)	↓
Erythrocyte	51, 53–55	↓	↓
Platelet	56	↑ $[Ca^{2+}]_i$ and ↑ aggregation	

↑ increased, ↓ decreased, ↔ unaltered, *ER* endoplasmic reticulum

tions in tissues responsible for the neurogenic or humoral control of vascular contraction (Fig. 1). Another question which requires further analysis in Dahl-type genetic hypertension is—what is the correct control? After all, the genetic defect may be present in these rats when not fed salt, but it may only result in hypertension when a salt load is imposed.

Putting together the evidence obtained collectively from this and other laboratories, a hypothesis of a generalized membrane defect as the primary cause of hypertension is presented in Fig. 6, and this variety of membrane defects present in SHR is also summarized in Table 2. Indeed, this hypothesis has recently received increasing experimental support [see reviews—3–6, 40, 47]. As an extension of this membrane hypothesis, membrane defects other than Ca^{2+} handling, such as Na^+ and K^+ handling, have been reported to exist in many tissues in genetic hypertension [48].

Conclusions and Future Perspectives

There is strong evidence of defective Ca^{2+}-membrane interactions in the plasma membrane of vascular smooth muscle in hypertension, and this membrane deficit could be a part of the causative mechanism for hypertension of both genetic and experimental origin. When genetic in origin, the Ca^{2+}-handling defect is not confined to the cardiovascular system; it represents a general membrane defect in ion handling by many cells. The multiplicity of membrane defects provides a reasonable working hypothesis toward the understanding of several putative functional mechanisms postulated by a variety of investigators to account for the initiation and pathogenesis of hypertension. It is desirable to explore further the relationship between: (a) various forms of ion dysfunction in vascular muscle membranes (e.g., Na^+, K^+, Cl^-, Ca^{2+}, and Mg^{2+}); (b) functional changes in ion handling and structural alterations in membranes (e.g., lipid metabolism, protein composition, and membrane fluidity); (c) vascular muscle membrane defects and structural changes in vascular muscle wall (e.g., hypertrophy, hyperplasia, and extracellular connective tissue metabolism); (d) membrane changes in nonvascular tissues involved in blood pressure regulation (e.g., relating to neural and humoral control of vascular tone); and (e) alterations in ion-membrane interactions and membrane receptor changes (e.g., for catecholamine and vasoactive peptides).

Acknowledgment. This work was supported by the Heart and Stroke Foundation of Ontario.

References

1. Tobian L, Binion JT (1952) Tissue cations and water in arterial hypertension. Circulation 5:754–758.
2. Dahl LK, Heine M, Tassinari L (1962) Effects of chronic salt ingestion: evidence that genetic factors play an important role in susceptibility to experimental hypertension. J Exp Med 115:1173–1190
3. Robinson BP (1984) Altered calcium handling as a cause of primary hypertension. J Hypertension 2:453–460
4. McCarron DA (1985) Is calcium more important than sodium in the pathogenesis of essential hypertension? Hypertension 7:607–627
5. Kwan CY (1985) Calcium-handling defects and smooth muscle pathophysiology. In: Grover AK, Daniel EE (eds) Calcium and contractility: smooth muscle. Humana,Clifton, pp 299–325
6. Sprenger KBG (1985) Alteration of cellular calcium metabolism as primary cause of hypertension. Clin Physiol Biochem 3:208–218
7. Aoki K, Kondo S, Mochizuki A, Yoshida T, Kato S, Kato K, Takikawa K (1978) Antihypertensive effects of cardiovascular Ca^{2+}-antagonist in hypertensive patients in the absence and presence of beta-adrenergic blockade. Am Heart J 96:218–226
8. Triggle DJ (1984) Some aspects of the chemical pharmacology of calcium channel antagonists. In: Ong HH, Lewis JC (eds) Hypertension: physiological basis and treatment. Academic, Orlando, pp 223–268
9. Fleckenstein A (1984) Calcium antagonism: History and prospects for a multifaceted pharmacodynanic principle. In: Opie HL (ed) Calcium antagonists and cardiovascular disease. Raven, New York, pp 9–28
10. Lederralle Pederson O (1983) Calcium blockade in arterial hypertension: Review. Hypertension 5 (Suppl II) II74–II79
11. Schroeder HA (1960) Relation between mortality from cardiovascular disease and treated water supplies: Variations in states and 163 largest municipalities of the United States. JAMA 172:1902–1908
12. McCarron DA, Morrid CD, Cole C (1982) Dietary calcium in human hypertension. Science 217:267–269
13. Kesteloot H, Geboers J (1982) Calcium and blood pressure, Lancet 1:813–815
14. Ayachi S (1979) Increased dietary calcium lowers blood pressure in the spontaneously hypertensive rat. Metabolism 28:1234–1238
15. McCarron DA (1982) Blood pressure and calcium balance in the Wistar-Kyoto rat. Life Sci. 30:683–689
16. Webb RC, Bohr DF (1981) Recent advances in the pathogenesis of hypertension: Consideration of structural functional and metabolic vascular abnormalities resulting in elevated arterial resistance. Am Heart J 102:251–264
17. Bohr DF (1963) Vascular smooth muscle: Dual effect of calcium. Science 139:597–599
18. Daniel EE, Kwan CY (1981) Control of contraction of vascular muscle—relation to hypertension. Trends Pharmacol Sci 2:270–273

19. Daniel EE, Grover AK, Kwan CY (1983) Calcium. In: Stephens NL (ed) Biochemistry of smooth muscle, vol III. CRC Press, Boca Raton, pp 1–88
20. Kwan CY, Garfield RE, Daniel EE (1979) An improved procedure for the isolation of plasma membranes from rat mesenteric arteries. J Mol Cell Cardiol 11:639–659
21. Kwan CY, Lee RMKW, Daniel EE (1981) Isolation of plasma membranes from mesenteric veins: A comparison of their physical and biochemical properties with arterial membranes. Blood Vessels 18:171–186
22. Wei JW, Janis RA, Daniel EE (1976) Isolation and characterization of plasma membrane from rat mesenteric arteries. Blood Vessels 13:279–292
23. Kwan CY, Belbeck L, Daniel EE (1980) Abnormal biochemistry of vascular smooth muscle plasma membrane isolated from hypertensive rats. Mol Pharmacol 17:137–140
24. Aoki K, Ikeda N, Yamashita K, Tomita N, Tazumi N, Hotta K (1974) ATPase activity and Ca^{2+} binding ability of subcellular membrane of arterial smooth muscle in spontaneously hypertensive rat. Jpn Heart J 2:180–181
25. Moore L, Hurwits L, Davenport GR, Landon EJ (1975) Energy-dependent calcium uptake activity of microsomes from the aorta of normal and hypertensive rats. Biochem Biophys Acta, 413–432
26. Webb RC, Bhalla RC (1976) Altered calcium sequestration by subcellular fractions of vascular smooth muscle from spontaneously hypertensive rats. J Mol Cell Cardiol 8:651–660
27. Grover AK, Kwan CY, Daniel EE (1981) Na-Ca exchange in rat myometrium membrane vesicles highly enriched in plasma membranes. Am J Physiol 240:C175–C182
28. Grover AK, Kwan CY, Daniel EE (1982) Ca^{2+} concentration dependence of Ca^{2+} uptake by rat myometrium plasma membrane enriched fraction. Am J Physiol 242:C278–C282
29. Grover AK, Kwan CY, Daniel EE (1983) High affinity pH dependent passive Ca binding by myometrial plasma membrane vesicles. Am J Physiol 244:C61–C67.
30. Wei J-W, Janis RA, Daniel EE (1976) Calcium accumulation and enzymatic activities of subcellular fractions from aortas and ventricles of genetically hypertensive rats. Circ Res 39:133–140
31. Kwan CY, Belbeck L, Daniel EE (1979) Abnormal biochemistry of vascular smooth muscle plasma membrane as an important factor in the initiation and maintenance of hypertension in rats. Blood Vessels 16:259–268
32. Holloway ET, Bohr DF (1981) Reactivity of vascular smooth muscle in hypertensive rats. Circ Res 33:678–685
33. Kwan CY, Daniel EE (1981) Biochemical abnormalities of venous plasma membrane fraction isolated from spontaneously hypertensive rats. Eur J Pharmacol 75:321–324
34. Blaustein MP (1980) How does sodium cause hypertension? A hypothesis. In: Zumkley H, Losse H (eds) Intracellular electrolytes and arterial hypertension. Thieme, Stuttgart, pp 151–157
35. Daniel EE, Grover AK, Kwan CY (1982) Isolation and properties of plasma membrane from smooth muscle. Fed Proc 41:2898–2904
36. Matlib MA, Schwartz A, Yamori Y (1985) Studies on a Na^+/Ca^{2+} exchange process in isolated sarcolemmal membranes of mesenteric arteries from Kyoto normotensive and spontaneously hypertensive rats. Am J Physiol 249:C166–C172
37. Van Breemen C, Aaronson P, Loutzenhiser R (1979) Na-Ca interactions in mammalian smooth muscle. Pharmacol Rev 30:167–205
38. Kwan CY, Grover AK, Daniel EE (1984) On the ouabain-sensitive potassium activated p-nitrophenyl phosphatase activity of vascular muscle plasma membranes. Arch Int Pharmacoldy Ther 272:245–255
39. Kwan CY, Daniel EE (1982) Arterial muscle membrane abnormalities of hydralazine-treated spontaneously hypertensive rats. Eur J Pharmacol 82:187–190
40. Kwan CY (1985) Dysfunction of calcium handling by smooth muscle in hypertension. Can J Physiol Pharmacol 63:366–374
41. Kwan CY, Grover AK, Sakai Y (1982) Abnormal biochemistry of subcellular membranes isolated from non-vascular smooth muscles of spontaneously hypertensive rats. Blood Vessels 19:273–283
42. Kwan CY, Grover AK (1983) Membrane abnormalities occur in vascular smooth muscle but

not in non-vascular smooth muscle from rats with deoxycorticosterone-salt induced hypertension. J Hypertension 1:257–265

43. Sakai Y, Kwan CY, Daniel EE (1984) Contractile responses of vasa deferentia from rats with genetic and experimental hypertension. J Hypertension 2:631–638

44. Kwan CY, Sakai Y, Daniel EE (1984) On the abnormalities of contractile responses of rat vasa deferentia. Clin. Expt. Hypertension A6:1257–1265

45. Kwan CY, Belbeck L, Daniel EE (1980) Characteristics of arterial plasma membrane in renovascular hypertension in rats. Blood Vessels 17:131–140

46. Kwan CY, Triggle CR, Grover AK, Daniel EE (1986) Subcellular membrane properties in vascular and nonvascular smooth muscles of Dahl hypertensive rats. J Hypertension 4:49–55

47. Bohr DF, Harris AL, Guthe CC, Webb RC (1984) Hypertension multiple membrane malfunctions. In: Villareal H, Sambhi MP (eds) Topics in pathophysiology of hypertension. Nijhoff, Boston, pp 100–111

48. Swales JD (1982) Ion transport in hypertension: review. Biosci Report 2:969–990

49. Kravtsov GM, Orlov SN, Pokudin, NI, Postnov YV (1983) Calcium transport in synaptosomes and subcellular membrane fractions of brain tissue in spontaneously hypertensive rats. Clin Sci 65:127–135

50. Limas CJ, Cohn JN (1979) Defective calcium transport by cardiac sarcoplasmic reticulum in spontaneously hypertensive rats. Circ Res 40 (5) (Suppl I): 162–169

51. Devynck MA, Pernollet MG, Nunez AM, Meyer P (1981) Calcium binding alteration in plasma membrane from various tissues of spontaneously hypertensive rat. Clin Exp Hypertension 3:797–808

52. Postnov YV, Orlov SN (1980) Evidence of altered calcium accumulation and calcium binding by membranes of adipocytes in spontaneously hypertensive rat. Pfluger's Arch 385:85–89

53. Postnov YV, Orlov SN, Pokudin NI (1979) Decrease of calcium binding by the red blood cell membrane in spontaneously hypertensive rats and in essential hypertension. Pfluger's Arch. 379:191–195

54. Postnov YV, Orlov, SN, Reznikova MF, Rjazhsky GG, Pokudin NI (1984) Calmodulin distribution and Ca transport in the erythrocytes of patients with essential hypertension. Clin Sci 66:459–463

55. Devynck MA, Pernollet MG, Nunez AM, Meyer P (1981) Analysis of calcium handling in erythrocyte membranes of genetically hypertensive rats. Hypertension 3:397–403

56. Bruschi G, Bruschi ME, Caroppo M, Orlandini G, Spaggiari M, Cavatorta A (1985) Cytoplasmic free [Ca^{2+}] is increased in the platelets of spontaneously hypertensive rats and essential hypertensive patients. Clin Sci 68:179–184

Actions of Calcium Antagonists on Smooth Muscle Cells of Vascular Tissues

Current Knowledge on Actions of Ca Antagonists

Y. Ohya, K. Terada, S. Satoh, T. Fujiwara, T. Nagao, K. Komori, M. Nozaki, and H. Kuriyama

Department of Pharmacology, Faculty of Medicine, Kyushu University, Fukuoka, 812 Japan

Summary. The actions of Ca antagonists, organic compounds which prevent the influx of Ca, were studied in various regions of vascular beds excised from several species using the micro-electrode and whole-cell voltage clamp methods. In relation to the actions of Ca antagonists on the membrane, the effects of these drugs on mechanical responses evoked by the Ca spike and depolarizations induced by high K or agonists were studied using the isometric tension recording method. In vascular smooth muscle, most Ca antagonists inhibited the voltage-dependent Ca channel to a greater extent than the receptor-operated Ca channel. However, some Ca antagonists inhibited not only the influx of Ca but also the Ca mobilization in smooth muscle cells. Since individual Ca antagonists possess different features on inhibition of the smooth muscle activity, we tentatively classified the Ca antagonists from their actions on the Ca-dependent and receptor-operated Ca channels, sarcoplasmic reticulum, and contractile proteins. The inhibitory actions of Ca antagonists on cardiac muscle are briefly discussed in comparison to those on vascular smooth muscle.

Key words: Ca antagonists—Vascular smooth muscle—Vasodilatation—Voltage-dependent Ca channel—Receptor-operated Ca channel—Regional differences in action of Ca antagonists

Ca antagonists (Ca slow channel blockers, Ca entry blockers, Ca overload blockers) have been used to identify inhibitory aspects of the Ca channel and clinically employed in the treatment and prevention of hypertension, angina pectoris, and other Ca-related diseases. In general, systemic experiments indicate that Ca antagonists show a stronger affinity for vascular smooth muscle than for other excitable tissues, including cardiac muscle [15, 17, 18, 25, 83]. The chemical structures of Ca antagonists vary markedly, for example, there are verapamil derivatives [verapamil, methoxyverapamil (D600), tiapamil, gallopamil], dihydropyridine derivatives (nifedipine, nimodipine, niludipine, nitrendipine, nisoldipine, nicardipine), benzothiazepine derivatives (diltiazem, KB-944), prenylamine derivatives (prenylamine), bepridil derivatives (bepridil), and diphenylpiperazine derivatives (cinnarizine, flunarizine, lidoflazine).

The Ca influx plays an essential role in the contraction-relaxation cycle in vascular smooth muscles. In most vascular tissues, the minimum concentration of Ca required to produce the contraction, as estimated from skinned muscle preparations, was 0.1 μM [45]. The Ca influx appears in a passive form due to the Ca concentration gradient between the intra- and extracellular fluids, voltage-dependent influx of Ca after depolarization of the membrane (Ca spike, electrically, and high K-induced depolarization), and receptor-operated Ca influx [7], which is composed of the voltage-dependent influx of Ca due to the receptor-operated depolarization of the membrane, such as increased Na permeability and the so-called receptor-operated Ca influx. In vascular smooth muscle, most Ca antagonists show the strongest potency in the case of the voltage-dependent Ca influx, especially agents which act on the high K-induced contraction rather than the Ca spike [45]. Despite the evidence that Ca antagonists have inhibitory actions on voltage-dependent Ca channels, individual Ca antagonists show marked differences in individual vascular tissues and species.

This paper is concerned with observations on the actions of Ca antagonists (diltiazem, nifedipine, nicardipine, nisoldipine, verapamil, bepridil, and flunarizine) on vascular tissues (including dispersed single cell fragments). The microelectrode and voltage-clamp methods were used for measurements of membrane potential and current; isometric tension in intact and skinned muscle tissues was measured. To explain the molecular mechanism, attention will be directed toward observations on cardiac muscles, as investigations on vascular smooth muscles are ongoing.

Calcium Antagonists As Inhibitors of the Voltage-Dependent Calcium Channel

The K-induced contraction

Many investigators have studied the effects of Ca antagonists on K-depolarized muscles using different procedures. The K-induced contraction in various vascular tissues is composed of a transiently developed phasic contraction (response) and a subsequently developed tonic contraction (sustained response). Some investigators have observed the effects of Ca antagonists from changes in the amplitude of the phasic contraction and others have noted changes in the amplitude of the tonic contraction. However, in some vascular tissues (elastic vascular tissues), clarification of both components was difficult. Given our current knowledge, there is no consensus as to the elucidation of the nature of phasic and tonic responses of the K-induced contraction. Ca antagonists (diltiazem, dihydropyridine, verapamil, bepridil, and flunarizine) inhibit both components but the tonic is more extensively inhibited than the phasic component. Furthermore, Ca antagonists had a more direct action on the tonic rather than on the phasic response, as estimated from the Lineweaver-Burk plot [36, 37].

As an example, the actions of Ca antagonists on the phasic and tonic responses of the K-induced contractions in the rabbit mesenteric artery were investigated using nisoldipine and Bay K 8644 (a derivative of dihydropyridine; this latter agent possesses the property of an accelerator of Ca entry, a Ca agonist such as YC-170 or CGP 28392) on the K-induced contraction. When amplitudes of contraction evoked by various concentrations of Ca in 39 mM K-containing solution in the presence or absence of nisoldipine were plotted (Lineweaver-Burks plot), the lines crossed at the same point on the vertical axis in the case of the tonic response but not in the case of the phasic response. Much the same relationship was observed in the presence of both Bay K 8644 and nisoldipine. Thus, nisoldipine competitively acts on the Ca entry during the generation of the tonic but not the phasic response. The above observations indicate that Bay K 8644 acts on the same site as nisoldipine (see below). The ID_{50} value of nisoldipine on the tonic response evoked by 128 mM K was much smaller than that on the phasic response (10^{-12} M vs. 10^{-9} M). Moreover, when various concentrations of Ca were subsequently applied after application of 128 mM K in Ca-free solution containing 1 mM EGTA, both tonic and phasic contractions occurred in a concentration-dependent manner. When nisoldipine was applied with 128 mM K, the phasic contraction was more resistant to nisoldipine than was the tonic response [36]. We postulated that generation of the phasic response of the K-induced contraction closely depended on the amount of Ca sequestered in intracellular stores. When a comparison was made in the presence or absence of stored Ca (depletion of Ca was prepared by repetitive applications of 10 mM caffeine in Ca-free 128 mM K solution containing 1 mM EGTA), the onset of the contraction was markedly delayed and the peak amplitude of the contraction was reduced after depletion of the stored Ca in the cells. After a long exposure to 2.6 mM Ca with 128 mM K, the amplitude of the tonic contraction reached the same value seen in the presence or absence of the stored Ca [36].

Much the same responses of vascular smooth muscle tissues to Ca antagonists were observed with other dihydropyridine derivatives (nifedipine, nimodipine, nitrendipine, and nicardipine) with different potencies and with diltiazem, verapamil, and bepridil [15, 17, 18, 25].

The Ca spike and the Ca spike-induced contraction
Other voltage-dependent influxes of Ca occur during the generation of the action potential. In smooth muscle cells of the portal vein of various species, spontaneous action potentials are generated due to the influx of Ca. However, no spontaneous spike generation is observed in other regions of vascular tissues, except for evoked spike generation due to perivascular stimulation or direct muscle stimulation. In smooth muscles of various elastic arteries, neither spontaneous nor evoked action potentials were generated, yet the spike potential or graded response was generated under treatment with tetraethylammonium (TEA) or TEA with procaine. Therefore, these observations indicate that smooth muscle cells of some elastic arteries possess the voltage dependent Ca channel which contributes toward generation of the action potential, even when electrical stimulation fails to produce the action potential under physiological conditions [45].

The concentration of nisoldipine required to inhibit the Ca spike was, however, higher than that required to inhibit the K-induced contraction in vascular smooth muscles: To inhibit the Ca spike to half the amplitude, concentrations of nisoldipine 10–100 times higher than those which inhibited the K-induced contraction were required [36]. Much the same effects as those observed with the application of nisoldipine were obtained on other dihydropyridine derivatives—diltiazem, verapamil, bepridil and fulnarizine, [21, 31, 36, 40, 48, 73, 74].

Holman's group noted different actions of nifedipine on the Ca spike, i.e., the sensitivity of the Ca spike evoked by electrical stimulation in the presence of TEA differed from that evoked in the absence of TEA [72]. In the rabbit mesenteric artery, Makita et al. [48] reported that dihydropyridine derivatives inhibited the action potential, in the presence or absence of TEA, with the same potency.

To analyze the action of Ca antagonists on the voltage-dependent Ca channel, a voltage-clamp method was used to study dispersed single smooth muscle cell fragments. The membrane potential of this fragment was about -40 mV and when the membrane potential was held at -60 mV, the outward current pulse provoked the generation of action potentials and also the inward and subsequently generated outward currents provoked by the depolarizing voltage step. As determined from the current-voltage relationship and drug actions using the voltage-clamp method, the inward current was due to the voltage dependent influx of Ca. Nisoldipine, in the order of 1 nM, inhibited the inward current and 100 nM nisoldipine halted the generation of the inward current [61].

In a solution containing Ca below 0.1 mM, the inward current could not be observed, however, when Ca concentrations were reduced to below 1 μM in the presence of 137 mM Na, the action potential (slow raising phase and prolonged duration) was recorded by outward current pulses, and the inward current could be recorded by the voltage clamp method, i.e., in the absence of Ca; a voltage-dependent Na influx occurred and this current ceased with the application of low concentrations of nisoldipine [61]. These observations indicate that the voltage dependent Ca channel required the presence of Ca to preserve ion selectivity and that nisoldipine possesses a specificity for the channel but not for the ions. Nicardipine (a photoresistant dihydropyridine derivative), diltiazem, and flunarizine also blocked the inward current and the latter two substances had to be used in much higher concentrations that the dihydropyridine derivatives to inhibit the inward current (Terada, unpublished observations).

Sites of Ca channels and actions of Ca antagonist
It is important to clarify whether the Ca antagonists act on the surface of the cell membrane or on the internal side of the membrane to block the voltage-dependent Ca channel. When nicardipine, diltiazem, or flunarizine were injected into the fragmented smooth muscle cell by the cell-perfusion method, the inward current was not affected by concentrations similar to those of the Ca antagonists mentioned above which inhibited the inward currents when applied extracellularly (Ohya and Terada, unpublished observations). Therefore, these agents may act on the channel from the extracellular side. In cardiac and skeletal muscles (transverse tubular structures), these agents applied from the intracellular side to the Ca channel have inhibitory actions. However, for potent inhibition of the Ca channel, extremely high concentrations applied intracellularly are required [50], except in the case of verapamil derivatives, i.e., verapamil and D600 are reported to inhibit the Ca channel from the inside of the sarcolemmal membrane in cardiac muscles (in comparison with the action of D600 against D890) [28, 77].

Pang and Sperelakis [63, 64] studied the permeation of Ca antagonists in various muscle cells and found that verapamil, bepridil, and nitrendipine were permeable but that diltiazem and nifedipine were less so.

In cardiac muscles, the number of Ca channels distributed on the membrane was calculated from the whole current of the isolated cell using the voltage-clamp method. The number of Ca channels was estimated to be $0.1-0.5/\mu m^2$ or $0.5-5/\mu m^2$ and the total number in a cell was 10^3-10^4 [4, 66].

The binding of Ca antagonists to the Ca channel has been investigated using [^{3}H]nitrendipine and [^{3}H]verapamil. Boger et al. [6] observed specific binding of nitredipine to the microsomal membrane fraction of guinea pig ileal longitudinal muscles. The dissociation constant was 0.18 nM and the maximum binding was 1.14 pmol/mg protein. In the transverse tubule membrane of rabbit skeletal muscle, the dissociation constant of the nitrendipine-receptor complex was 1.8 nM and the maximum binding capacity was 50 pmol/mg protein. Verapamil, amiodarone, and bepridil were noncompetitive inhibitors for the [^{3}H]nitrendipine binding to the Ca channel [19]. Curtis and Catterall [11] observed [^{3}H]nitrendipine binding on the receptor protein extracted from rat brain and concluded that the nitrendipine concentration that gave half the maximal amount of the soluble [^{3}H]nitrendipine-receptor complexes was identical to the K_d for specific nitrendipine binding to the brain membrane. They also reported that verapamil increased and diltiazem inhibited the dissociation rate to a similar extent. Thus, the solubilized receptor contains both the dihydropyridine- and diltiazem/verapamil-binding sites. From the sucrose gradient sedimentation measurement, Curtis and Catterall [11] estimated the coefficient value to be 19.2 for the receptor-digitonin complex. In skeletal muscle transverse tubule membrane, [^{3}H]verapamil binding to the membrane showed the K_d value to be 27 nM and the maximum binding capacity was 50 pmol/mg protein; a 1:1 stoichiometry of binding was found for verapamil vs. nitrendipine. D600, diltiazem, and bepridil are competitive inhibitors of [^{3}H]verapamil binding with the K_d values between 40 and 200 nM, while dihydropydidine derivatives appear as noncompetitive inhibitors of [^{3}H]verapamil binding with a half-maximum inhibition value of between 1 and 5 nM [23]. These experiments indicate that the site of action on the Ca channel between dihydropyridine derivatives against other Ca antagonists (diltiazem, verapamil, or bepridil) may differ.

The mechanism of inhibitory actions induced by Ca antagonists

Detailed experiments on the action of Ca antagonists on the Ca channel have been done mainly on the cardiac muscle membrane (Ba was used instead of Ca) using the voltage- and patch-clamp methods and the main results can be summarized as follows.

Ca antagonists have no effect on the resting membrane potential and rate of rise of the action potential but do inhibit the slow Ca inward current [42, 44, 57, 60].

Ca antagonists possess the property of a use-dependent (frequency-dependent) inhibition of the Ca channel. The potency of these inhibitory actions differed with individual agents in the order of D600, diltiazem, nitrendipine [12, 46, 49, 52, 53, 77, 85]. There are two hypotheses concerning the use-dependent inhibition according to modes of the Ca channel, i.e., an open channel block hypothesis [46] and an inactivated channel block hypothesis [39].

Charges of the Ca antagonists play an important role in Ca-channel blocking actions: D600, verapamil, and diltiazem are tertiary amines, while nifedipine has a noncharged structure. Hescheler et al. [28] postulated that Ca antagonists might penetrate the cell in a noncharged lipophilic form and act from inside the cell membrane, as deduced from the actions of D600 and D890 [51–53]. Differences in the use-dependent inhibition of the Ca channel among Ca antagonists may, in part, be explained by such differences (verapamil and diltiazem vs. nifedipine). On the other hand, in skeletal muscles, Pang and Sperelakis [64] reported that verapamil, bepridil, and nitrendipine entered and accumulated inside the muscle cells (mainly) sarcoplasmic reticulum, whereas nifedipine and diltiazem did not readily permeate the cell.

Hess et al. [29] noted the inhibitory mechanism of Ca channels by Ca antagonists using patch-clamp techniques, i.e., nifedipine and nimodipine did not modify the amplitude of the Ca channel current (a unit current) and decreased the channel-open probability by increasing the percentage of sweeps. While nitrendipine seems to be a partial antagonist, i.e., the mean open time is actually increased, the net effect was inhibitory because of a predominant shift toward no detectable opening of the Ca channel (at mode 0 in the classification of Hess et al.). Diltiazem and verapamil possess much the same effect on the Ca channel [46].

When the inhibitory actions of Ca antagonists were compared in the case of the Ca current (inward current) against the K current (outward current), the potency required to inhibit the Ca channel was in the order—nisoldipine, D600, diltiazem; the ratios of K_d values for inhibition of the Ca current against the K current $(K_d(I_k)/K_d(I_{Ca}))$ were 2.2×10^3 (D600), 10^3 (nisoldipine) and 7.6×10 (diltiazem), respectively [30]. In smooth muscle tissues, T. Terada (personal communication) confirmed the above conclusion concerning the difference in the inhibitory potency of nicardipine, verapamil, flunarizine, and diltiazem on the $K_d(I_k)/K_d(I_{Ca})$ using the voltage-clamp method.

We postulate that since individual Ca antagonists possess different moieties, the inhibitory mechanism of these agents on the voltage-dependent Ca channel may differ with individual agents.

Effects of Calcium Antagonists on the Receptor-Operated Calcium Channel

Various agonists will contract vascular smooth muscles, but in general, Ca antagonists possess a much weaker action on the agonist-induced contraction in comparison with the K-induced contraction. The agonist-induced contraction is caused by an increased free Ca concentration in the cells due to increased Ca influx following activation of the receptor-operated Ca influx [7] and voltage-dependent influx of Ca due to depolarization of the membrane induced by activation mainly of the Na channel. Activation of receptors accelerates the release of Ca from cellular stores through synthesis of inositol 1,4,5-trisphosphate, as demonstrated in vascular smooth muscle tissues [27, 69, 71]. Further, activation of receptors by agonists modifies the synthesis of cyclic nucleotides, e.g., alpha$_2$-agonists inhibited the synthesis of cyclic AMP, muscarinic agonists accelerated the synthesis of cyclic GMP [5, 33, 38, 43, 54, 59, 67, 70], and 5-hydroxytryptamine (5-HT) synthesized prostanoids in the basilar artery [20]. Therefore, the contraction evoked by agonists may occur as a sum of many factors contributing to Ca mobilization and modifications of contractile proteins [phosphorylation of myosin modified by cyclic nucleotide A and G, and C kinases) [5, 38, 59, 65].

Dihydropyridine derivatives (nifedipine, nisoldipine, nimodipine, nitrendipine and nicardipine), diltiazem, and verapamil showed much weaker actions on the agonist-induced contraction than those induced on the K-induced contraction. In smooth muscle cells of the guinea pig basilar artery, 5-HT depolarized the membrane by reduction in the ionic permeability of the membrane and contraction occurred. The 5-HT-induced contraction ceased in a Ca-free solution containing 1 mM EGTA and this contraction was not modified by the application of nicardipine. We, therefore, postulated that the 5-HT-induced contraction was mainly due to activation of the receptor operated Ca channel. Since nicardipine mainly inhibited the voltage-dependent influx of Ca, the inhibitory actions of this agent on the receptor-operated influx of Ca were negligibly small [22].

Flunarizine, in the rabbit mesenteric artery, inhibited the K- and noradrenaline-induced contractions to the same extent; thus, the receptor-operated Ca influx and Ca release from the intracellular storage together with the voltage-dependent influx of Ca may be inhibited (Sato et al., unpublished data). In the rabbit basilar and ear arteries, flunarizine inhibited the K-, transmural stimulation-, and noradrenaline-induced contractions and the potency to inhibit the contraction was higher for the former two conditions than the latter [55]. These observations differed somewhat from the observations made by Van Neuten et al. [80, 81]. Nevertheless, the inhibition brought about by flunarizine on the noradrenaline-induced contraction was more potent than that seen with other Ca antagonists [55]. It has also been reported that this agent inhibited the stretch-induced contraction in the basilar artery [56]. This means that the actions of flunarizine differ from those of other Ca antagonists (dihydropyridine, verapamil, and diltiazem derivatives) with regard to agonist-induced contraction. Compared with other Ca antagonists, flunarizine requires a much longer latency for initiation of the inhibition of contractions evoked by high concentrations of K or agonists (30–60 min to reach maximum action). The underlying mechanisms of action of flunarizine require further study.

Effects of Calcium-Calmodulin Phosphodiesterase Inhibitors in Relation to Calcium Antagonistic Actions

Phenotiazine derivatives (trifluoperazine, chlorpromazine, pimozide or penfluridol) are antipsychotic agents and inhibit Ca-calmodulin interactions through the mediation of phosphodiesterase [47]. These agents inhibit the contractile machinery in smooth muscles as the Ca-calmodulin inhibitor in relation to the activation of myosin light chain kinase [1, 2, 26]. One of these derivatives, chlorpromazine, inhibits the Ca influx in lower concentrations than those required to inhibit the contractile machinery, as concluded from the Ca-induced contraction in skinned muscles [35].

The ID_{50} of chlorpromazine on Ca-calmodulin phosphodiesterase is 42 μM [84], that of W-7, a specific calmodulin antagonist is 26 μM [75] and that of trifluoperazine 5.7 μM [78]. In comparison, calmidazolium (R24571) [78] has much lower values (0.5–1.0 nM). Ca antagonists are also Ca-calmodulin phosphodiesterase inhibitors, i.e., the ID_{50} value of nifedipine was over 50 μM, but it was 37 μM for D600, 28 mM for verapamil [79], but 340 μM according to Volgi et al. [82], 3.5 μM for cinnarizine, 2.5 μM for flunarizine [79], 2 mM for nimodipine, and 1 μM for nicardipine [13]. Calmodulin acts as a secondary messenger in viable cells, therefore inhibitions of the voltage-dependent influx of Ca by Ca antagonists may have a causal relation to the Ca-calmodulin phosphodiesterase inhibition. However, nifedipine and nimodipine showed marked differences with regard to the Ca-calmodulin-phosphodiesterase inhibition. The underlying mechanisms thus remain to be clarified.

The activations of cyclic AMP and cyclic AMP-dependent protein kinase (A kinase) are closely related to the Ca channel in cardiac muscles [8, 9, 62, 66]. On the other hand, the intracellular application of cyclic AMP or extracellular application of dibutyryl cyclic AMP did not modify the Ca current in isolated fragmented smooth muscle cells (Ohya, unpublished data), as would be expected from the action of isoprenaline on vascular beds [33, 37]. This is clear evidence that there is a difference in the nature of the voltage-dependent Ca channel distributed on the cardiac and smooth muscle.

In skinned skeletal muscles, Fabiato and Fabiato [14] found that Ca antagonists have no effect on the Ca-induced contraction. In skinned vascular smooth muscle tissues, there were no interactions of Ca antagonists on the Ca-activated contraction: diltiazem, Suzuki et al. [73]; nifedipine, Kanmura et al. [40, 41]; verapamil, Ishikawa et al. [31]; nisoldipine, Itoh et al. [36]. On the other hand, it was also observed that bepridil [74] and flunarizine (Sato et al. unpublished data) slightly inhibited the Ca-induced contraction when the Ca concentrations were low (0.3–1 μM Ca), while flunarizine (1 μM) had no effect on the contraction evoked by high concentrations of Ca (over 1 μM), (Sato et al., unpublished data).

When the effects of diltiazem were observed on the Ca accumulation into or release from the cellular storage in the mesenteric artery, 1 μM diltiazem had no effect [73], while Saida and van Breemen [68] noted an inhibitory action on the Ca release with high concentrations of diltiazem (0.1 mM) in the same species of tissue. Presumably, the difference observed between the above observations may be due to different concentrations of this agent. Nifedipine, nisoldipine, and verapamil, in concentrations required to inhibit the K- or agonist-induced contractions, had no effect on the Ca accumulation into and release from the Ca storage in vascular smooth muscle tissues [31, 36, 40 41]. Much the same effect was observed with applications of flunarizine as with applications of other Ca antagonists, i.e., in Ca-free solution in intact and skinned muscles, the caffeine-induced contraction was not affected. Furthermore, the inositol 1,4,5-trisphosphate-induced contraction (5 μM) in skinned muscles was not affected by 1 μM flunarizine (Satoh et al., unpublished data). On the other hand, bepridil depolarized the membrane mainly by inhibition of the K permeability and inhibited the Ca spike and K-induced contraction (5–10 μM). In high concentrations (0.1 mM), this agent blocked the caffeine-induced contraction in Ca-free solution in intact and skinned muscle tissues.

Conclusion

Many drugs have been reevaluated as Ca antagonists, e.g., an antispastic agent, eperison, has a Ca antagonistic action on the basilar artery, i.e., this agent blocks the Ca spike evoked by an electric current in the presence of TEA and inhibits the K- and 5-HT-induced contractions. In addition, this agent partly inhibits the Ca-induced contraction in skinned muscle tissues of the basilar artery [20]. Verapamil was initially synthesized as a beta-adrenoceptor blocker [16], cinnarizine as an anti-histamic agent [24], and bepridil as a beta-adrenoceptor blocker [10]. If we reinvestigate the action of commercially available agents, no doubt some of them would be found to possess Ca antagonistic actions.

From the standpoint of basic research, Ca antagonistics are defined as follows: (1) diminished contractile force without a major change in membrane potential; (2) reduced high-energy phosphate utilization of the contractile system; (3) lowered extra oxygen consumption during activity; (4) readily neutralized by administration of additional Ca, beta-adrenergic catecholamine, or cardiac glycoside, i.e., by measures which restore the supply of Ca to the contractile system [17]. Recently, Fleckerstein classified Ca antagonists into selective and nonselective groups from the Ca-influx inhibitory action, relative to the fast Na-influx inhibitory action [18]. On the other hand, Godfraind [25] suggested that Ca antagonists might be defined as drugs able to interact with the function of Ca during activation by physiological or pathological processes. The former mainly concerns the action of the Ca antagonist on cardiac muscles [in cardiac muscles, the fast Na inward current (I_{Naf}) contributes to the spike generation, but not in the case of smooth muscles], but the latter extends to external and internal Ca antagonists. As a consequence, phenothiazine derivatives, local anesthetics and others are included in the category of Ca antagonists.

We tentatively categorize Ca antagonists as organic substrates that selectively inhibit the voltage-dependent Ca channel at the sarcolemma, which is a main action in both cardiac and smooth muscles. Since Ca antagonists are used to treat cardiovascular diseases and the Na influx is not closely related to excitation of the membrane in smooth muscle cells, the inhibition of the Ca influx, compared with that of the Na influx, may not be an essential factor [45]. Phenothiazine derivatives inhibit the voltage-dependent influx of Ca, Ca-calmodulin interaction, and phosphorylation of myosin [33]. Therefore, the inhibitory action of this group of Ca antagonists may be related to the Ca-calmodulin-phosphodiesterase interactions. Furthermore, actions of local anesthetics vary with the tissue. In nerve fibers and smooth muscles, these agents inhibit the Na or K permeability, respectively, and some local anesthetics inhibit the release of stored Ca and also the breakdown of phosphatidyl inositol 4,5-bisphosphate [27, 32, 34; Ueno, personal communication].

Individual Ca antagonists possess different actions, even though these agents act on the voltage dependent Ca channel, as described in this paper, i.e., dihydropyridine derivatives possess a potent inhibitory action on the voltage-dependent Ca channel compared with the action of verapamil, diltiazem, bepridil, or flunarizine in equimolar concentrations. Furthermore, verapamil and diltiazem have different properties from the dihydropyridine derivatives, as determined from

Ca-binding, permeation, and voltage-clamp experiments. Flunarizine possesses stronger inhibitory actions on the receptor operated Ca influx than other Ca antagonists (K-induced contraction vs. agonist-induced contraction). Bepridil and eperison also possess different properties from other Ca antagonists.

It is evident that the voltage-dependent Ca channel, analyzed using the voltage-clamp method, is composed of more than two different channels in cardiac muscle [3, 58] and Ca antagonists possess different sensitivities to these two channels. Therefore, the nature of the voltage-dependent Ca channel may differ not only in the same cell but also in different tissues, e.g., the sensitivity of the Ca channel to vascular smooth muscle differed from that at the nerve terminal regulating the release of chemical transmitters (diltiazem vs. nifedipine) [40, 41, 73]. The extra-cellular application of dibutyryl cyclic AMP and intracellular injection of cyclic AMP did not modify the Ca current measured using the voltage-clamp method in smooth muscle tissues (Ohya, unpublished data). This nature of the channel differed from that observed in cardiac muscle [76]. The Ca channel distributed in central and peripheral nerves, skeletal, cardiac, and smooth muscles, secretory glands and other tissues may differ in nature and, as a consequence, the actions of Ca antagonists may be different in individual tissues. The actions of Ca antagonists on Ca channels require further attention.

Ca antagonists have been used to treat cardiac arrhythmia, vasospastic angina, stable and unstable angina, hypertension, hypertrophic cardiomyopathy, preservation of the myocardium against ischemic damage, peripheral vascular disorders, cerebrovasospasm, cerebral ischemia, and migraine [25]. Further investigations may well extend the indication of Ca antagonists for clinical applications. The clinical trials of Ca antagonists intended for therapeutic purposes lag behind the detailed in vivo and in vitro investigations, including the mode of action of these agents.

References

1. Adelstein RS, Eisenberg E (1980) Regulation and kinetics of the actin-myosin-ATP interaction. Ann Rev Biochem 49:921–956
2. Aksoy MO, Mras S, Kamm KE, Murphy RA (1983) Ca^{2+}, cAMP and changes in myosin phosphorylation during contraction of smooth muscle. Am J Physiol 245:c255–c270
3. Bean BP (1985) Two kinds of calcium channels in canine artial cells. J Gen Physiol 86:1–30
4. Bean BP, Nowycky MD, Tsien RW (1983) Electrical estimates of Ca channel density in heart cell membranes. Biophys J 41:295 a
5. Berridge JM, Irvine RF (1984) Inositol triphosphate, a novel second messenger in cellular signal transduction. Nature 312:315–321
6. Boger GT, Gengo PJ, Luchowski EM, Siegel H, Triggle DJ, Janis RA (1982) High affinity binding of a calcium channel antagonist to smooth and cardiac muscle. Biochem Biophys Res Commun 120:481–485
7. Bolton TB (1979) Mechanisms of action of transmitters and other substances on smooth muscle. Physiol Rev 59:606–718
8. Brum G, Flockerzi V, Hofmann F, Osterrieder W, Trautwein W (1983) Injection of catalytic subunit of c-AMP-dependent protein kinase into isolated cardiac myocytes. Pflugers Arch 398:147–154
9. Brum G, Osterrieder A, Trautwein W (1984) β-Adrenergic increase in the calcium conductance of cardiac myocytes studies with the patch clamp. Pflugers Arch 401:111–118

10. Cosnier D, Duchenne-Marullaz P, Rispat G, Streichenberger G (1977) Cardiovascular pharmacology of bepridil (1[3 isobutoxy 2 (benzylphenyl) amino] propyl pyrrolidine hydrochloride) a new potential anti-anginal compound. Arch Int Pharmacodyn 225:113-151
11. Curtis BM, Catterall WA (1983) Solubilization of the calcium antagonist receptor from rat brain. J Biol Chem 258:7280-7283
12. Ehara T, Kaufman R (1978) The voltage- and time dependent effects of (−)-verapamil on the slow inward current in isolated cat ventricular myocardium. J Pharmacol Exp Ther 207:49-55
13. Epstein PM, Fiss K, Hachisu R, Andrenyak DM (1982) Interaction of calcium antagonists with cyclic AMP phosphodiesterases and calmodulin. Biochem Biophys Res Commun 105:1142-1149
14. Fabiato A, Fabiato F (1979) Calcium and excitation-contraction coupling. Ann Rev Physiol 41:473-484
15. Flaim SF, Zelis R (1982) Calcium Blockers: Mechanisms of Action and Clinical Applications. Urban and Schwarzenberg, Baltimore
16. Fleckenstein A (1964) Die Bedeutung der energiereichen Phosphate für Kontraktilität und Tonus des Myokards. Verh Dtsch Ges Inn Med 70:81-99
17. Fleckenstein A (1977) Specific pharmacology of calcium in myocardium, cardiac pacemaker and vascular smooth muscle. Ann Rev Pharmacol Toxicol 17:149-166
18. Fleckenstein A (1983) Calcium Antagonism in Heart and Smooth Muscle. Wiley, New York
19. Fosset M, Jaimovich E, Delpont E, Lazdunski M (1983) [^{3}H] nitrendipine receptors in skeletal muscle properties and preferential localization in transverse tubules. J Biol Chem 258:6086-6092
20. Fujioka M, Kuriyama H (1986) Eperison, an anti-spastic agent, possesses vasodilating actions on smooth muscle cells of the guinea-pig basilar artery. J Pharmacol Exp Ther 235:757-763
21. Fujiwara S, Kuriyama H (1983) Nicardipine actions on smooth muscle cells and neuromusclar transmission in guinea-pig basilar artery. J Pharmcol Exp Ther 225:447-455
22. Fujiwara S, Kuriyama H (1984) Hemolysate-induced contraction in smooth muscle cells of the guinea pig basilar artery. Stroke 15:503-510
23. Gallizi JP, Fosset M, Lazdunski M (1984) [^{3}H]verapamil binding sites in skeletal muscle transverse tubule membranes. Biochem Biophys Res Commun 118:239-245
24. Godfraind T, Kaba A (1969) Blockade or reversal of contraction induced by calcium and adrenaline in deporalized arterial smooth muscle. Br J Pharmacol 36:549-560
25. Godfraind T (1985) Calcium and Cell Physiology. Springer, Berlin Heidelberg New York Tokyo, pp 204-226
26. Hartshorne DJ, Gorecka A (1980) Biochemistry of the contractile proteins of smooth muscle. In: Handbook of physiology, The cardiovascular system, vol 2: Vascular smooth muscle. Am Physiol Soc, Bethesda, pp 93-120
27. Hashimoto T, Hirata M, Itoh T, Kanmura Y, Kuriyama H (1985) Inositol 1,4,5-triphosphate activates pharmacomechanical coupling in smooth muscle of the rabbit mesenteric artery. J Physiol (Lond) 370:605-618
28. Hescheler J, Pelzer D, Trube G, Trautwein W (1982) Does the organic calcium channel blocker D600 act from inside or outside on the cardiac cell membrane? Pflugers Arch 393:287-291
29. Hess P, Lansman JB, Tsien RW (1984) Different modes of Ca channel gating behavior favored by dihydropyridine Ca agonists and antagonists. Nature 311:538-544
30. Hume JR (1985) Comparative interactions of organic Ca^{++} channel antagonists with myocardial Ca^{++} and K^+ channels. J Pharmacol Exp Ther 234:134-140
31. Ishikawa S, Izumi H, Satoh S, Kanmura Y, Itoh T (1985) Regional differences in the actions of verapamil and isosorbide dinitrate on rabbit and dog vascular smooth muscle. Naunyn-Schmiedeberg's Arch Pharmacol 331:376-383
32. Itoh T, Kajiwara M, Kitamura K, Kuriyama H (1981) Effects of vasodilator agents on smooth muscle cells of the coronary artery of the pig. Br J Pharmacol 74:455-468
33. Itoh T, Izumi H, Kuriyama H (1982a) Mechanisms of relaxation induced by activation of β-adrenoceptors in smooth muscle cells of guinea-pig mesenteric artery. J Physiol (Lond) 326:475-493
34. Itoh T, Kajiwara M, Kitamura K, Kuriyama H (1982b) Roles of stored calcium on the

mechanical response evoked in smooth muscle cells of the porcine coronary artery. J Physiol (Lond) 322:107–125

35. Itoh T, Kuriyama H, Suzuki H (1982c) Effects of chlorpromazine on the electrical and mechanical properties of intact and skinned muscle cells of guinea-pig mesenteric artery. Br J Pharmacol 75:513–523

36. Itoh T, Kanmura Y, Kuriyama H, Suzuki H (1984) Nisoldipine-induced relaxation in intact and skinned smooth muscles of rabbit coronary arteries. Br J Pharmacol 83:243–258

37. Itoh T, Kanmura Y, Kuriyama H, Sasaguri T (1985) Nitroglycerine- and isoprenaline-induced vasodilation: assessment from the actions of cyclic nucleotide. Br J Pharmacol 84:393–406

38. Kamm KE, Stull JT (1985) The function of myosin and myosin light chain kinase phosphorylation in smooth muscle. Ann Rev Pharmacol Toxicol 25:593–620

39. Kanaya S, Arlock BG Katzung BG, Hondeyhem LM (1983) Diltiazem and verapamil preferentially block inactivated cardiac calcium channels. J Mol Cell Cardiol 15:145–148

40. Kanmura Y, Itoh T, Suzuki H, Ito Y, Kuriyama H (1983a) Effects of nifedipine on smooth muscle cells of the rabbit mesenteric artery. J Pharmacol Exp Ther 226:238–248

41. Kanmura Y, Itoh T, Suzuki H, Ito Y, Kuriyama H (1983b) Nifedipine actions on smooth muscle cells of pig and rabbit skinned and intact coronary arteries. In: Hashimoto K, Kawai C (eds) Asian pacific adalat symposium. New therapy of ischemic heart disease and hypertension. Medical Tribune, Tokyo, pp 3–30

42. Kass RS, Tsien RW (1975) Multiple effects of calcium antagonists on plateau currents in cardiac Purkinje fibers. J Gen Physiol 66:169–192

43. Kerrick WGL, Hoar PE (1981) Inhibition of smooth muscle tension by cyclic AMP-dependent protein kinase. Nature 292:253–255

44. Kohlhardt M, Baver B, Krause H, Fleckenstein A (1972) Differentiation of the transmembrane Na and Ca channels in mammalian cardiac fibers by the use of specific inhibitors. Pflugers Arch 355:309–322

45. Kuriyama H, Ito Y, Suzuki H, Kitamura K, Itoh T (1982) Factors modifying contraction-relaxation cycle in vascular smooth muscles. Am J Physiol 243:H641–H662

46. Lee KS, Tsien RW (1983) Mechanism of calcium channel blockade by verapamil, D600, diltiazem and nitrendipine in single dialysed heart cells. Nature 302:790–794

47. Levin RM, Weiss B (1976) Mechanism by which psychotropic drugs inhibit adenosine cyclic 3'5'monophosphate phosphodiesterase of brain. Mol Pharmacol 12:581–589

48. Makita Y, Kanmura Y, Itoh T, Suzuki H, Kuriyama H (1983) Effect of nifedipine derivatives on smooth muscle cells and neuro-muscular transmission in the rabbit mesenteric artery. Naunyn-Schmiedeberg's Arch Pharmacol 324:302–312

49. McCans JL, Lindenmayer GE, Munson EG, Evans RW, Schwarz A (1974) A dissociation of positive staircase (Bowditch) from ouabain-induced positive inotropism; use of verapamil. Circ Res 35; 439–447

50. McCleskey EW (1985) Calcium channel and intracellular calcium release are pharmacologically different in frog skeletal muscle. J Physiol (Lond) 361:231–249

51. McDonald TF, Pelzer D, Trautwein W (1980) On the mechanism of slow calcium channel block in heart. Pflugers Arch 385:175–179

52. McDonald TF, Pelzer D, Trautwein W (1984a) Cat ventricular muscle treated with D600: Effects on calcium and potassium currents. J Physiol (Lond) 352:203–216

53. McDonald TF, Pelzer D, Trautwein W (1984b) Cat ventricular muscle treated with D600: Characteristics of calcium channel block and unblock. J Physiol (Lond) 352:217–241

54. Miller JR, Silver PJ, Stull JT (1983) The role of myosin light chain kinase phosphorylation in β adrenergic relaxation of tracheal smooth muscle. Mol Pharmacol 24:235–242

55. Nagao T, Suzuki H, Kuriyama H (1986) Effects of flunarizine on smooth muscle cells and on neuromuscular transmission in the rabbit basilar and ear artery. Naunyn-Schmiedeberg's Arch Pharmacol (in press)

56. Nakayama K, Kasuya Y (1980) Selective abolition of Ca-dependent responses of smooth and cardiac muscles by flunarizine. Japan J Pharmacol 30:731–742

57. Nawrath H, Ten Eick RE, McDonald TF, Trautwein W (1977) On the mechanism underlying the action of D600 on slow inward current and tension in mammalian myocardium. Circ Res 40:408–414

58. Nilius B, Hess P, Lansman JB, Tsien RW (1985) A novel type of cardiac calcium channel in ventricular cells. Nature 316:443–446
59. Nishizuka Y (1984) The role of protein kinase C in cell surface signal transduction and tumor promotion. Nature 308:693–698
60. Noma A, Trautwein W (1978) Relaxation of the ACh-induced potassium current in the rabbit sinoatrial node cell. Pflugers Arch 377:193–200
61. Ohya Y, Terada K, Kitamura K, Kuriyama H (1986) Membrane currents recorded from a fragment of rabbit intestinal smooth muscle. Am J Physiol (in press)
62. Osterrieder W, Brum G, Hescheler J, Trautwein W, Flockerzi V, Hofmann F (1982) Injection of subunits of cyclic AMP-dependent protein kinase into cardiac myocytes modulates Ca^{2+} current. Nature 298:576–578
63. Pang DC, Sperelakis N (1982) Differential actions of calcium antagonists on calcium binding to cardiac sarcolemma. Eur J Pharmacol 81:403–409
64. Pang DC, Sperelakis N (1984) Uptake of calcium antagonistic drugs into muscles as related to their lipid solubilities. Biochem Pharmacol 33:821–826
65. Rasmussen H, Barrett PQ (1984) Calcium messenger system: An integrated view. Physiol Rev 64:938–984
66. Reuter H (1983) Calcium channel modulation by neurotransmitters, enzymes and drugs. Nature 301:569–574
67. Ruegg JC, Sparrow MP, Mrwa U (1981) Cyclic AMP-mediated relaxation of chemically skinned fibers of smooth muscle. Pflugers Arch 390:198–201
68. Saida K, van Breemen C (1983) Inhibiting effect of diltiazem on intracellular Ca^{2+} release in vascular smooth muscle. Blood Vessels 20:105–108
69. Sasaguri T, Hirata M, Kuriyama H (1985) Dependence of Ca^{2+} of the activities of phosphatidylinositol 4,5-bisphosphate phosphodiesterase and inositol 1,4,5-triphosphate in smooth muscles of the porcine coronary artery. Biochem J 231:497–503
70. Scheid CR, Honeyman TW, Fay FS (1979) Mechanism of β-adrenergic relaxation of smooth muscle. Nature 277:32–36
71. Suematsu E, Hirata M, Hashimoto T, Kuriyama H (1984) Inositol 1,4,5-triphosphate releases calcium from intracellular store sites in skinned single cells of porcine coronary artery. Biochem Biophys Res Commun 120:481–485
72. Suprenant AM, Neild TO, Holman ME (1983) Effects of nifedipine on nerve-evoked action potentials and consequent contractions in rat tail artery. Pflugers Arch 396:342–349
73. Suzuki H, Itoh T, Kuriyama H (1982) Effects of diltiazem on smooth muscles and neuromuscular junction in the mesenteric artery. Am J Physiol 242:H325–H336
74. Suzuki H, Itoh T, Kuriyama H (1986) Mechanisms of the bepridil-induced vasodilation of the rabbit mesenteric artery. J Pharmacol Exp Ther 235:749–756
75. Tanaka T, Ohmura T, Hidaka H (1982) Hydrophobic interaction of the Ca^{2+}-calmodulin complex with calmodulin antagonists. Mol Pharmacol 22:403–407
76. Trautwein W, Brum G, Osterrieder W (1985) Effects of cAMP or catalytic subunit of protein kinase on cardiac calcium channels. In: Proceedings of the 16th FEBS congress, part B. pp 385–390
77. Trautwein W, Pelzer D, McDonald TF (1983) Interval- and voltage-dependent effects of the calcium channel blocking agents D600 and AQA 39 on mamalian ventricular muscle. Circ Res 52 (Suppl I) 60–68
78. Van Belle H (1981) R24571: A potent inhibitor of calmodulin-activated enzymes. Cell Calcium 2:483–494
79. Van Belle H (1984) The effects of drugs on calmodulin and its interaction with phosphodiesterase. In: Greengard P et al. (eds) Advances in cyclic nucleotide and protein phosphorylation research, vol 17. Raven, New York
80. Van Neuten JM, Van Beek J, Janssen AA (1978) Effect of flunarizine on calcium-induced responses of peripheral vascular smooth muscle. Arch Int Pharmacodyn Ther 232:42–52
81. Van Neuten JM, Vanhoutte PM (1981) Selectivity of calcium-antagonism and serotonin-antagonism with respect to venous and arterial tissues. Angiology 32:476–484
82. Volgi M, Shaafi RI, Epstein PM, Andrenyak DM, Feinstein MB (1981) Local anaesthetics, mepcrine and propranolol are antagonists of calmodulin. Proc Natl Acad Sci USA 78:795–799

83. Weiss GB (1981) New Perspectives on Calcium Antagonists. American Physiological Society, Maryland
84. Weiss GB, Prozialeck WC, Wallace TL (1982) Interaction of drugs with calmodulin. Biochem Pharmacol 31:2217–2226
85. Wit AL, Cranefield PF (1974) Effect of verapamil on the sinoatrial and atrioventricular nodes of the rabbit and the mechanism by which it arrests reentrant atrioventricular nodal tachycardia. Circ Res 35:413–425

Myogenic Activity of Vascular Tissues and the Effects of Calcium Agonists and Antagonists

K. Nakayama

Department of Pharmacology, Shizuoka University of Pharmaceutical Sciences, Oshika, Shizuoka, 422 Japan

Summary. The effects of Ca agonists and antagonists on the stretch-induced contraction in arterial smooth muscles were studied. The stretch-induced contraction was potentiated by promotors of influx of Ca such as high K, cardiac glycosides, and BAY k 8644, a 1,4-dihydropyridine Ca agonist, while the potentiated responses were inhibited by Ca antagonists. The significance of myogenic tone of vascular tissues in physiological and pathological conditions is discussed.

Key words: Coronary artery—Cerebral artery—Saphenous artery—Hypertension—Vasospasm—Myogenic tone—Stretch activation—Ca antagonists—BAY k 8644—Spontaneously hypertensive rat

The contractile reaction of the vascular smooth muscle in response to mechanical stretch, first reported by Bayliss [2] from his study on an isolated segment of the canine carotid artery, has been often postulated as an intrinsic mechanism of control of blood flow. Our previous reports [9, 11–13] demonstrated that the arteries isolated from certain vascular beds, such as those in the brain, heart, kidney, and somatic periphery, were particularly sensitive to mechanical stimulation, and this may be related to spastic vasoconstriction, e.g., vasospasm and hypertension. The contraction produced by stretch is largely influenced by promotors and inhibitors of Ca influx. Among these, it was found that Bay k 8644 (methyl-1, 4-dihydro-2, 6-dimethyl 3-nitro-4-[2-trifluoromethylphenyl]-pyridine-5-carboxylate), a putative activator of the voltage-dependent Ca channel in smooth and cardiac muscles [14], strongly potentiated the stretch-induced contraction, indicating a good pharmacological alternative for analysis of the Ca-dependent mechanism of contraction produced by stretch. In the present paper, the characteristic properties of the stretch-induced contraction are described, and the significant role of myogenic vascular tone in physiological and pathological conditions is briefly discussed.

Methods

Helical strips (about 10 mm long) of basilar and coronary arteries of rabbits, dogs, and pigs and the saphenous artery of old spontaneously hypertensive rats (SHR; male, 54–60 weeks old) were mounted in an organ bath maintained at 35°C and containing Tyrode solution (containing in mM: NaCl, 158.3; KCl, 4; CaCl$_2$, 2; MgCl$_2$, 1.05; NaHCO$_3$, 10; NaH$_2$PO$_4$, 0.42; glucose, 5.6) through which 97% O$_2$ and 3% CO$_2$ were bubbled to give a pH of 7.35.

The stretch activation of the artery was carried out by the following procedures. The arterial strip was stretched with an electromagnetic puller, which moved a force-transducer upward. The degree and velocity of stretch could be varied. Static stretch (excessive elongation of the preparation in increments up to a final basal tension of 100 mg in the pig coronary artery and 1.5 g in the dog basilar artery) or dynamic stretch (quick stretch at a rate of 10 cm/s, the amount of stretch being equivalent to 140% of the initial muscle length, with a duration of 30 s separated by 20-min intervals) was given to the preparation. In a separate series of experiments, a segment of the dog basilar artery was separately perfused, i.e., intra- and extraluminally with Tyrode solution. The small branches of the artery were sutured with thin silk thread. The perfusion pressure could be varied by changing the height of the reservoir containing the perfusion solution. Intraluminal flow was recorded by means of a drop counter.

All measurements were displayed on a pen recorder. Further experimental details on stretch activation are given in earlier publications [8, 9].

Drugs
Nifedipine, nimodipine, nisoldipine, and BAY k 8644 were supplied by Bayer Yakuhin, Japan, dissolved in Cremophor (BASF, West Germany) and used under a sodium lamp. Nicardipine hydrochloride (Yamanouchi, Japan), verapamil hydrochloride (Eisai, Japan), and diltiazem hydrochloride (Tanabe, Japan) were dissolved in physiological saline. All drugs used were expressed as molar concentrations in the organ bath.

Results

Physiological properties of stretch-induced contraction
Figures 1 and 2 show the mechanical responses of arteries to various types of stretch. The responses to stretch were myogenic in nature and were independent of neural elements. The saphenous artery of old SHR produced an initial tension rise coincident with a quick stretch (Fig. 1A) at a rate of 10 cm/s, the amount of stretch being 140% of the initial muscle length (= 100%) and duration (30 s); the subsequent tension fall at the completion of stretch was followed by delayed tension development, which reached a maximum 4–6 s after the application of stretch. The contractile response of vascular tissues to quick stretch depends on three main parameters—the magnitude and rate of stretch and the duration of the interval between stretches. Figure 1B shows the effect of varying the degree of stretch on tension development in the saphenous artery from an old SHR. In normal Tyrode solution containing 2 mM Ca, the stretch-induced contraction was reproducible when the preparation was stretched at 20-min intervals. Ca antagonists, such as verapamil and nifedipine, or the removal of Ca inhibited the contraction only after successive trials of quick stretching during the observation period of 90 min. Excessive elongation of vascular tissue by static stretch also

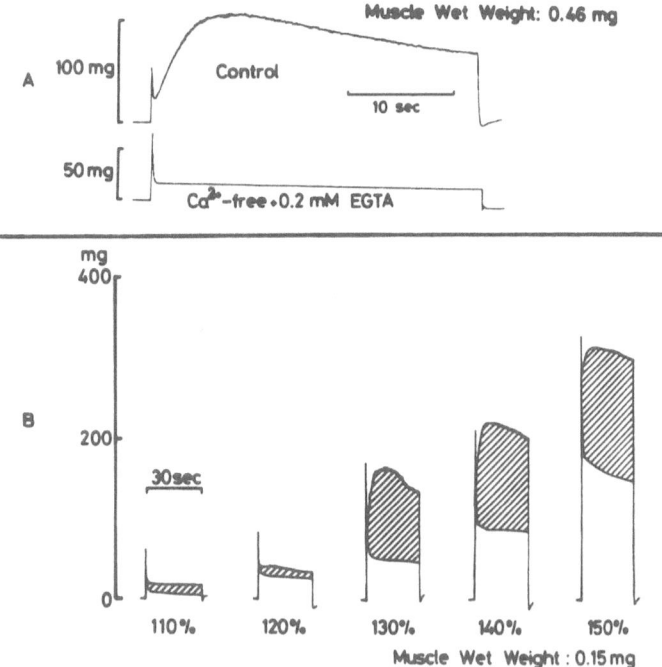

Fig. 1A, B. Effect of quick stretch on tension development in the saphenous artery of an SHR. **A** Time-course of tension development of a saphenous strip after quick stretch at a rate of 10 cm/s, the amount of stretch being 140% of initial muscle length (=100%) and duration of stretch, 30 s. Note that in Ca-free medium containing 0.2 mM EGTA the stretch-induced contraction disappeared after successive trials of stretches during the observation time of 90 min. **B** Effect of varying the amount of stretch on tension development. *Hatched area* of mechanogram shows active tension which is superimposed on passive increase in tension. The initial muscle length of the preparation was 10 mm

produced contraction. In Fig. 2A, a helically cut small coronary artery (outer diameter, 150 μm) from a pig produced contraction, while nifedipine (3×10^{-8} mol) inhibited the augmented response.

A sudden increase in perfusion pressure expressed as hydrostatic pressure (cmH_2O) produced contractile activation of the dog cerebral artery, which led to a decrease in intraluminal flow (Fig. 2B). This contraction disappeared after administration of Ca antagonists or removal of Ca.

Promotors and inhibitors of stretch-induced contraction
Previous reports have demonstrated that the contractile response to stretch is largely potentiated by promotors of Ca influx such as cardiac glycosides, high K, tetraethylammonium, and vasoconstrictor amines such as norepinephrine, histamine, and serotonin [9]. Figure 3 shows that xylazine, an α_2 adrenergic agonist, augmented the stretch-induced contraction of a saphenous artery segment of an old SHR, and nicardipine, a 1,4-dihydropyridine Ca antagonist, inhibited the

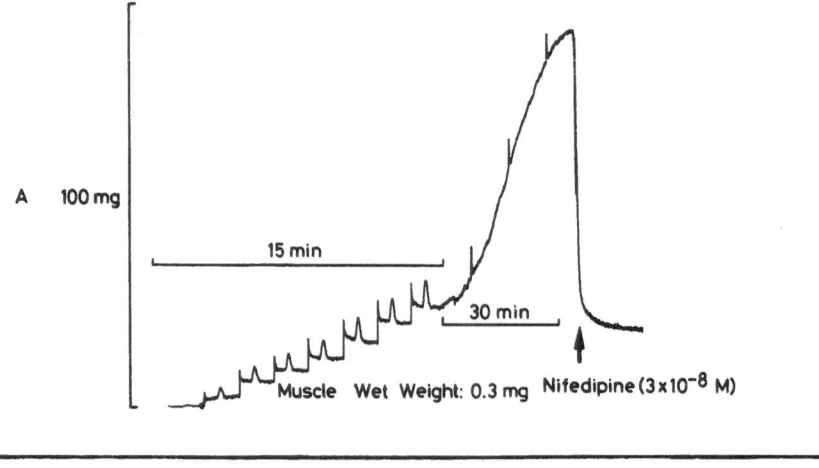

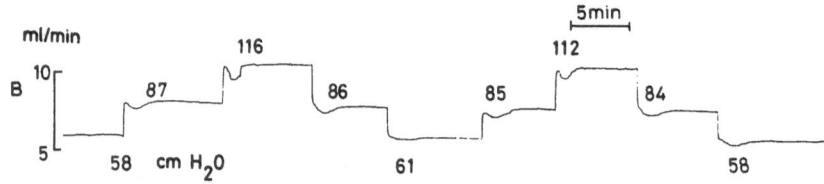

Fig. 2A, B. Effects of mechanical stimulation on tension development of vascular tissues. **A** Pig small coronary artery. Time-course of tension development after graded elongation (static stretch) of the preparation. The muscle strip, 10 mm long, was stretched seven times (1 mm every 2 min) and stimulated intermittently with rectangular alternating currents (10 V, 10 Hz, stimulus period 8 s) to secure contractile responsiveness. Nifedipine inhibited the stretch-induced contraction. **B** Dog basilar artery. The change in intraluminal flow was a measure of the contraction produced by varying the perfusion pressure expressed as cmH_2O

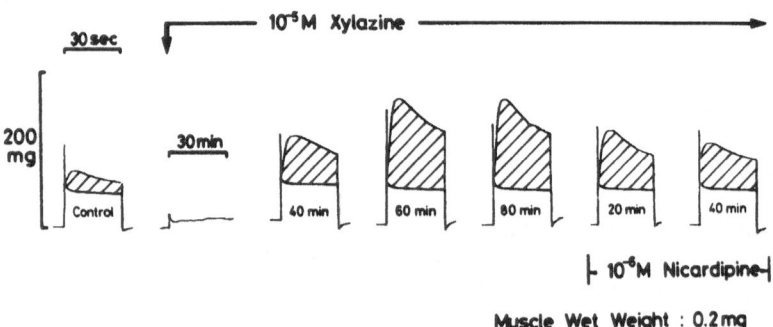

Fig. 3. Mechanical response of saphenous artery of SHR to quick stretch augmented by xylazine. Nicardipine inhibited the potentiating effect of xylazine

augmented response. Furthermore, in the cerebral artery, a small amount of hemolysate prepared from autologus blood containing oxyhemoglobin, which is widely accepted as a plausible spasmogen in subarachinoidal hemorrhage, potentiated the contraction in response to stretching. Hemolysate potentiates both mechanical and pharmacological stimulation [13]. The contractions produced by serotonin, histamine, and norepinephrine were potentiated by hemolysate. Dose-response curves for vasoactive amines were shifted to the right and the maximum responses were augmented. Contractile responses potentiated by xylazine and hemolysate were easily inhibited by Ca antagonists, such as nicardipine and nisoldipine, and by Ca withdrawal. Thus, the potentiating action of hemolysate on the contractile responses to both mechanical and pharmacological stimulation seems to be mainly attributable to augmentation of Ca influx.

Dual Ca components in stretch activation and the effect of BAY k 8644, a Ca agonist

With regard to the cellular mechanism involved, there is a well-known explanation given for the sequence of events which follows the stretching of vascular smooth muscle: Excitation-contraction coupling is improved by an increase in permeability to Ca concomitant with membrane depolarization [3]. However, the following experiments indicate that depolarization of the membrane due to stretch is unlikely to be the sole mechanism.

The contraction produced by stretch is quite resistant to Ca antagonists compared with that produced by a depolarizing high K solution. Table 1 compares the inhibitory action of such drugs on the K contracture with that on stretch-induced contraction in the saphenous artery. The contracture produced by high K was 300–8000 times more easily antagonized by Ca antagonists than the stretch-induced contraction. Furthermore, previous work [11] demonstrated that the phasic contractions due to electrical stimulation, which were strongly dependent on extracellular Ca [10], disappeared in Ca-free depolarizing medium, while the stretch-induced contraction still remained. This mechanical component was resistant to Ca antagonists and decreased with the number of stretches applied, while it was potentiated by ryanodine, which releases Ca from intracellular depots [11]. Thus, the stretch-induced contraction seems to be dependent on dual Ca

Table 1. Comparison of the inhibitory action of various drugs on the K contracture (80 mM K) with their inhibition of the contractile response to quick stretch in the saphenous artery of SHR

Drug	K	Q	Q/K
Diltiazem	$3.1 \times 10^{-7}\ M$ $n = 6$	1.1×10^{-4} $n = 5$	>350
Verapamil	1.1×10^{-7} $n = 7$	3.4×10^{-4} $n = 7$	>3000
Nicardipine	1.4×10^{-8} $n = 6$	1.2×10^{-4} $n = 8$	>8500

K K contracture ED_{50}, Q quick stretch ED_{50}, n number of experiments

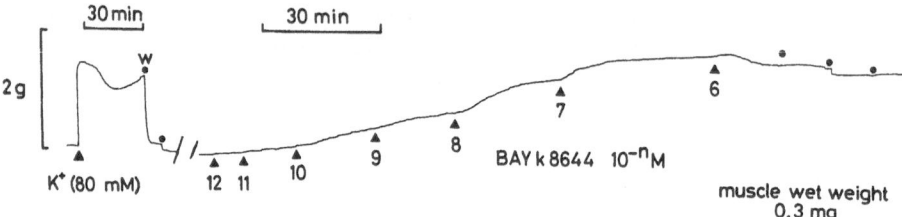

Fig. 4. Effect of increasing dose of BAY k 8644 on the basal tone of a dog basilar artery. Note that maximal tension developed by 10^{-6} M BAY k 8644 is almost equal to that produced by 80 mM K. *w* washout

components, i.e., influx of extracellular Ca, which is sensitive to Ca antagonists, and the release of intracellular Ca, possibly located on the inner surface of the plasma membrane [11], which is more susceptible to mechanical deformation.

The introduction of novel Ca channel activators, or "Ca agonists," have recently led to greater understanding of the mechanism of action of drugs on the Ca channel [15]. Of several Ca agonists, BAY k 8644 is the most potent. Thus, it is important to examine the effect of this Ca agonist on the stretch-induced contraction.

Figure 4 shows a typical tracing of the effect of increasing doses of BAY k 8644 on tension development in the dog basilar artery. Maximum tension developed at a dose of 10^{-6} M, which was almost equal to the full contracture produced by 80 mM K. In the cerebral artery, BAY k 8644 is effective without partial depolarization by high K as observed in the aorta [14], which seems to be attributable to the high dependency of excitation-contraction coupling on extracellular Ca in the cerebral artery [7]. The ethanol used as a solvent for BAY k 8644 acts as a constrictor at the same amount required to dissolve more than 10^{-5} M BAY k 8644. Thus, BAY k 8644 at a dose of more than 10^{-6} M would appear to have a Ca-antagonistic action.

BAY k 8644 potentiated the contractile response to stretch. Figure 5 shows the contractile responses to varying amounts of quick stretch; in this experiment, the rate and the stimulus period were 10 cm/s and 30 s, respectively. The direct effect of BAY k 8644 on basal tone was clamped to no measurable increase in tension by releasing the muscle strip, and the artery was quickly stretched. BAY k 8644 also sensitized the dog cerebral artery to static stretch, as shown in Fig. 6. The artery, which had shown no measurable active tension in response to static stretch in increments up to a final basal tension of 1.5 g, produced a remarkable increase in amplitude of delayed contraction after the administration of BAY k 8644. BAY k 8644 potentiated the delayed contraction in a dose-dependent manner. Both types of stretch-induced contraction potentiated by BAY k 8644 were easily inhibited by Ca antagonists, such as verapamil, diltiazem, and nimodipine. Figure 7A shows concentration-response curves to BAY k 8644 for the increase in amplitude of delayed contractions produced by static stretch in the presence or absence of nimodipine or by the removal of Ca. Figure 7B shows a Schild plot of the mean values, indicating the competitive antagonism of the inhibitory action of nimodipine by BAY k 8644 in the dog basilar artery.

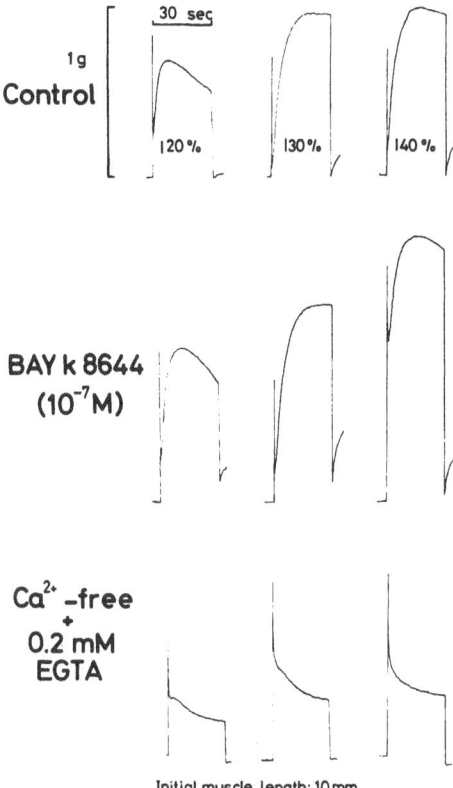

Fig. 5. Effect of varying the amount of quick stretch on tension development in the dog basilar artery before and after administration of BAY k 8644. Ca withdrawal suppressed the strech-induced contraction

Discussion

The present study has shown that vigorous contractile activation of cerebral, coronary, and saphenous arteries is produced by various types of mechanical stimulation. The properties of stretch-induced contraction and their modulation will now be discussed with special reference to the following two points: Ca-dependent mechanisms of stretch-induced contraction of vascular tissues and their implications under physiological and pathological conditions.

Dual Ca components or stretch-sensitive Ca channel?
Unlike the contraction produced by high K and direct electrical stimulation of muscle, which are totally dependent on extracellular Ca [8, 9], the stretch-induced contraction was much more resistant to Ca antagonists and Ca withdrawal. It was necessary to stretch the preparation repeatedly in Ca-free solution or in a Ca antagonist-containing solution in order to suppress the contractile response to stretch. This may be taken to indicate that the stretch-induced contraction is

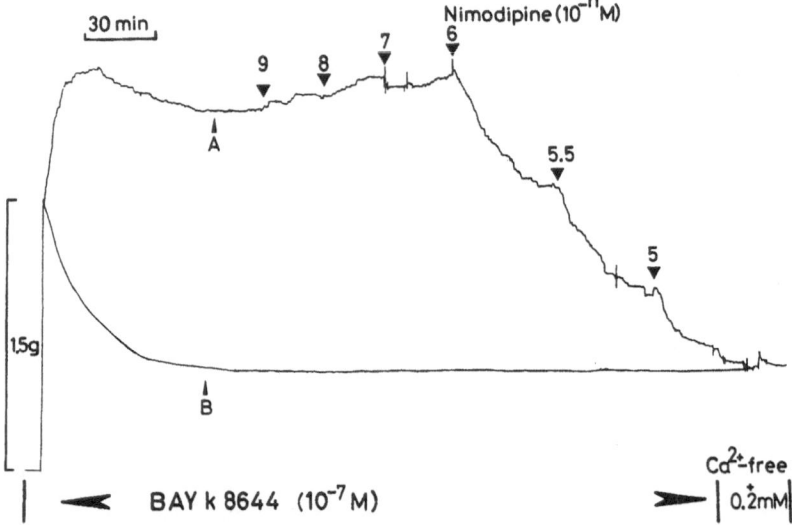

Fig. 6. Effect of BAY k 8644 on tension development produced by static stretch in the dog basilar artery. BAY k 8644 potentiated the stretch-induced contraction in normal Tyrode solution (*A*), while nimodipine suppressed the augmented contraction. BAY k 8644 showed no apparent effect on the tension development after static stretch in Ca-free medium (*B*)

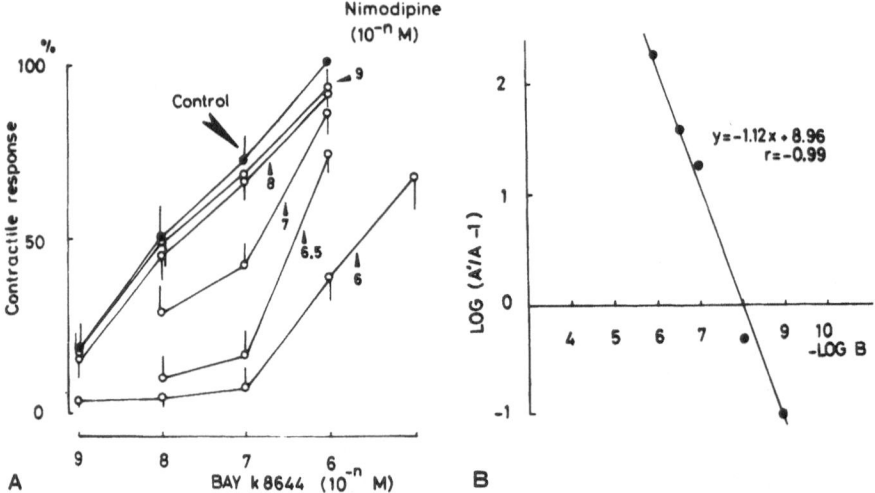

Fig. 7A. Contraction-response curves for the potentiating effect of BAY k 8644 on the contractile response of dog basilar artery to static stretch in the absence (●) or presence (○) of nimodipine. Each *point* and *bar* represents mean ± SE of four to six experiments. **B** Schild plot of mean values showing the competitive antagonism of the potentiating effect of BAY k 8644 on the stretch-induced contraction by nimodipine

produced not only by the influx of Ca but also by the release of intracellularly stored Ca from some structures such as the internal layer of the plasma membrane [12]. The transmembranous Ca supply was potentiated by promotors of influx of Ca through voltage-dependent and/or receptor-operated channels and was susceptible to Ca antagonists and Ca withdrawal, while the release of Ca was not primarily affected by Ca antagonists and Ca withdrawal.

Likewise, from a study on the mechanical stimulation of certain vascular smooth muscles, such as those in the basilar artery and facial vein of the rabbit, it was proposed that Ca influx was promoted through a stretch-sensitive channel [4]. The channel was sensitive to stretch but resistant to Ca antagonists such as diltiazem. In the present study, BAY k 8644, which is an activator of the voltage-dependent Ca channel strongly potentiated the stretch-induced contraction. Furthermore, nimodipine competitively antagonized the augmented response, indicating that both BAY k 8644 and nimodipine compete for the same binding sites, i.e., dihydropyridine receptors located in the channel structure. The low susceptibility of the stretch-induced contraction to Ca antagonists seems to be attributable to dual Ca supplies. Thus, it is unlikely that a new type of Ca channel, i.e., one which is stretch-sensitive but resistant to Ca antagonists, truely exists in vascular tissue such as the cerebral artery.

Significance of myogenic tone

The "myogenic theory" of control of blood flow has had a long history and has often been criticized in terms of its physiological significance, because the theory/mechanism lacks a so-called "break mechanism" [6]. The scheme in Fig. 8 shows a positive feedback loop, in which increasing myogenic tone leads to hypertension and vasospasm in a *circulus vitiosus* manner. Ca antagonists specifically interrupt Ca-dependent vasospastic constriction without affecting basic/intrinsic vascular tone produced by the primary stimulus. About 40% of the total amount of stretch-induced contraction under control conditions is susceptible to Ca antagonists, indicating the influx of extracellular Ca, while the rest (about 60%) is less sensitive to Ca antagonists [9]. These two Ca supplies seem to be involved in basic/intrinsic vascular tone. However, the tone once potentiated by promotors of influx of Ca becomes very sensitive to Ca antagonists, which indicates that the augmented tone/extrinsic tone is primarily dependent on promoted influx of Ca. It seems possible that activation of a gate mechanism or a use-dependent process of voltage-dependent Ca channels is accelerated in the presence of promotors of Ca influx, when the vascular tissues are subjected to stretch. In accordance with the present basic studies, Ca antagonists were more effective in hypertensive patients than in normotensive individuals in lowering systemic blood pressure [1]. Since Ca antagonists inherently have a slight effect on basal vascular tone, they are beneficial in relieving hypertension and vasospasm without causing circulatory disorders, such as orthostatic hypotension or luxurious perfusion syndrome.

The main therapeutic efforts in the treatment of primary/essential hypertension have long been focused on lowering central and peripheral sympathetic vascular tone, activity of the renin-angiotensin system, or blood volume in the systemic circulation. But now, it has been established that with the help of Ca antagonists

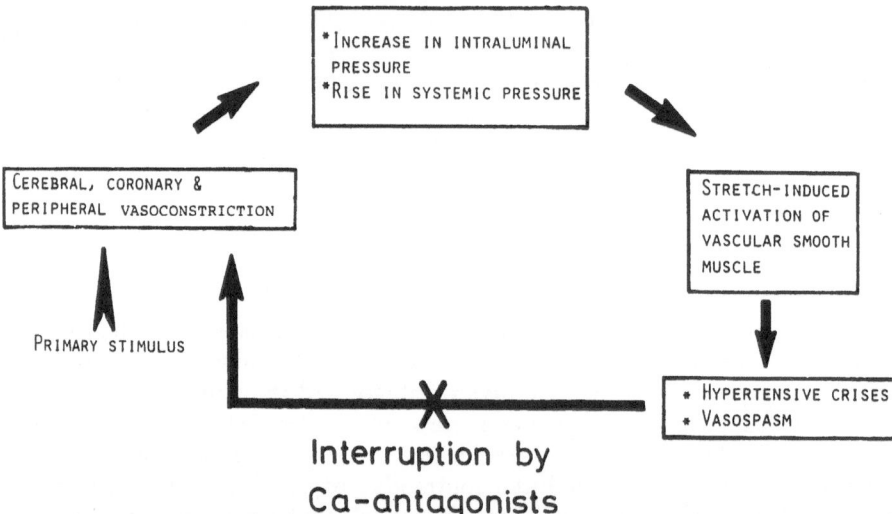

Fig. 8. Scheme of positive feedback loop of stretch-induced contraction. Ca antagonists interrupt the vicious circle, which is possibly the underlying mechanism of hypertensive crises and vasospasm. Modified after Fleckenstein [5]

a more direct intervention [5], i.e., the control of Ca kinetics at the plasma membrane level in resistance vessels, is possible. Further investigation of the pharmacological action of Ca agonists and antagonists will also open the way for understanding the mechanisms of vasospastic circulatory disorders, including hypertension and vasospasm.

Acknowledgments. The author expresses sincere thanks to Dr. K. Aoki, the president of the symposium, and the organizing committee for inviting him to attend the symposium and present this paper.

References

1. Aoki K, Kondo S, Mochizuki A, Yoshida T, Kato S, Kato K, Takikawa K (1978) Antihypertensive effect of cardiovascular Ca^{2+}-antagonist in hypertensive patients in the absence and presence of beta-adrenergic blockade. Am Heart J 96:218–226
2. Bayliss WM (1902) On the local reactions of the arterial wall to change of internal pressure. J Physiol (Lond) 28:220–231
3. Bohr DF (1964) (In discussion on the paper by Folkow B. Description of the myogenic hypothesis) Circ Res 15 (Suppl 1): 279–285
4. Bevan JA (1983) Diltiazem selectively inhibits cerebrovascular extrinsic but not intrinsic myogenic tone. A review. Circ Res 52, (Suppl I): 104–109
5. Fleckenstein A (1983) Calcium antagonism in heart and smooth muscle. In: Experimental facts and therapeutic prospects. Wiley, New York, p 311
6. Folkow B (1964) Description of the myogenic hypothesis. Circ Res 14–15 (Suppl I): 279–287
7. Harder DR (1984) Pressure-dependent membrane depolarization in cat middle cerebral artery. Circ Res 55:197–202

8. Nakayama K, Fleckenstein A, Byon YK, Fleckenstein-Gruen G (1978) Fundamental physiology of coronary smooth musculature from extramural stem arteries of pigs and rabbits (electric excitability, tension development, influence of Ca, Mg, H and K ions). Eur J Cardiol 8:319–335
9. Nakayama K (1982) Calcium-dependent contractile activation of cerebral artery produced by quick stretch. Am J Physiol 242 (Heart Circ Physiol 11): H760–H768
10. Nakayama K, Kasuya Y (1980) Selective abolition of Ca-dependent responses of smooth and cardiac muscles by flunarizine. Jpn J Pharmacol 30:731–742
11. Nakayama K, Ishii K, Kato H (1983) Effect of Ca-antagonists on the contraction of cerebral and peripheral arteries produced by electrical and mechanical stimuli. Gen Pharmacol 14:111–113
12. Nakayama K, Suzuki S, Sugi H (1986) Physiological and ultrastructural studies on the mechanism of stretch-induced contractile activation in rabbit cerebral artery smooth muscle. Jpn J Physiol 36:745–760
13. Nakayama K, Hashimoto K (1984) Blood components and cerebral vasospasm. Biblthca Cardiol 38:148–160
14. Schramm M, Thomas G, Towart R, Franckowiak G (1983) Activation of calcium channels by novel 1,4-dihydropyridines. A new mechanism for positive inotropics or smooth muscle stimulants. Arzneim-Forsch 33:1268–1272
15. Schramm M, Towart R (1985) Modulation of calcium channel function by drugs. Life Sciences 37:1843–1860

Effects of Diltiazem on Myogenic Tone in Pressurized Brain Arteries from Spontaneously Hypertensive Rats*

G. Osol, R. Osol, and W. Halpern

Department of Physiology and Biophysics, The University of Vermont, College of Medicine, Burlington, VT 05405, USA

Summary. The inhibitory effects of diltiazem on myogenic tone in resistance-sized branches of the posterior cerebral artery from 16- to 24-week-old hypertensive (SHRSP) and normotensive (WKY) rats were studied. Using a video-electronic technique, which permits measurement of the lumen diameter and wall thickness, freshly excised arteries were mounted on a microcannula and pressurized to 75 mmHg. During equilibration, or shortly thereafter, spontaneous tone developed, resulting in a 35% reduction of lumen diameter (180–118 μm, ID). When diltiazem was added cumulatively in concentrations from 10^{-8} to 10^{-5} M, progressive relaxation was observed. The calculated IC_{50} values, 7.7×10^{-7} M (SHRSP) and 8.9×10^{-7} M (WKY), were not significantly different. Arteries from hypertensive animals showed rhythmic diameter oscillations which were also suppressed by diltiazem. These results show that: (1) the level of spontaneous tone is similar in resistance-sized cerebral arteries taken from hypertensive and normotensive rats; (2) tone is dependent on the influx of extracellular calcium; and (3) the diltiazem sensitivity of the population of calcium channels responsible for maintaining this tone is not altered in this genetic model of hypertension.

Key words: Cerebral arteries—Hypertension—Pressurized vessels—Calcium blocker—WKY and SHRSP rats

Several studies have suggested that the smooth muscle cell membranes of arteries are modified in hypertension so that their handling of calcium ion transport into and out of the cells favors an elevated intracellular calcium level [1, 2]. The consequence of this for peripheral resistance arteries might then be a further mechanism through which they maintain an increased peripheral resistance. Similar ionic changes occurring in arteries that exhibit myogenic behavior could contribute to the modification of blood flow and pressure distribution in these vascular beds.

It is generally agreed that several membrane channels participate in calcium exchange of smooth muscle cells; these are the receptor- and potential-operated channels and the passive calcium leak channels [3–5]. A fourth channel, stretch dependent, has also been proposed for myogenic arteries [6]. Calcium channel blockers have been used to provide a means for understanding the sources of calcium which activate smooth muscle and the differential effectiveness of the various agents. These tools have been applied in many studies to determine the sensitivity of in vitro responses of different vessels [7–10] and perfused vascular

* Supported by National Institutes of Health Grant Number HL 17335.

beds [11] to various agonists. However, only a few studies have been concerned with the channels that might be responsible for arteries showing a spontaneous tone, such as those of the coronary and brain circulation. For example, intrinsic myogenic tone was found to be relatively resistant to the calcium entry blocker diltiazem in the basilar artery of the rabbit [12, 13]. This observation was also confirmed from in vivo studies of cat pial arteries in which nimodipine, a dihydropyridine type of calcium blocker, did not change basal cerebral blood flow, although autoregulation was impaired [14]. These results are interpreted as being in accord with other studies showing that spontaneous tone occurs as a result of calcium entry through either passive channels in the membrane or from the use of intracellular calcium stores, both of which are relatively insensitive to dihydropyridine blockers [3, 15].

   This study was undertaken to determine whether the spontaneous tone of isolated, pressurized small branches of the posterior cerebral artery from stroke-prone spontaneously hypertensive rats (SHRSP) was sensitive to diltiazem, a dihydropyridine class calcium blocker, and whether this sensitivity was different in vessels from normotensive Wistar-Kyoto rats (WKY).

Methods

SHRSP and WKY rats, 16–24 weeks of age, were obtained from the colony maintained at The University of Vermont. A standard rat chow diet was fed to both groups of rats. Systolic blood pressures were measured indirectly by tail cuff plethysmography during the week prior to an experiment. The animals were killed by decapitation under light ether anesthesia and the entire brain was immediately removed and placed in a dish containing oxygenated physiological saline solution (PSS) at room temperature. A 2- to 3-mm-long segment of the middle branch of the posterior cerebral artery was then carefully dissected out from the surrounding connective tissues and transferred to the experimental chamber of an arteriograph, which was also filled with oxygenated PSS at 25°C. The proximal end of the vessel was attached to a glass cannula of about 100 μm OD, and the distal end occluded. The cannula was connected to a pressure transducer and a motorized syringe filled with PSS. The transmural pressure was then brought to 75 mmHg (the estimated in situ transmural pressure of these arteries); the cannula was moved by means of a micrometer in the direction of the vessel axis to just remove any buckling of the artery and then lowered to 25 mmHg for equilibration. Detailed descriptions of the arteriograph and the procedure for mounting these vessels have been published elsewhere [16, 17].

   The arteriograph was placed on the stage of a compound microscope having a TV camera attached to the viewing tube. The signal derived from the vidicon image of the vessel was processed by an electronic system (Living Systems Instrumentation, Burlington, VT, USA) for continuous measurement and recording of the arterial lumen diameter and wall thickness [17]. A reservoir of physiological saline was bubbled with 95% O_2 and 5% CO_2 and circulated through the arteriograph. The temperature of this superfusate, measured with a thermistor probe, was adjusted to 37°C by flowing the solution through a heat exchanger, and the gassing rate was adjusted so that the pH of the solution surrounding the vessel was 7.40 ± 0.02. Under these conditions, the pCO_2 of the solution in the chamber was between 29 and 33 mmHg.

After a 1-h equilibration period, the artery was subjected to three pressure cycles between 25 and 120 mmHg at a rate of approximately 1 mmHg/s. The pressure was then set to 75 mmHg and the vessel allowed to stabilize again before dimensional measurements were taken. The responses of each vessel to cumulatively increasing concentrations of diltiazem (Marion Laboratories) in the superfusate from 10^{-8} to 10^{-5} M were then recorded. Measurements were made after a steady state response was observed, usually 5-10 min after each concentration change. After the last diltiazem concentration, EGTA-PSS was superfused in order to obtain the relaxed dimensions of the artery for evaluation of vessel tone. Tone was defined as the difference in diameters of the vessel in PSS and EGTA-PSS expressed as a percentage of the EGTA-PSS diameter. Relaxation responses resulting from the various diltiazem concentrations were calculated as the percentage difference in artery diameters in the presence of diltiazem and in its absence (PSS alone) referred to the latter. The diltiazem dose-response data were first normalized to the maximum relaxation obtained in each vessel and then fitted to the Hill equation for a sigmoid curve [18] in order to determine the IC_{50}, the concentration producing a 50% relaxation.

The composition of the PSS solution was in millimoles per liter: NaCl 119, $NaHCO_3$ 24, KCl 4.7, KH_2PO_4 1.18, $MgSO_4 \cdot 7H_2O$ 1.17, $CaCl_2$ 1.6, glucose 5.5, ethylene diamine tetraacetic acid (EDTA) 0.026. The relaxing solution (EGTA-PSS) consisted of PSS with a substitution of 1 mM ethyleneglycol-bis (β-aminoethyl ether) N,N,N',N'-tetraacetic acid (EGTA) for $CaCl_2$.

Data are expressed as mean values $\pm$ 1 SE. An unpaired Student's t-test was used for evaluating the statistical significance of the results between the two groups of rats.

Results

The systolic pressures of the WKY and SHRSP rats were 112 ± 11 ($n = 5$) and 157 ± 20 ($n = 4$) mmHg; these were significantly different ($P < 0.05$). The lumen diameters of the WKY and SHRSP arteries at 75 mmHg were not different when fully relaxed in EGTA-PSS or measured in PSS, and their tones were similar (Table 1). The average wall thickness and wall/radius ratios of SHRSP arteries ranged from 22% to 38% larger than those of WKY rats (Table 1).

A typical response of an SHRSP vessel to two concentrations of diltiazem is shown in Fig. 1. All SHRSP arteries possessed spontaneous diameter vasomotion in PSS which decreased in rate at increasing concentrations of diltiazem; at the higher concentrations, this vasoactivity was invariably lost. None of the WKY vessels were spontaneously active. The diameter relaxations to diltiazem were concentration-dependent for both the WKY and SHR arteries (Fig. 2). Although mean threshold relaxations (IC_{10}) were slightly greater for the SHRSP vessels, they were not significantly different from those of WKY rats. The mean IC_{50} concentrations (± 1 SE) were 7.7 (10.1 and 5.9) $\times$ 10^{-7} M for SHRSP and 8.9 (10.8 and 7.3) $\times$ 10^{-7} M for WKY rats. At the highest concentration of diltiazem used, 10^{-5} M, the vessels were approximately within 10% of their fully relaxed size.

Table 1. Vessel data at 75 mmHg transmural pressure

	WKY	SHRSP
Lumen diameter (μm)		
EGTA-PSS	176 ± 10	184 ± 13
PSS	117 ± 8	118 ± 15
Tone (%)	33 ± 2	37 ± 4
Wall thickness (μm)		
EGTA-PSS	12 ± 1	16 ± 1**
PSS	18 ± 1[a]	22 ± 1*
Wall/radius		
EGTA-PSS	0.14 ± 0.00	0.18 ± 0.01***
PSS	0.29 ± 0.02	0.40 ± 0.04

Values are means ± SE
Number of vessels = number of rats = five except[a] where number = four
Differences in mean values were evaluated using unpaired Student's *t*-test
* $P < 0.05$
** $P < 0.01$
*** $P < 0.001$
Other differences were not significant

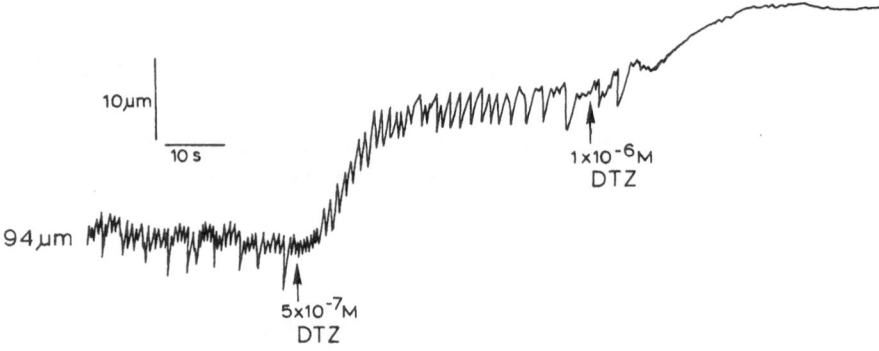

Fig. 1. Typical diameter response of an SHRSP posterior cerebral artery branch to two concentrations of diltiazem. Mean vessel lumen sizes were 85 μm in PSS, 94 μm at 10^{-7} *M*, 115 μm at 5×10^{-7} *M*, and 130 μm at 10^{-6} *M* diltiazem. Relaxed diameter was 175 μm. The normal vasomotion seen in these vessels was decreased in rate by 5×10^{-7} *M* diltiazem and lost following 10^{-6} *M* diltiazem. *DTZ*, diltiazem

Discussion

The key results of this study are: (1) myogenic tone in resistance-sized cerebral arteries is primarily dependent on the influx of extracellular calcium; (2) diltiazem is effective in inhibiting the calcium channels of the smooth muscle cells that are responsible for the maintenance of spontaneous tone in these brain arteries; (3) the sensitivity of these channels to inhibition by diltiazem is similar in arteries from normotensive and hypertensive rats; and (4) there may be a common membrane pathway for calcium exchange that is involved with tone, myogenicity, and spontaneous vasomotion, suggesting that intracellular calcium handling

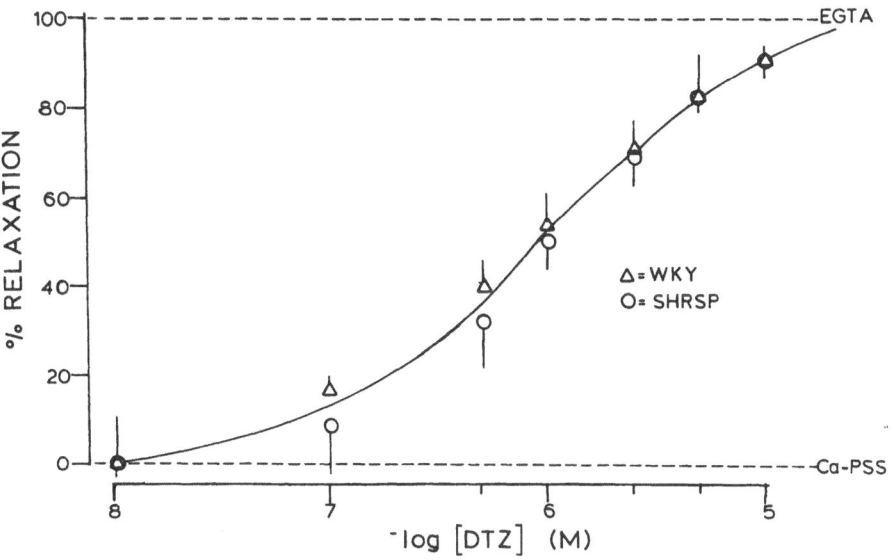

Fig. 2. Concentration-dependent diltiazem relaxation of spontaneous tone in WKY and SHRSP posterior cerebral artreries. Ca-PSS (PSS) mean lumen diameters for WKY and SHRSP are 117 and 118 μm, respectively; the corresponding mean EGTA (EGTA-PSS) diameters are 176 and 184 μm. *DTZ* diltiazem

related to the latter two types of phenomenon is differentially modulated as a result of hypertension.

Our results are at variance with the only other study that we are aware of concerning calcium blockers and brain vessels possessing spontaneous tone. In that study of the rabbit basilar artery, the IC_{50} for diltiazem was 4×10^{-4} M, which is more than three orders of magnitude higher than the diltiazem IC_{50} $(10^{-7}–10^{-8}$ $M)$ found to be effective against tone induced by potential-operated channel (POC) and receptor-operated channel (ROC) activation [12]. Since spontaneous tone developed in our vessels without extrinsic receptor or depolarization activating agents, calcium may enter the cells through passive leak channels, which have been reported to be relatively insensitive to diltiazem and other calcium channel blockers in different vessels [3, 13, 19]. On the other hand, both nifedipine and nimodopine reduce basal tone in isolated rat coronary resistance vessels at very low concentrations (IC_{50} about 10^{-9} M) [20]. Several in vivo experiments have also demonstrated that calcium entry blockers are effective in dilating resistance vessels of the coronary [21, 22] and cerebral pial vascular beds [14], which are generally considered to have a basal tone. The diltiazem IC_{50} values reported here ($7.7–8.9 \times 10^{-7}$ M) are similar to those found with POC and ROC activators, as described above, and in other vessels not possessing spontaneous tone, such as isolated pig coronary arteries, which were also relatively sensitive to diltiazem (IC_{50} of 10^{-7} M) when activated by potassium depolarization [23]. Thus, while the issue of which channels permit calcium to enter the cells and give rise to the basal tone is not resolved, it is certain that the spontaneous tone in resistance-sized rat cerebral arteries is sensitive to diltiazem.

Relaxed WKY and SHRSP arteries have similar diameters, and in PSS they contract to smaller, essentially equal, diameters (Table 1). The calcium responsible for these tones is clearly extracellular since no tone is evident in the absence of external calcium (unpublished data), and diltiazem is equally effective in reducing these spontaneous tones (Fig. 2). These data suggest that the sensitivity of the calcium channels to inhibition by diltiazem is similar in arteries from both rat strains. Thus, our results do not indicate greater leakage or permeability of calcium through the membrane of vascular smooth muscle from hypertensive animals. The fact that the SHRSP vessels have thicker walls (Table 1) but do not achieve smaller luminal diameters than those of the WKY may be related to the reduced smooth muscle cell myosin and actin content in hypertension [24, 25].

The brain arteries studied have four combined characteristics distinguishing them from most other vessels used in calcium blocker experiments: (1) They are resistance-sized; (2) they develop a spontaneous tone; (3) they respond myogenically to pressure changes [26]; and (4) those from the SHRSP are spontaneously vasoactive. Removal of calcium from the external medium and high concentrations of diltiazem suppresses all three types of behavior. Although we did not study the myogenic responses of the vessels at less than maximal concentrations of diltiazem, the rate of the diameter vasoactivity of the SHRSP was reduced along with the degree of diminished tone before it was lost completely (Fig. 1). Hence, there may be a common link between these mechanically expressed phenomena, specifically, a pathway through which calcium ions enter and leave the smooth muscle cells. This does not, however, rule out other membrane or intracellular changes brought about in these vessels by hypertension. One example is the lack of spontaneous vasomotion in WKY vessels found in the present study. Another concerns the elevation of the myogenic pressure range and reduction of the strength of the myogenic response consequent to high blood pressure [16, 26].

In conclusion, the differences between the results of this study and others may lie in the well-recognized individuality of vessels from different vascular beds and animal species, or in the methodology. These experiments were done using pressurized resistance arteries which were allowed to develop a spontaneous tone isobarically. The small size of these vessels and the closer similarity to in situ conditions that our in vitro pressurized vessel technique allows (natural geometric configuration, transmural pressure, intact endothelium, isotonic contraction) has provided another insight into the complexity of ionic calcium transfer and the action of calcium blockers in the cerebral vasculature.

References

1. Suzuki A, Yanagawa T, Higashino H, Tajiri T (1979) The reactivity of vascular smooth muscle in Stroke-Prone SHR, especially from the standpoint of aging. Jap Heart J 20 (Suppl I): 715
2. Mochizuki A, Aoki K, Mizuno T Hotta K (1979) Specificity of tension development and calcium flux of the arterial smooth muscle in SHR. Jpn Heart J 20 (Suppl I): 225
3. Van Breemen C, Mangel A, Fahim M, Meisheri K (1982) Selectivity of calcium antagonistic action in vascular smooth muscle. Am J Cardiol 49: 507–510
4. Bou J, Llenas J, Massingham R (1983) Calcium entry blocking drugs, 'calcium antagonists' and vascular smooth muscle function. J Auton Pharmac 3: 219–232

5. Nayler WG, Poole-Wilson PH (1981) Calcium antagonists: definition and mode of action. Basic Res Cardiol 76:1–15
6. Bevan JA, Hwa JJ, Owen MP, Winquist RJ (1985) Calcium and myogenic or stretch-dependent vascular tone. In: Rubin RP, Weiss GB, Putney JW Jr (eds) Calcium in biological systems. Plenum, New York, pp 391–398
7. Godfraind T, Miller RC (1982) Actions of prostaglandin F_{2a} and noradrenaline on calcium exchange and contraction in rat mesenteric arteries and their sensitivity to calcium entry blockers. Br J Pharmac 75:229–236
8. Van Neuten JM, Vanhoutte PM (1980) Calcium entry blockers and vascular smooth muscle heterogeneity. Fed Proc 40:2862–2865
9. Schümann HJ, Görlitz BD, Wagner J (1975) Influence of papaverine, D-600, and nifedipine on the effects of noradrenaline and calcium on the isolated aorta and mesenteric artery of the rabbit. Naunyn-Schmiedeberg's Arch Pharmacol 289:409–418
10. Towart R (1981) The selective inhibition of serotonin-induced contractions of rabbit cerebral vascular smooth muscle by calcium antagonistic dihydropyridines. Circ Res 48:650–657
11. Kondo K, Suzuki H, Okuno T, Suda M, Saruta T (1980) Effects of nifedipine, diltiazem and verapamil on the vasoconstrictor responses to norepinephrine and potassium ions in the rat mesenteric artery. Archiv Int Pharm Ther 245:211–217
12. Bevan JA (1982) Selective action of diltiazem on cerebral vascular smooth muscle in the rabbit: Antagonism of extrinsic but not intrinsic maintained tone. Am J Cardiol 49:519–524
13. Bevan JA, Bevan RD, Hwa JJ, Owen MP, Tayo FM Winquist RJ (1982) Calcium, extrinsic and intrinsic (myogenic) vascular tone. In: Godfraind T, Albertini A, Paoletti R (eds) Calcium modulators. Elsevier/North Holland, Amsterdam, pp 125–132
14. Haws CW, Heistad DD (1984) Effects of nimodipine on cerebral vasoconstrictor responses. Am J Physiol 247:H170–H176
15. Droogmans G, Casteels R (1980) Effect of Ca-antagonists on the contractile response and on the ^{45}Ca exchange in vascular smooth muscle cells of the rabbit ear artery. Archiv Int Physiol Biochim 88:P25
16. Osol G, Halpern W (1985) Myogenic properties of cerebral blood vessels from normotensive and hypertensive rats. Am J Physiol 249 (Heart Circ Physiol 18): H914–H921
17. Halpern W, Osol G, Coy GS (1984) Mechanical behavior of pressurized in vitro prearteriolar vessels determined with a video system. Annals Biomed Eng 12:463–479
18. Hill A (1913) The combinations of haemoglobin with oxygen and with carbon monoxide. Biochem J 7:471–480
19. Godfraind T (1982) Pharmacology of calcium entry blockers. In: Godfraind T, Albertini A, Paoletti R (eds) Calcium modulators. Elsevier/North Holland, Amsterdam, pp 51–66
20. Nyborg NCB, Mikkelsen EO (1985) Effects of nifedipine and nimodipine on basal tone, 5-HT, and potassium response in isolated rat coronary resistance arteries. (abstract) IUPHAR 9th Int Congress of Pharmacol
21. Vanhoutte PM, Cohen RA (1983) Calcium-entry blockers and cardiovascular disease. Am J Cardiol 52:99A–103A
22. Vatner SF, Hintze TH (1982) Effects of a calcium-channel antagonist on large and small coronary arteries in conscious dogs. Circ Res 66:579–588
23. Schwartz A (1983) Calcium channel inhibitors. The Physiologist 26:200–205
24. Brayden JE, Halpern W, Brann LR (1983) Biochemical and mechanical properties of resistance arteries from normotensive and hypertensive rats. Hypertension 5:17–25
25. Winquist RJ, Bohr DF (1983) Structural and functional changes in cerebral arteries from spontaneously hypertensive rats. Hypertension 5:292–297
26. Osol G, Halpern W (1986) Effect of antihypertensive treatment on myogenic properties of brain arteries from the stroke prone rat. J Hypertension 4 (Suppl 3) (in press)

Growth Factors and Vascular Smooth Muscle Cells in Spontaneously Hypertensive Rats

Role of Ca^{2+} in Cellular Proliferation

Y. Hirata[1,2], M. Tomita[2], and T. Fujita[2]

[1] Hypertension Division, National Cardiovascular Center Research Institute, Suita, Osaka, 565 Japan
[2] Third Division, Department of Medicine, Kobe University, School of Medicine, Kobe, 650 Japan

Summary. Vascular structural changes induced by hypertension are represented by the abnormal proliferation of vascular smooth muscle cells (VSMC) associated with increased synthesis of collagen and noncollagen protein. Cultured VSMCs from rat aorta appear to be a suitable in vitro system to study the mechanism of cellular proliferation of VSMC, because they are completely free from mechanical and neurohumoral influence. Therefore, the present study was designed to define serum-derived growth factors responsible for stimulating synthesis of DNA by cultured rat aortic VSMC, to compare the responses of VSMC from spontaneously hypertensive rats (SHR) and normotensive Wistar-Kyoto (WKY) control rats, and to study the role of intracellular Ca^{2+} ions in the regulation of cell growth.

Among a variety of serum-derived growth factors tested, platelet-derived growth factor (PDGF) and epidermal growth factor (EGF), both well-characterized polypeptide mitogens, were capable of stimulating DNA synthesis by cultured VSMC as assessed by incorporation of [^{3}H]thymidine into the cells. VSMC from SHR displayed significantly greater incorporation of [^{3}H]thymidine than those from age-matched WKY rats in response to both EGF ($0.1-10\,nM$) and PDGF ($0.1-1$ U/ml). DNA synthesis stimulated by EGF, PDGF, or fetal calf serum (FCS) was significantly inhibited by a variety of Ca^{2+}-antagonists, such as verapamil, diltiazem, and nicardipine, in a dose-dependent manner ($10^{-6}-10^{-5}\,M$); nicardipine, a dihydropyridine derivative, was the most potent in inhibiting stimulated DNA synthesis, followed by diltiazem and verapamil. Trifluoperazine and W-7, both specific calmodulin (CaM) inhibitors, similarly inhibited DNA synthesis stimulated by EGF, PDGF, or FCS in a dose-dependent fashion ($10^{-6}-10^{-4}\,M$), whereas W-5, a less specific CaM inhibitor, was minimally effective. Tetradecanoyl phorbol acetate (TPA), a potent tumor promotor, induced a significant stimulation of DNA synthesis in a dose-dependent manner ($10^{-10}-10^{-8}\,M$), while β-phorbol, an inactive compound, was without effect.

These findings indicate that PDGF and EGF, both localized in human platelets, are the major serum-derived mitogens for cultured VSMC, and suggest that both of these growth factors, released from the platelets at the sites of blood vessel injury, participate in the process of repairing the damaged tissues. The present study revealed that VSMC from SHR are more responsive to PDGF and EGF than are those from WKY, suggesting that VSMC of SHR have intrinsically greater sensitivity to both growth factors, which may in part contribute to the abnormal proliferation of VSMC in SHR independently of blood pressure. The inhibitory effects of both Ca^{2+} antagonists and CaM inhibitors on stimulated DNA synthesis strongly suggest that the Ca^{2+}-CaM system is involved in the mechanism of cellular proliferation of VSMC. Furthermore, the potent stimulatory effect of TPA, a compound substituting for diacylglycerol, on DNA synthesis suggests the possible additional involvement of the C-kinase system in the regulation of cell growth.

Key words: Vascular smooth muscle cell—Serum-derived growth factors—DNA synthesis—Ca^{2+}-antagonists—Calmodulin inhibitors

Vascular structural changes are important in the pathogenesis of hypertension [1]. The principal features underlying such vascular lesions are represented by medial hypertrophy of the arterial walls resulting from the abnormal proliferation of vascular smooth muscle cells (VSMC) associated with increased synthesis of collagenous and noncollagenous protein. Hypertensive vascular changes are largely ascribed to the consequence of raised blood pressure [1]. However, the thickening of the arterial walls in spontaneously hypertensive rats (SHR) has been observed during the prehypertensive stage [2]. Therefore, it is suggested that factors other than mechanical load, such as neural, humoral, and genetic factors, may also be involved in the development of the hypertensive vascular changes [2, 3]. In fact, it has recently been reported that cultured VSMC from SHR have intrinsically greater growth activity than those from normotensive Wistar-Kyoto (WKY) rats independent of blood pressure [4].

Several serum-derived growth factors, such as platelet-derived growth factor (PDGF) [5, 6], epidermal growth factor (EGF) [7, 8], insulin [9, 10], somatomedin(s) [10–12], fibroblast growth factor (FGF) [12], and low-density lipoprotein [13, 14], are capable of stimulating proliferation of VSMC in culture. Among them, PDGF and EGF are well-defined polypeptide mitogens localized in human platelets [15, 16], which play a pivotal role in the process of blood coagulation and repair of tissue damage.

Using cultured VSMC isolated from the rat aorta, we have studied the effects of serum-derived growth factors on DNA synthesis, compared the responses of VSMC from SHR and WKY rats to these growth factors, and elucidated the molecular mechanism by which growth factors stimulate DNA synthesis in relation to intracellular Ca^{2+} ions.

Materials and Methods

Cell culture

VSMC were obtained from the thoracic aortas of 20-week-old male Wistar rats by the explant method of Ross [17]. Cells were grown and maintained in Dulbecco's modified Eagles' Medium (DMEM) containing 10% fetal calf serum (FCS; Flow Laboratories: McLean, VA) and antibiotics (100 U/ml penicillin, 100 μg/ml streptomycin, 2.5 μg/ml fungizone) under a humidified atmosphere of 5% CO_2-95% air. VSMC from 9-week-old SHR and age-matched WKY rats were also obtained and cultured in the same manner. Cells from the sixth to tenth passage were used in the experiments.

Synthesis of DNA by cultured VSMC

The effect of growth factors on DNA synthesis was assessed by the incorporation of [³H]thymidine into VSMC as described elsewhere [18]. In brief, subconfluent cells ($1-5 \times 10^5$ cells/well) that had become quiescent in the presence of 0.5% FCS were stimulated by EGF (1.7 nM), PDGF (0.5 U/ml), and 10% FCS with or without Ca^{2+} antagonists or calmodulin (CaM) inhibitors. The cells were incubated at 37°C for 20 h, after which 1 μCi [³H]thymidine (specific activity— 6.7 Ci/mmol, New England Nuclear: Boston, MA) was added and further incubated for 4 h. After incubation, ice-cold 10% trichloroacetic acid (TCA) was added and TCA-insoluble protein was solubilized with 0.5 N NaOH. An aliquot was removed, neutralized with 0.5 N HCl, and its radioactivity was determined in a liquid scintillation counter.

Drugs

Mouse EGF, bovine FGF, multiplication-stimulating activity (MSA), insulin (all from Collaborative Research Inc. Waltham, MA), PDGF from human platelets (specific activity—10 000 U/mg; Kor Inc.: Cambridge, MA), verapamil (Knoll Pharmaceutical Co.: Whipanny, NJ), diltiazem (Tanabe Pharmaceutical Co.: Osaka, Japan), nicardipine (Yamanouchi Pharmaceutical Co.: Tokyo, Japan), W-7, W-5 (Biochemical Co.: Tokyo, Japan) [19], trifluoperazine (TFP), tetradecanoyl phorbol acetate (TPA), and β-phorbol (all from Sigma Chemical: St. Louis, MO) were used in the experiments.

Results

EGF significantly stimulated DNA synthesis and cell proliferation of VSMC in a dose-dependent manner (0.01–1 nM); approximately half-stimulation was induced with 0.15 nM and maximal stimulation with 1 nM. A binding study using ^{125}I-labeled EGF revealed the presence of a single class of binding sites for EGF in cultured VSMC; the apparent dissociation constant was 0.25 nM and the maximal binding capacity was $\sim 70\,000$ sites/cell. PDGF also stimulated DNA synthesis and cell proliferation of VSMC in a dose-responsive manner (0.1– 1 U/ml). The simultaneous addition of EGF and PDGF in maximal doses induced an additive effect on DNA synthesis by cultured VSMC, although the effect was about two-thirds that by 10% FCS (Fig. 1). Other growth factors, such as insulin (1 μg/ml), MSA (100 ng/ml), and FGF (100 ng/ml), failed to affect DNA synthesis.

The effects of EGF and PDGF on DNA synthesis in cultured VSMC from aged-matched SHR and WKY rats are shown in Figs. 2 and 3, respectively. VSMC from SHR have significantly greater incorporation of [3H]thymidine than those from WKY in response to both EGF (0.1–10 nM) and PDGF (0.1– 1 U/ml), suggesting that VSMC from SHR have intrinsically greater sensitivity to both growth factors than WKY control rats.

To determine the role of intracellular Ca^{2+} ions on DNA synthesis stimulated by growth factors, the effects of a variety of Ca^{2+} antagonists were studied. Verapamil, diltiazem, and nicardipine all inhibited DNA synthesis stimulated by EGF, PDGF, or 10% FCS in a dose-dependent manner (10^{-6}–10^{-5} M). The inhibitory effects of these Ca^{2+} antagonists (10^{-5} M) on stimulated-DNA synthesis are compared in Fig. 4. Nicardipine, a dihydropyridine derivative, was the most potent in inhibiting stimulation of DNA synthesis (56%–79%), followed by diltiazem (50%–70%) and verapamil (26%–56%). Such inhibitory effects were more evident when stimulated by EGF (56%–79%) and PDGF (50%–70%), but less by FCS (26%–56%), depending on the degree of stimulation achieved.

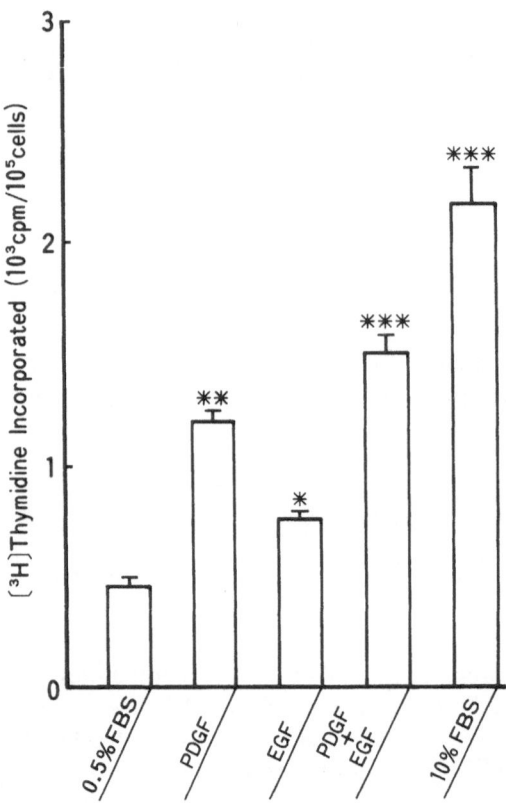

Fig. 1. Effects of PDGF, EGF, and fetal bovine serum (*FBS*) on DNA synthesis by cultured VSMC from rat aorta [18]. VSMC (5×10^5 cells) were pre-incubated for 20 h in 1 ml Dulbecco's modified Eagles' medium (DMEM) containing 0.5% FBS, PDGF (1 U/ml), EGF (1.7 nM), PDGF plus EGF, and 10% FBS. [^{3}H]Thymidine (1 μCi) was added and further incubated for 4 h. Radioactivity of trichloroacetic acid insoluble proteins was measured. Each *column* represents the mean of three samples; *bar* indicates SE. *Asterisks* show statistically significant differences from control: *$P < 0.02$, **$P < 0.005$, ***$P < 0.001$)

To investigate the role of CaM, an intracellular Ca^{2+}-binding protein, on DNA synthesis stimulated by growth factors, the effects of specific CaM inhibitors were studied. TFP and W-7 similarly inhibited DNA synthesis stimulated by EGF, PDGF, or FCS in a dose-dependent fashion (10^{-6}–10^{-4} M), whereas W-5, a less specific CaM inhibitor, was minimally effective at 10^{-4} M. The inhibitory effects of these CaM inhibitors (10^{-4} M) on stimulated-DNA synthesis are compared in Fig. 5. Both TFP (70%–84%) and W-7 (74%–80%) were equipotent in inhibiting stimulation of DNA synthesis, whereas W-5 was minimally (23%–30%) effective.

TPA, a potent tumor promotor, induced a significant stimulation of DNA synthesis by cultured VSMC in a dose-dependent manner (10^{-10}–10^{-8} M), while β-phorbol, an inactive compound, was without effect (Fig. 6).

Discussion

It is generally accepted that the medial hypertrophy of the arterial walls observed in hypertension is basically secondary to mechanical loads, i.e., raised blood pressure [1]. However, evidence has recently accumulated suggesting that such hyper-

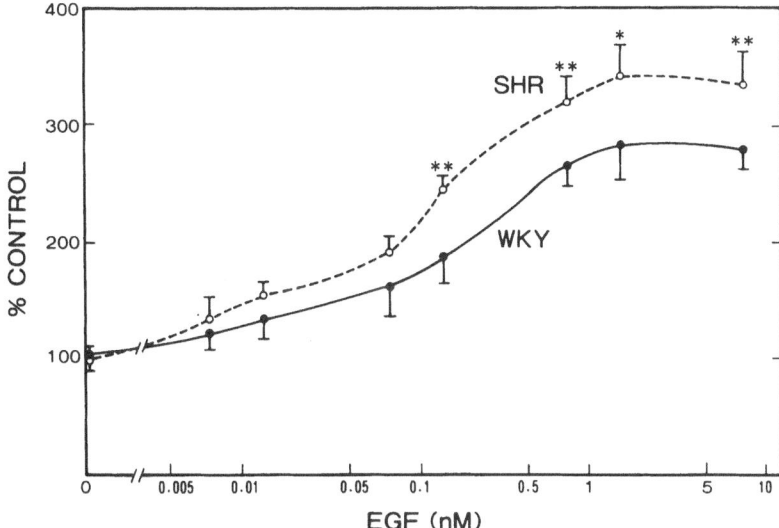

Fig. 2. Effects of EGF on DNA synthesis by cultured VSMC from 9-week-old SHR and age-matched WKY control rats. VSMC (5×10^5 cells) from SHR (o) and WKY rats (●) were incubated in DMEM containing 0.5% FCS with or without EGF in concentrations as indicated. Incorporation of [^{3}H]thymidine into DNA was determined as in Fig. 1. Each *value* is the mean of three samples and expressed as a percentage of control; *bar* indicates SE. *Asterisks* show statistically significant differences between SHR and WKY: * $P < 0.05$, ** $P < 0.02$

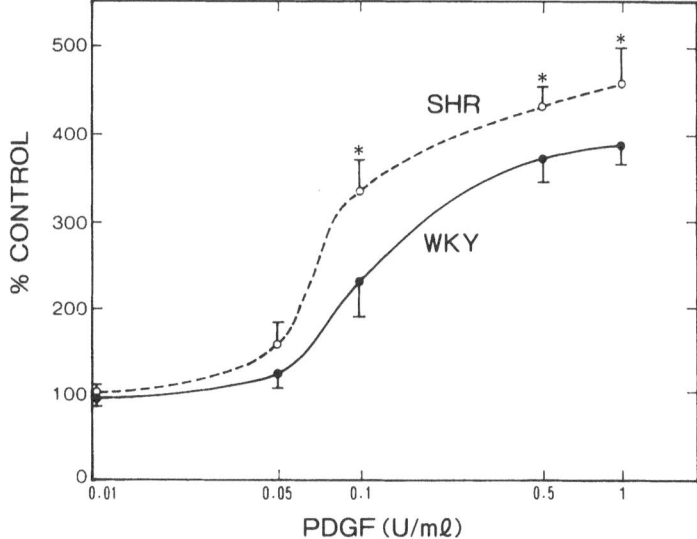

Fig. 3. Effect of PDGF on DNA synthesis by cultured VSMC from 9-week-old SHR and age-matched WKY control rats. VSMC (5×10^5 cells) from SHR (o) and WKY rats (●) were incubated in DMEM containing 0.5% FCS with or without PDGF in concentrations as indicated; [^{3}H]thymidine incorporated into DNA was determined. The results are shown as in Fig. 2. *Asterisks* show statistically significant differences between SHR and WKY: * $P < 0.05$

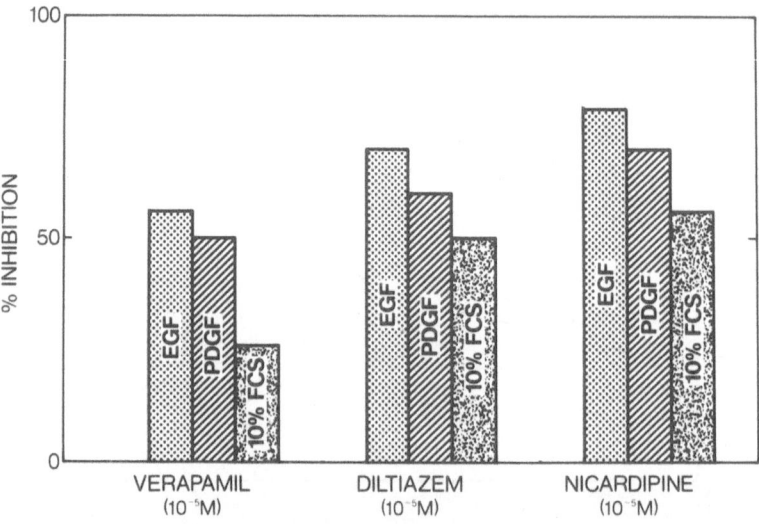

Fig. 4. Effects of Ca^{2+} antagonists on DNA synthesis stimulated by EGF, PDGF, and FCS by cultured VSMC. Quiescent VSMC ($1-5 \times 10^5$ cells) stimulated by EGF ($1.7\ nM$), PDGF, (0.5 U/ml), and 10% FCS in the presence or absence of verapamil, diltiazem, and nicardipine (10^{-5} M) were incubated for 20 h and [^{3}H]thymidine incorporated into DNA for 4 h was determined. Each *value* is the mean of three samples and expressed as percentage inhibition of control

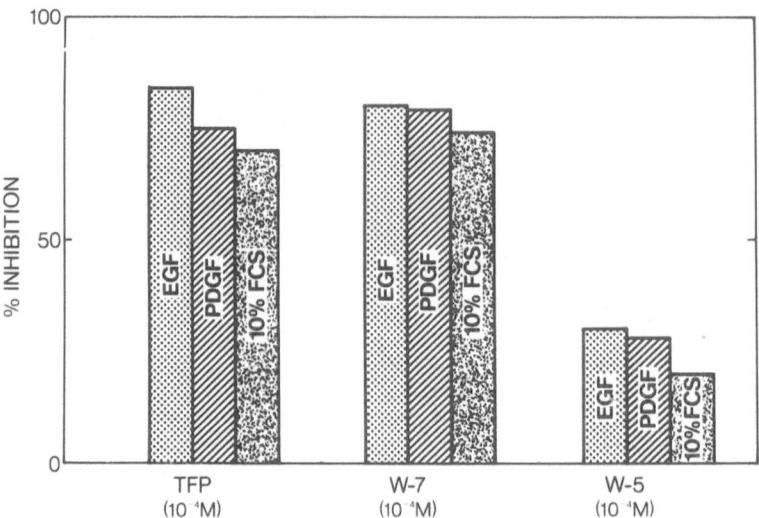

Fig. 5. Effects of calmodulin inhibitors on DNA synthesis stimulated by EGF, PDGF, and FCS by cultured VSMC. Quiescent VSMC ($1-5 \times 10^5$ cells) stimulated by EGF ($1.7\ nM$), PDGF (0.5 U/ml), and 10% FCS in the presence or absence of trifluoperazin (TFP), W-7, and W-5 ($10^{-4}\ M$) were incubated for 20 h and [^{3}H]thymidine incorporated into DNA for 4 h was determined. The results are shown as in Fig. 4

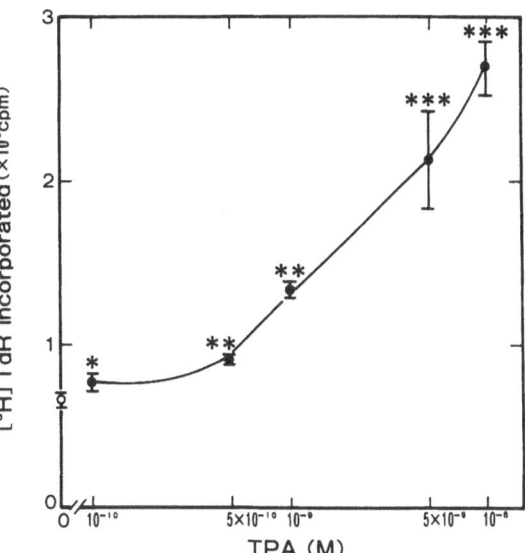

Fig. 6. Effect of tetradecanoyl phorbol acetate (TPA) on DNA synthesis by cultured VSMC. VSMC (5×10^5 cells) were incubated for 20 h in DMEM containing 0.5% FCS with (●) or without (○) TPA in concentrations as indicated, and [³H]thymidine incorporated into DNA for 4 h was determined. Each *point* is the mean of three samples; *bar* indicates SE. *Asterisks* show statistically significant differences from control: $*P < 0.05$, $**P < 0.01$, $***P < 0.001$

tensive vascular changes are influenced not only by mechanical factors but also by neurohumoral and genetic factors [2–4]. Thus, cultured VSMC from rat aortas which are completely isolated from mechanical and neurohumoral influences should provide a suitable in vitro model for studying the mechanism of cellular proliferation of VSMC.

Among a variety of serum-derived growth factors tested, the present study shows that PDGF and EGF are the major growth factors for cultured VSMC. Both PDGF and EGF are well-characterized and potent polypeptide mitogens for mesenchymal cells, including fibroblasts and VSMC in culture [5–8]. In addition to the localization of PDGF in the platelet α-granule [15], EGF has been shown to be associated with human platelets [16]. Therefore, it is suggested that both PDGF and EGF are released from the platelets during blood clotting or at the sites of blood vessel injury, thereby repairing the damaged tissue by replicating fibroblasts and VSMC. However, other serum-derived factors may also play a part in the proliferation of VSMC [11, 12] because the stimulatory effect on DNA synthesis by the simultaneous addition PDGF and EGF in maximal doses did not reach that induced by 10% FCS.

The present study demonstrates that VSMC from SHR have greater incorporation of [³H]thymidine into DNA than VSMC from age-matched WKY rats in response to EGF and PDGF. These results appear to be comparable with those of a previous report in which cultured VSMC from SHR have intrinsically greater growth activity than those from WKY independent of blood pressure [4]. Taken together, these data suggest that VSMC of SHR have intrinsically greater sensitivity to humoral trophic factors, such as serum-derived growth factors, which may partly contribute to the abnormal proliferation of VSMC in SHR. Whether such altered sensitivity of growth factors observed in VSMC of SHR is due to a primary abnormality of cell membranes that is genetically predetermined in SHR awaits further study.

It has long been implicated that intracellular Ca^{2+} functions as a second messenger in the control of cell growth [20, 21]. In this study, Ca^{2+} antagonists significantly inhibited DNA synthesis stimulated by EGF, PDGF, or FCS in cultured VSMC; nicardipine is the most potent in inhibiting DNA synthesis, followed by diltiazem and verapamil. It has recently been shown that growth factors (EGF, PDGF) as well as FCS immediately raise the cytoplasmic free Ca^{2+} concentration—$[Ca^{2+}]i$—in cultured fibroblasts [22, 23]. Since Ca^{2+} antagonists act on voltage-dependent Ca^{2+} channels to inhibit Ca^{2+} influx, these data suggest that an increase of $[Ca^{2+}]i$ stimulated by serum-derived growth factors is essential for stimulation of DNA synthesis in cultured VSMC. This is clinically important because treatment of hypertension with Ca^{2+} antagonists not only reduces high blood pressure but may prevent hypertensive vascular changes in the long run. The same inhibitory effect of β-adrenergic antagonist on β-agonist-induced ornithine decarboxylase activity in cultured VSMC has been reported [3].

It is now apparent that CaM, an intracellular Ca^{2+}-binding protein [24], plays a central role in the regulation of a variety of cellular functions including cell proliferation [19, 25]. The present experiments clearly show that specific CaM inhibitors, TFP and W-7, significantly inhibited DNA synthesis stimulated by EGF, PDGF, or FCS in cultured VSMC. These results complement the inhibitory effects by Ca^{2+} antagonists on stimulated-DNA synthesis and provide evidence that the Ca^{2+}-CaM system is involved in the regulation of DNA synthesis in VSMC.

It has recently been proposed that a Ca^{2+}-activated phospholipid-dependent protein kinase, so-called C-kinase, plays a crucial role in the mechanism of cellular functions and proliferation [26, 27]. PDGF [28, 29] and EGF [30] have been shown to stimulate phosphatidylinositol (PI) turnover, whereby endogenous diacylglycerol (DG), one of the products of signal-induced inositol phospholipid breakdown, is produced, which, in turn, activates C-kinase; inositol 1,4,5-triphosphate (IP_3), another breakdown product from PI turnover, may mobilize intracellular Ca^{2+} ions [26, 27]. In this study, TPA, a potent tumor promotor substituting for DG, stimulated DNA synthesis in cultured VSMC, whereas β-phorbol, an inactive compound, was ineffective. These data are consistent with the involvement of C-kinase in the regulation of cellular proliferation of VSMC [26, 27]. Taken together, it is suggested that Ca^{2+}-CaM as well as the DG-C-kinase system is critical for the initiation of DNA synthesis by VSMC as originally proposed by Nishizuka [26] (Fig. 7). However, the questions of whether C-kinase activation and Ca^{2+} mobilization act synergestically to stimulate DNA synthesis, how activation of Ca^{2+}-dependent C-kinase and the CaM system leads to initiation of DNA synthesis, and what role(s) the tyrosin-specific protein kinases by these growth factors plays in the cell growth, remain unresolved.

Acknowledgments. This study was supported in part by Research Grants from the Ministry of Education, Science and Culture, and the Ministry of Health and Welfare, Japan.

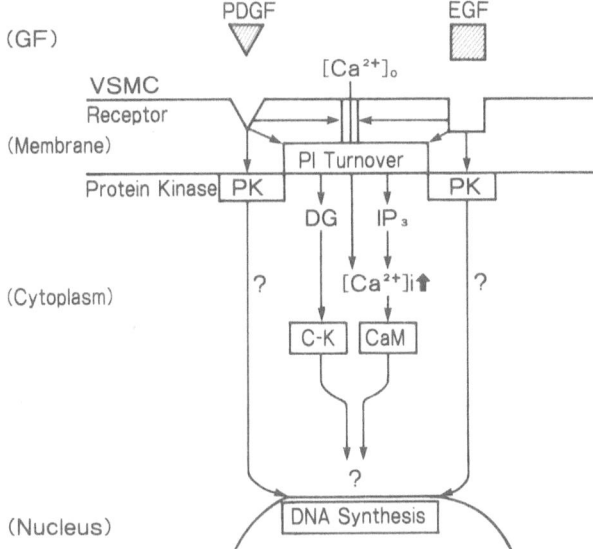

Fig. 7. Possible mechanism of PDGF and EGF actions on DNA synthesis in VSMC. *GF* growth factor, *PDGF* platelet-derived growth factor, *EGF* epidermal growth factor, *VSMC* vascular smooth muscle cell, *PI* phosphatidylinositol, *DG* diacylglycerol, *IP₃* inositol 1,4,5-triphosphate, $[Ca^{2+}]_o$ extracellular Ca^{2+} concentration, $[Ca^{2+}]i$ intracellular Ca^{2+} concentration, *CaM* calmodulin, *C-K* protein kinase C, *PK* tyrosin-specific protein kinase

References

1. Folkow B, Hallbäck M, Lundgren Y, Siversson R, Weiss L (1973) Importance of adaptive changes in vascular design for establishment of primary hypertension: studies in man and spontaneously hypertensive rats. Cir Res 32/33 (Suppl I): I-2–I-6
2. Yamori Y (1976) Interaction of neural and nonneural factors in the pathogenesis of spontaneous hypertension. In: Julius A, Esler M (eds) The nervous system in arterial hypertension. Thomas, Springfield, pp 17–50
3. Kanbe T, Nara Y, Tagami M, Yamori Y (1983) Studies of hypertension-induced vascular hypertrophy in cultured smooth muscle cells from spontaneously hypertensive rats. Hypertension 5:887–892
4. Yamori Y, Igawa T, Tagami M, Kanbe T, Nara Y, Kihara M, Horie R (1984) Humoral trophic influence on cardiovascular structural changes in hypertension. Hypertension 6 (Suppl III): III-27–III-32
5. Ross R, Glomset J, Kariya B, Harkar (1974) A platelet-dependent serum factor that stimulates the proliferation of arterial smooth muscle cells in vitro. Proc Natl Acad Sci USA 71:1207–1210
6. Rutherford RB, Ross R (1976) Platelet factors stimulate fibroblasts and smooth muscle cells quiescent in plasma to proliferate. J Cell Biol 69:196–202
7. Carpenter G, Cohen S (1979) Epidermal growth factor. Ann Rev Biochem 48:193–216
8. Bhargava G, Rifas L, Markman (1979) Presence of epidermal growth factor receptors and influence of epidermal growth factor on proliferation and aging in cultured smooth muscle cells. J Cell Physiol 100:365–374

9. Pfeifle B, Ditschuneit HH, Ditschuneit H (1980) Insulin is a cellular growth regulator of rat arterial smooth muscle cells in vitro. Horm Metab Res 12:381–385
10. Pfeifle B, Ditschuneit H (1980) The effect of insulin and insulin-like growth factors on cell proliferation of human smooth muscle cells. Artery 8:336–341
11. Clemmons DR (1984) Interaction of circulating cell-derived plasma growth factors in stimulating cultured smooth muscle cell replication. J Cell Physiol 121:425–430
12. Gospodarowicz D, Hirabayashi K, Giguere L, Tauber J-P (1981) Factors controlling the proliferative rate, final density, and life span of bovine vascular smooth muscle cells in culture. J Cell Biol 89:568–578
13. Brown G, Mahley R, Assman G (1976) Swine aortic smooth muscle cells in tissue culture: Some effect of purified swine lipoproteins on cell growth and morphology. Cir Res 39:415–424
14. Fisher-Dzoga K, Fraser R, Wissler RW (1976) Stimulation of proliferation in stationary primary cultures of monkey and rabbit aortic smooth muscle cells: I. Effects of lipoprotein fractions of hyperlipemic serum and lymph. Exp Mol Pathol 24:346–359
15. Witte LD, Kaplan KL, Nossel HL, Lages BA, Weiss HJ, Goodman DS (1978) Studies of the release from human platelets of the growth factor for cultured human arterial smooth muscle cells. Cir Res 42:402–409
16. Oka Y, Orth DN (1983) Human plasma epidermal growth factor/β-urogastrone is associated with blood platelets. J Clin Invest 72:249–259
17. Ross R (1971) The smooth muscle cells: II. Growth of smooth muscle cells in culture and formation of elastic fibers. J Cell Biol 50:172–186
18. Tomita M, Hirata Y, Uchihashi M, Fujita T (1986) Characterization of epidermal growth factor receptors in cultured vascular smooth muscle cells of rat aorta. Endocrinol Jpn 33:177–184
19. Hidaka H, Sasaki Y, Tanaka T, Endo T, Ohno S, Fujii Y, Nagata T (1981) N-(6-Aminohexyl)-5-chloro-1-naphthalenesulfonamide, a calmodulin antagonist, inhibits cell proliferation. Proc Natl Acad Sci USA 78:4354–4357
20. MacManus JP, Boynton AL, Whitfield JF (1978) Cyclic AMP and calcium as intracellular regulators in the control of cell proliferation. Adv Cyclic Nucleotide Res 9:485–491
21. Whitfield JF, Boynton AL, MacManus JP, Rixox RH, Siroska H, Tsang B, Walker PR, Swierenga SHH (1980) The roles of calcium and cyclic AMP in cell proliferation. Ann NY Acad Sci 339:216–262
22. Moolenaar WH, Tertoolen LGJ, DeLaat SW (1984) Growth factors immediately raise cytoplasmic free Ca^{2+} in human fibroblasts. J Biol Chem 259:8066–8069
23. Morris JDH, Metcalfe JC, Smith GA, Hesketh TR, Taylor MV (1984) Some mitogens cause rapid increases in free calcium in fibroblasts. FEBS Lett 169:180–188
24. Cheung WY (1980) Calmodulin plays a pivotal role in cellular regulation. Science 207:19–27
25. Chafouleas JG, Bolton WE, Hidaka H, Boyd AEIII, Means AR (1982) Calmodulin and the cell cycle: Involvement in regulation of cell-cycle progression. Cell 28:41–50
26. Nishizuka Y (1984) The role of protein kinase C in cell surface signal transduction and tumour promotion. Nature 308:693–698
27. Berridge MJ (1984) Inositol triphosphate and diacylglycerol as second messengers. Biochem J 220:345–360
28. Habenicht AJR, Glomset JA, King WC, Nist C, Mitchell CD, Ross R (1981) Early changes in phosphatidylinositol and arachidonic acid metabolism in quiescent Swiss 3T3 cells stimulated to divide by platelet-derived growth factor. Proc Natl Acad Sci USA 256:12329–12335
29. Berridge MJ, Heslop JP, Irvine RF, Brown KD (1984) Inositol triphosphate formation and calcium mobilization in Swiss 3T3 cells in response to platelet-derived growth factor. Biochem J 222:195–201
30. Sawyer ST, Cohen S (1981) Enhancement of calcium uptake and phosphatidylinositol turnover by epidermal growth factor in A-431 cells. Biochemistry 20:6280–6286

Calcium and Calcium Antagonists on Vascular Damage in Spontaneously and Dahl Hypertensive Rats

S. Kazda

Institute of Pharmacology, Bayer AG, 5600 Wuppertal 1, Federal Republic of Germany

Summary. Increased cellular availability of calcium ions is the decisive step in increased tone of vascular smooth muscle in hypertension. Long-term inhibition of transmembrane calcium influx by nifedipine prevented the genetically determined hypertension, cardiac hypertrophy, and renal ischaemia in Aoki spontaneously hypertensive rats. In salt-sensitive Dahl rats, nifedipine and its calcium antagonistic dihydropyridine derivatives prevented vascular fibrinoid necrosis and improved the survival rate parallel to their effective control of high blood pressure. Enhancement of calcium influx by the calcium agonistic dihydropyridine BAY k 8644 accelerated the development of salt-induced hypertension and vascular damage in Dahl rats. In some sensitive Dahl rats on a low-salt diet, BAY k 8644 induced renovascular lesions without sustained hypertension. In adult stroke-prone spontaneously hypertensive rats (SHR SP), a high-salt diet resulted in severe lesions with high mortality without any additional increase in blood pressure. Treatment with the calcium antagonistic dihydropyridines nitrendipine or nimodipine markedly increased survival and the reduced vascular lesions without decreasing the high blood pressure in SHR SP. Similar pressure-independent prevention of vascular lesions has been achieved by parathyroidectomy in salt-loaded SHR SP. Obviously, an excessive increase in the cellular calcium content is the cause of vascular lesions in malignant or accelerated hypertension. It is suggested that the deleterious calcium overload may be prevented by calcium antagonistic drugs independently of their effect on systemic high blood pressure.

Key words: Hypertension—Calcium overload—Vascular lesions—Calcium antagonists—Parathyroidectomy

Calcium antagonists have been introduced in the therapeutic armamentarium because of their specific effects on myocardial contractility, myocardial blood supply, and oxygen consumption. During the past two decades, broad clinical experience has demonstrated that calcium antagonists are highly effective in all forms of angina pectoris and other ischemic heart diseases.

As the calcium antagonists also decrease peripheral vascular resistance, their trial in hypertension treatment seemed to be a logical step. Apart from some earlier episodic experimental and clinical studies, the systematic investigation of the antihypertensive effect of these drugs was stimulated by the clinical work of Aoki et al. [1]. In their experimental work, Aoki with his team [2] focused attention on the pathogenetic role of calcium ions in hypertension. The sarcoplasmic reticulum in arterial smooth muscle (and heart) from spontaneously hypertensive rats has limited capacity to bind calcium ions in comparison with that from normotensive rats [2]. This finding stimulated a number of experimental studies. Presently, it seems to be established that an increased availability of cytoplasmic free calcium ions in vascular smooth muscle is the limiting step in increased vascular tone and elevated peripheral resistance in hypertension. Calcium ions seem to be the messenger realizing the translation of a genetically determined stimulus to the contraction of vascular smooth muscle.

In this report, it is suggested that an excessive increase in cellular calcium availability is the crucial step in the progressive hypertension which results in tissue damage and mortality.

Long-Term Effects of Calcium Antagonists in Spontaneously Hypertensive Rats

The antihypertensive effect of calcium antagonists has been confirmed in experiments with long-term treatment of genetically hypertensive rats. Using the Okamoto-Aoki rats with spontaneous hypertension [3], Fleckenstein et al. were able to prevent the hereditary hypertension with chronic treatment with verapamil or nifedipine for 5 months [4]. In these experiments, the concomitantly elevated content of calcium ions in the aortic and mesenteric vessels was blocked by the treatment with these drugs [5].

In our experiments, Aoki spontaneously hypertensive rats (SHR) remained normotensive for nearly the entire life span when treated by the calcium antagonist nifedipine (Fig. 1) [6] or nitrendipine [7] and their survival rate was increased [7]. Whereas the untreated controls developed hypertension with cardiac hypertrophy [6, 7] and subsequent heart failure [8], the weight of the heart ventricle and cardiac performance of the treated rats remained normal even in advanced age [6–8].

With the progression of hypertensive disease, plasma renin activity (PRA) increased in the control SHR, reaching two and a half times higher levels at the age of 17 months (Fig. 2). This continuous elevation of PRA was prevented by the treatment with nifedipine.

Calcium antagonists do not only have a prophylactic effect in hereditary hypertension: Treatment of adult SHR with established hypertension with nifedipine or nitrendipine decreased blood pressure, reduced heart weight, and decreased PRA [7, 9].

The effect of chronic treatment with nifedipine on PRA contrasts with the stimulatory effect on renin release after single administration in rat kidneys [10] as well as in humans [1]. This effect is also in sharp contrast to the effect of nonspecific vasodilators even in chronic administration. Minoxidil reduced high blood pressure in young [11] and old [9] SHR but resulted in elevated PRA even after long-term treatment. The degree of cardiac hypertrophy was also aggravated in the minoxidil-treated SHR despite effective control of blood pressure [9, 12].

In SHR, the renin release is stimulated in the late stage of the disease by the nephrosclerotic renovascular disease [13]. In 16-month-old SHR, a two fold increase in PRA was observed parallel to the increase in plasma volume [13].

It is apparent that chronic treatment with nifedipine—but not with minox-

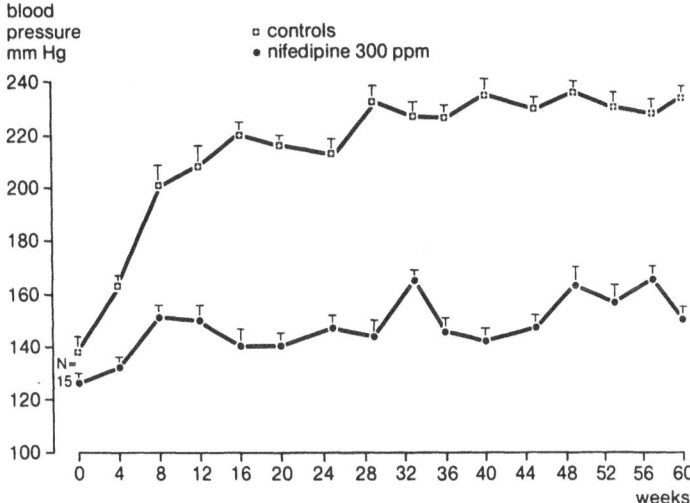

Fig. 1. Development of hypertension in male spontaneously hypertensive rats from the age of 8 weeks (=0). Chronic feeding with nifedipine for 60 weeks prevented hypertension. Values are ± SEM

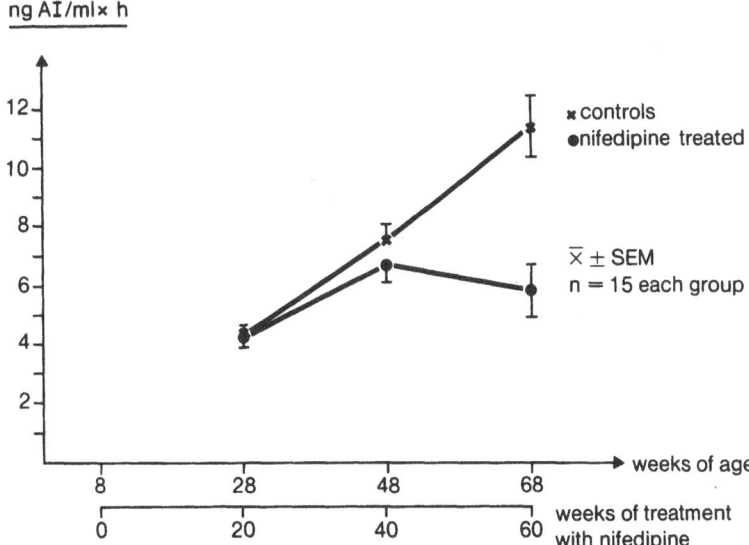

Fig. 2. Increase of plasma renin activity in control SHR. The late increase between weeks 40 and 60 was completely inhibited in the nifedipine-treated SHR

idil—suppressed the secondary increase in PRA by preventing the ischemic renovascular damage in SHR. In this way, the decreased volume load together with decreased arterial afterload contributes to the prevention or regression of hypertensive cardiac hypertrophy [14].

Calcium and Calcium Antagonists in Experimental Malignant Hypertension

For the further evaluation of the presumably renovascular protective effect of calcium antagonists, we used salt-sensitive (S) and salt-resistant (R) Dahl rats. When loaded with a high-salt diet, the S rats developed malignant hypertension within a few weeks, whereas the R strain remained normotensive and survived for a long period of time [15].

In the S rats, the high-salt diet resulted in vascular damage usually described as hypertensive vasculopathy. Especially in the renal vessels, subendothelial fibrin deposition, medial hypertrophy, and periarteritis were observed. Fibrinoid necrosis of the vasa afferentia led to regressive glomerular changes, including collapse and hyalinization (Fig. 3) [16]. Excessive intracellular deposition of calcium ions in the smooth muscle cells of renal arteries of the salt-loaded S rats was observed by electron-microscopic investigations; this deposition was absent in the vessels of the R rats (J. Staubesand, personal communication, 1985).

In vascular smooth muscle, calcium overload is a pathogenic factor leading to necrotization similar to that in heart muscle fibers. The crucial reaction consists of high-energy phosphate exhaustion, which is brought about by excessive activation of calcium-dependent intracellular adenosine triphosphatase and by calcium-induced impairment of mitochondrial functions [5].

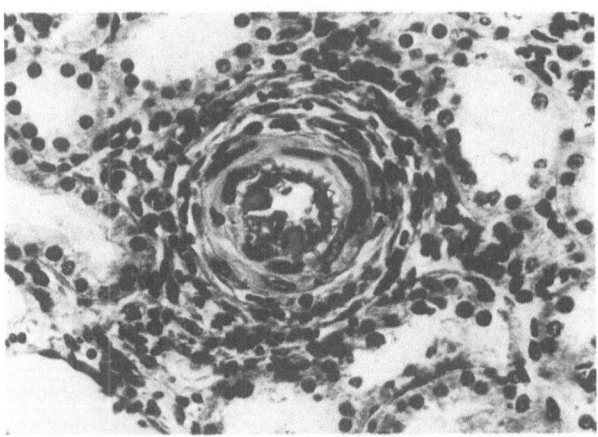

Fig. 3. Interlobular artery of the kidney with considerable subendothelial fibrin deposition causing a luminal stenosis. The media is thickened. The adventitia is markedly infiltrated by round cells (periarteritis). Malignant hypertension; salt-loaded S rat. After Luckhaus et al. [16], with permission of Editio Cantor. H and E, × 400

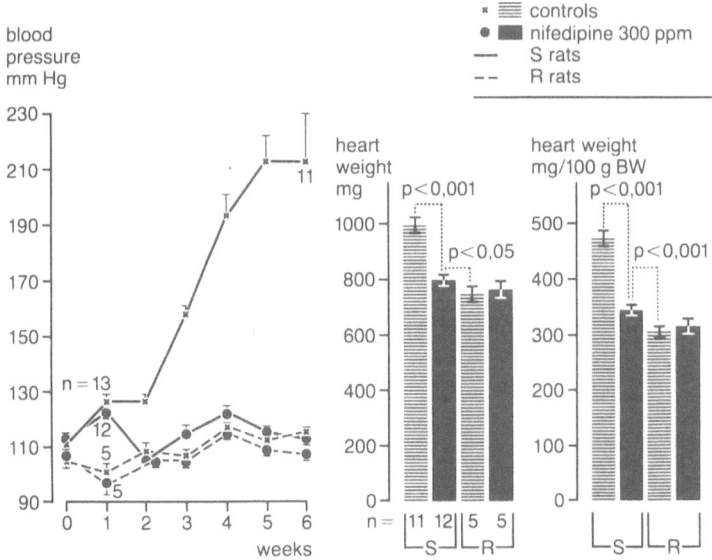

Fig. 4. Prevention of fulminant hypertension, mortality, and cardiac hypertrophy in salt-loaded (8% NaCl diet) S-Dahl rats with nifedipine. No effect of nifedipine in R-Dahl rats. Values shown are $\pm$ SEM

Treatment of S rats on a high-salt diet with nifedipine prevented the increase in blood pressure and reduced cardiac hypertrophy and mortality (Fig. 4). Moreover, no morphological vascular changes were recorded in S rats after the chronic nifedipine treatment [16]. Similar preventive effects were described for nisoldipine [17] and nitrendipine [18] but not for captopril [19].

In electron-microscopic studies, the calcium deposits in renal vascular cells were completely absent in S rats treated by nifedipine (J. Staubesand, personal communication, 1985). Obviously, the sodium challenge in S rats results in hypertensogenic vasoconstriction and tissue damage by an excessive increase in the cellular content of calcium ions.

The specific calcium antagonistic drugs, such as nifedipine and its analogues, prevent the calcium overload of the vascular smooth muscle, which is the ultimate cause of cellular death.

Promotion of Calcium Influx by the Calcium Agonist and Tissue Damage

This hypothesis was supported by our experiments with the calcium agonistic compound BAY k 8644 in Dahl rats. BAY k 8644 is a dihydropyridine derivative structurally close to nifedipine (Fig. 5). However, the pharmacological properties of BAY k 8644 are exactly the reverse of those of nifedipine [20]. In contrast to nifedipine, BAY k 8644 enhances the influx of calcium ions via the stimulated membrane, enhances vascular and myocardial contraction, and increases the

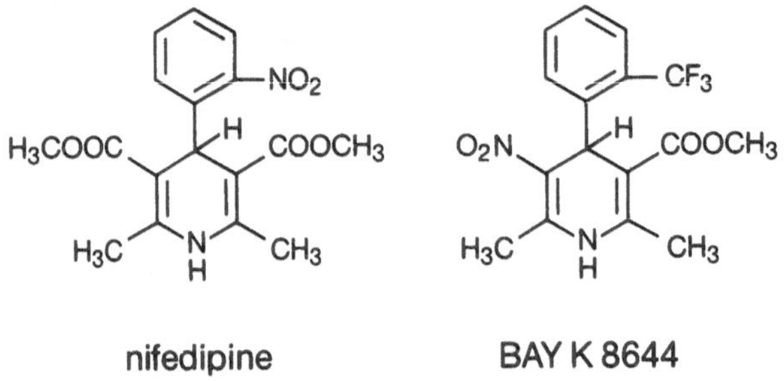

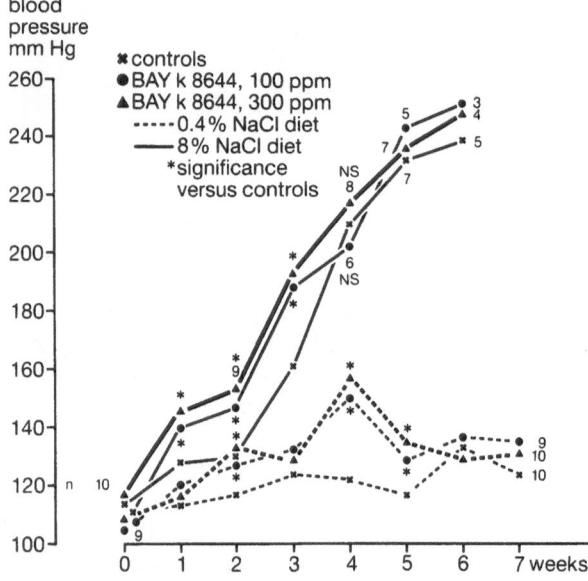

Fig. 5. Structure of nifedipine and BAY k 8644

Fig. 6. Effect of the calcium agonist BAY k 8644 on blood pressure and survival rate (*numbers over the curves*) in S rats of the John Rapp colony on a high- and low-sodium diet

arterial blood pressure, at least in acute experiments [21]. Because of this, BAY k 8644 has been called a calcium agonist [20, 21].

In the sensitive Dahl rats of the John-Rapp colony (S/JR), chronic feeding with BAY k 8644 in addition to the high-salt diet accelerated the development of salt-induced hypertension, especially in the first 3 weeks of administration, precipitated mortality (Fig. 6), and aggravated vascular lesions [22]. Feeding of the resistant Dahl-rats (R/JR) with BAY k 8644 in the diet in addition to 8% NaCl for 7 weeks did not result in any increase of blood pressure or in any morphological changes. However, in S rats on a low-salt diet (0.4% NaCl), which normally remain normotensive for a long period of time, feeding with BAY k 8644 produced a transient increase in blood pressure during the 4th and 5th weeks of the experiment. During the further course of observation, the blood pressure of these agonist-treated S rats returned to normal (Fig. 6). At the end of the experiment, four of these agonist-treated, low-salt rats had a high serum creatinine concentration and a high plasma renin activity. These four animals developed slight renovascular morphological changes, which were never observed in S rats on a low-salt diet [16]. Vasculopathy was normally observed only in severely hypertensive rats on a high-salt diet. In the present experiment, vasculopathy developed in some calcium agonist-treated animals without a sustained increase in blood pressure.

Calcium Overload and High Blood Pressure

These findings suggest that development of vascular lesions in hypertension-prone animals is not merely dependent on the high intravascular pressure. We also obtained a dissociation between blood pressure and tissue damage in experiments with stroke-prone SHR (SHR SP).

In adult male SHR SP with established hypertension, the dietary salt load (8% NaCl) did not produce any additional increase in blood pressure (Fig. 7). It did, however, drastically accelerate the mortality and produced severe cerebro- and renovascular lesions. After 9 weeks on a high-salt diet, 11 of the 16 animals died. All the animals that died and those that had been killed had severe hypertensive arteriopathy, localized mainly in the kidneys, brain, and heart [23].

Simultaneous treatment with nitrendipine produced only a small decrease in

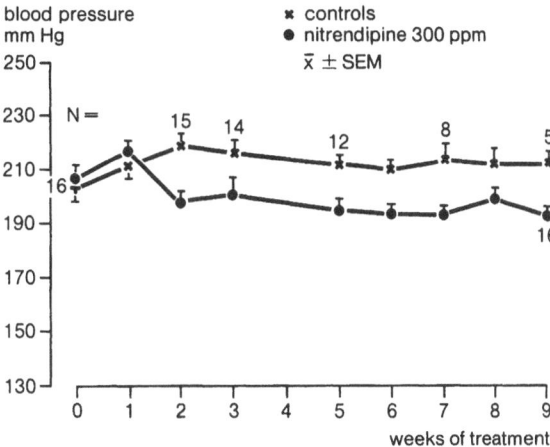

Fig. 7. High-salt diet accelerated the mortality in adult SHR SP (males, 5 month old) without an additional increase in blood pressure. Treatment with nitrendipine slightly decreased blood pressure but completely prevented mortality (*numbers over the curves* represent number of surviving animals)

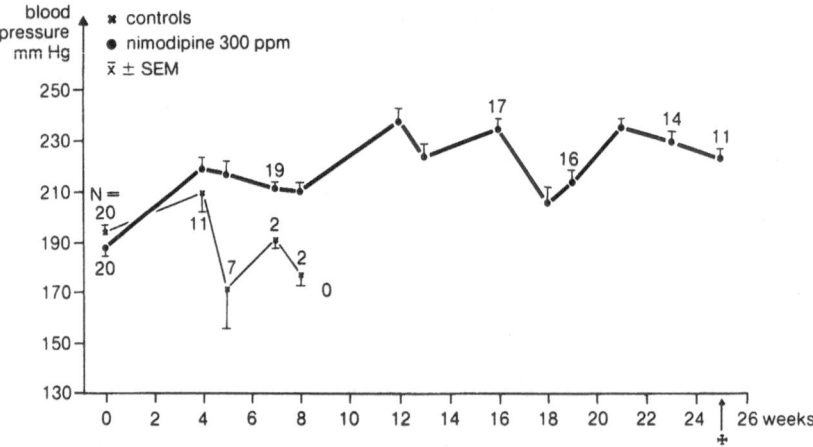

Fig. 8. Chronic treatment with nimodipine increased the survival rate (*numbers over the curves*) in salt-loaded (8% Nacl diet) SHR SP (males) without decreasing the high blood pressure. (With permission of Elsevier Biomedical Press)

the high blood pressure. However, all the nitrendipine-treated animals survived and the incidence and degree of lesions were markedly reduced.

A dramatic increase in the survival rate and a reduction of vascular lesions in SHR SP were achieved with nimodipine. In this experiment, all control rats died within 9 weeks on the high-salt diet, having severe cerebro- and renovascular lesions [23]. More than half of the treated animals survived 25 weeks. Nimodipine is a calcium antagonist dihydropyridine derivative with very weak peripheral vascular effects. In this experiment, the high blood pressure was not decreased by nimodipine (Fig. 8). In contrast, in the very sick controls, the blood pressure dropped *ante finem*; on average, it was lower than that of the nimodipine-treated animals.

Conclusions

Obviously, other factors in addition to the high blood pressure are involved in the vascular damage in the present experimental conditions. The mechanism of the tissue-protective and life-saving effect of calcium antagonists also seems to be complex. There are a number of clinical and experimental observations indicating that the activity of the parathyroid gland is stimulated in some forms of hypertension. Parathormone has been shown to promote calcium influx and to increase the cellular concentration of calcium ions in the brain, kidney, and heart [24–26], resulting in cellular death. The parathormone-induced calcium overload could be enhanced by calcium ionophore and inhibited by some calcium antagonists. In DOCA-salt hypertensive rats, renovascular lesions have been ameliorated by parathyroidectomy but without influencing the high blood pressure [27].

In our preliminary experiments [28], surgical parathyroidectomy largely prevented vascular lesions in the kidneys, brain, and heart in salt-loaded SHR SP without substantially changing the high blood pressure. In this sense, parathyroidectomy mimics the tissue-protective effect of the dihydropyridine calcium antagonists in preventing the malignancy of the hypertensive disease. Therefore, it can be postulated that the detrimental factors in advanced hypertension operate by inducing the deleterious calcium overload of the cell.

References

1. Aoki K, Yoshida T, Kato J, Tazumi K, Sato J, Takikawa K, Hotta T (1976) Antihypertensive action and plasma renin activity by Ca^{2+}-antagonist (nifedipine) in hypertensive patients. Jap Heart J 17:479–482
2. Aoki K, Yamashita K, Suzuki A, Takikawa K, Hotta K (1976) Uptake of calcium ions by sarcoplasmic reticulum from heart and arterial smooth muscles in the spontaneously hypertensive rat (SHR). Clin Exp Pharmacol Physiol 3:27–30
3. Okamoto K, Aoki K (1963) Development of a strain of spontaneously hypertensive rats. Jap Circ J 27:282–293
4. Von Witzleben H, Frey M, Keidel J, Fleckenstein A (1980) Normalization of blood pressure in spontaneously hypertensive rats by long-term oral treatment with verapamil and nifedipine. Pflügers Arch Ges Physiol 384 (Suppl) R9
5. Fleckenstein A, Frey M, von Witzleben H (1983) Vascular calcium overload—a pathogenic factor in arteriosclerosis and its neutralization by calcium antagonists. In: Kaltenbach M, Neufeld HN (eds) New therapy of ischaemic heart disease and hypertension, 5th International Adalat Symposium. Excerpta Medica, Amsterdam Oxford Princeton, pp 36–52
6. Garthoff B, Kazda S, Knorr A, Thomas G (1983) Factors involved in the antihypertensive action of calcium antagonists. Hypertension 5 (Suppl II): 34–38
7. Kazda S, Garthoff B, Luckhaus G (1984) Mode of antihypertensive action of nitrendipine. J Cardiovasc Pharmacol 6:S956–S962
8. Motz W, Ploeger M, Ringsgwandl G, Goedel N, Garthoff B, Kazda S, Strauer BE (1983) Influence of nifedipine on ventricular function and myocardial hypertrophy in spontaneously hypertensive rats. J Cardiovasc Pharmacol 5:55–61
9. Kazda S, Garthoff B, Thomas G (1982) Antihypertensive effect of a calcium antagonistic drug: Regression of hypertensive cardiac hypertrophy by nifedipine. Drug Develop Research 2:313–323
10. Marré M, Misumi J, Raemsch KG, Corvol P, Menard J (1982) Diuretic and natriuretic effects of nifedipine on isolated perfused rats kidneys. J Pharm Exp Therap 223:263–270
11. Tarazi RC, Sen S (1972) Renin and cardiac hypertrophy in SHR. Clinical Research 20:772–776
12. Sen S, Tarazi RC, Bumpus FM (1977) Cardiac hypertrophy and antihypertensive therapy. Cardiovasc Res 11:427–433
13. Bagby SP, McDonald WJ, Mass RD (1979) Serial renin-angiotensin studies in spontaneously hypertensive and Wistar-Kyoto normotensive rats. Hypertension 1:347–354
14. Kazda S, Garthoff B, Luckhaus G (1983) Calcium antagonists in hypertensive disease: experimental evidence for a new therapeutic concept. Postgraduate Med J 59 (Suppl 2) 78–83
15. Dahl LK, Heine M, Tassinari L (1962) Role of genetic factors in susceptibility to experimental hypertension due to chronic salt ingestion. Nature (Lond) 194:480–482
16. Luckhaus G, Garthoff B, Kazda S (1982) Prevention of hypertensive vasculopathy by nifedipine in salt-loaded Dahl rats. Arzneim Forsch/Drug Res 32:1421–1425
17. Garthoff B, Kazda S (1982) Prevention and reversal of salt induced hypertension in DS-Dahl rats by nisoldipine. Federation Proc 41:1664
18. Kazda S, Garthoff B, Knorr A (1983) Nitrendipine and other calcium entry blockers (calcium antagonists) in hypertension. Federation Proc 42:196–200

19. Rapp JR (1982) Dahl salt-susceptible and salt-resistant rats: a review. Hypertension 4: 753–763
20. Schramm M, Thomas G, Towart R, Franckowiak G (1983) Novel dihydropyridines with positive inotropic action through activation of Ca^{2+} channels. Nature 303:535–537
21. Schramm M, Thomas G, Towart R, Franckowiak G (1983) Activation of calcium channels by novel 1,4 dihydropyridines. Arzneim Forsch/Drug Res 33:1268–1272
22. Garthoff B, Kazda S, Luckhaus G (1983) "Calcium agonist" in salt-dependent hypertension, hints at calcium mediated blood pressure increase. J Hypertension 2 (Suppl 3): 503–505
23. Kazda S, Garthoff B, Luckhaus G, Nash G (1983) The calcium antagonist nifedipine and its analogues preserve tissue integrity and increase life span in experimental malignant hypertension. In: Hashimoto K, Kawai C (eds) Asian Pacific Adalat Symposium. Medical Tribune, Tokyo, pp 50–62
24. Borle AB (1968) Effect of purified parathyroid hormone on the calcium metabolism of monkey kidney cells. Endocrinology 83:1361–1322
25. Bogin E, Massry SG, Harary J (1981) Effect of parathyroid hormone on rat heart cells. J Clin Invest 67:1215–1227
26. Arieff AI, Massry SG (1974) Calcium metabolism of brain in acute renal failure. J Clin Invest 53:387–392
27. Nickerson PA, Conran RM (1981) Parathyroidectomy ameliorates vascular lesions induced by deoxycorticosterone in the rat. Am J Pathol 105:185–190
28. Kazda S, Garthoff B, Hirth C, Preis W, Stasch JP (1986) Parathyroidectomy mimics the protective effect of the calcium antagonist nimodipine in salt loaded stroke prone SHR. J Hypertension (in press)

Use of Isolated Membranes of Smooth Muscle to Study Calcium Channels*

C. Y. Kwan, A. K. Grover, and E. E. Daniel

Department of Neurosciences, McMaster University, Hamilton, Ontario, L8N 3Z5 Canada

Summary. Studies of binding to isolated uterine muscle membranes show that dihydropyridine Ca-channel antagonists bind specifically to plasma membranes. Furthermore, other studies show that binding of these antagonists correlates with their functional effects in the same tissue. However, the agents have no effect detected to date on Ca fluxes into or out of isolated vesicles from the same tissue. Thus, it is possible that Ca^{2+} channels are inactivated during or after membrane isolation and that correlations between binding and functional antagonism by these antagonists may be irrelevant. However, other studies using an irreversible ligand of the dihydropyridine type for Ca channels applied to isolated cells found a similar locus of binding to plasma membranes, but binding characteristics were not studied. Thus, the relationship between binding of these antagonists to plasmalemmal sites and their functional effects needs further study.

Key words: Smooth muscles—Ca channels—Ligands for Ca channels—Nitrendipine—Diltiazem—Verapamil

The presence of Ca channels in smooth muscle has been established first by studies showing that many responses of smooth muscle are dependent on extracellular Ca [3, 4, 8, 10] and prevented by agents which we will call Ca-channel antagonists (CCA) [21]. These responses have been shown in some cases to be associated with entry of external Ca as measured using ^{45}Ca cellular uptake [5; reviews in 8, 10] or inward currents [29, 30]. However, the methods for and results of assessing inward currents are controversial [22]. An unresolved question is how many types of Ca channels exist in smooth muscle. The usual opinion is that there are leakage channels, voltage (or potential)-dependent channels (POC), opened by a decrease in transmembrane potential, and separate receptor-operated channels (ROC), opened by occupation of certain receptors by effective agonists [3, 4, 5]. Potential-dependent Ca channels are postulated to explain the occurrence of Ca^{2+} entry and contraction on depolarization of the cell membrane [3, 4, 8, 10]. The distinction between these POC and other Ca channels (leakage channels or ROC) is based upon the following observations: (1) leakage channels are postulated to explain that external Ca uptake proceeds in normal polarized resting

---

* Supported by the Medical Research Council of Canada, the Ontario Heart Foundation, and Miles Laboratories Inc., New Haven, Conn.

muscle and is unaffected by CCA; (2) ROC are postulated because external Ca-dependent responses can be elicited by agonists after complete depolarization of the membrane by high potassium [8, 10], because in some tissues certain agonists elicit Ca-dependent contractions without membrane depolarization [3, 4] and also because in some tissues, some agonists induce Ca entry which is much less sensitive to verapamil, nitrendipine, and related CCA than are voltage-dependent channels [5]. However, there is no consistency in different tissues as to the nature of the channels present or their sensitivity to CCA [4].

Recently, a number of studies in guinea pig ileum [2, 31] and bladder [36] have found good correlation between inhibition of external Ca-entry dependent contractions, induced both by a muscarinic agonist and by high Ca, and binding of dihydropyridine-type CCA. In these muscles there was also good correlation between log IC_{50} values for antagonism of initial phasic component and the later tonic component of contractions to both stimuli by verapamil and diltiazem, as well as by a series of dihydropyridine. However, the tonic component was always more sensitive to CCA than the phasic component, especially in high K^+-induced contractions, suggested by Yousif et al. [36] to be related to the "use dependence" of a single class of Ca channels which are resting or "open" during the phasic contraction and become "inactivated" during the tonic contraction. It seems likely that this "inactivation" does not imply a complete channel closure, since Ca^{2+} entry proceeds during the tonic phase of contraction; however, it does imply greater affinity for Ca^{2+}-channel antagonists. Similarly, the greater sensitivity of tonic contraction responses to high K^+ compared with tonic contractile responses to muscarinic agonists to various Ca^{2+}-channel antagonists (which nevertheless showed good correlation between log IC_{50} values for the two responses) was also attributed to possibly greater depolarization and Ca-channel inactivation by high K^+. The alternate explanation—two different classes of Ca^{2+} channels (for tonic vs phasic contractions or for high K^+ vs muscarinic agonist as stimulus)—is more complex, and inconsistent with the finding that only a single class of binding for CCA has been identified [see 2, 36 for discussion]. To date, comparable detailed studies of correlations between function and binding of Ca channels in vascular smooth muscles have not been reported. As noted in several reviews [21, 23], binding of CCA to vascular muscle membranes suggests the existence of fewer binding sites than in other smooth muscles.

Since other classes of CCA often do not interact competitively with the dihydropyridine ligands for binding, and may even enhance it [see 21, 33], but do inhibit Ca-channel function, it is evident that there may be several interacting sites on, or associated with, the Ca channels which, when occupied, inhibit their function. The nature of these sites or interactions remain to be determined.

The approach of our laboratory has been to study Ca handling, including Ca channels, in highly purified plasma membrane vesicle preparations from a variety of smooth muscles. These include a number of vascular smooth muscles, but we have so far used these membranes for study of Ca^{2+} channels only in a limited way [31; references to isolation and characterization of the membranes are given in 1, 6, 7, 14–17, 19, 23–28, 31].

Our studies of Ca channels have focussed on the locus of these channels, i.e., what cellular membranes are involved [19, 20]. In striated muscles, this locus may not be the plasma membrane [11, 35]. They have also focussed on whether these channels were functioning in isolated membrane vesicles, a problem not yet resolved. Recently, since we have extensively characterized the Ca-handling properties of membranes from rat myometrium [see 9, 10 for review], studies of the correlation between the binding and the function of dihydropyridine and other CCA have been carried out [20].

Methods

Our methods for isolation of plasma membrane fractions and for their utilization in Ca-handling studies are detailed in references in Table 1 and summarized in reviews [9, 10]. In brief, they depend upon careful, histologically characterized dissection of as pure smooth muscle as possible, followed by homogenization using Polytron, optimizing of the yield of plasma membrane, minimizing of the damage to subcellular membranes, preparation of mitochondrial and microsomal fractions by differential centrifugation, and subfractionation of microsomes, first by continuous and later routinely by discontinuous sucrose gradients. All fractions are characterized by marker enzymes, e.g., K^+-activated ouabainsensitive p-nitrophenylphosphatase, 5'-nucleotidase, phosphodiesterase-1, alkaline phosphatase for plasma membrane, NADPH-cytochrome c reductase for endoplasmic reticulum, and various NADH-cytochrome c reductases, succinatedependent cytochrome c reductase, and cytochrome c oxidase for mitochondrial membranes. Our plasma membranes are estimated to be 70%–95% pure, with the chief contaminant from outer mitochondrial membrane broken off during homogenization and fractionation procedures. Some endoplasmic reticulumderived membrane is also present in some preparations [8, 10]. Ligand binding of neurotransmitters—alpha-adrenergic [1], neurotensin [23], and hormones (oxytocin, angiotensin II [6, 18]—correlate closely with the distribution of plasma membrane markers, as does the ATP-dependent Ca^{2+} uptake [8, 10].

Table 1. Nitrendipine-binding parameters for some subcellular fractions

Subcellular fraction	B_{max} (pmol/mg)	K_d (nM)
Rat fundus [25]		
Mitochondrial (MIT II)	0.07	0.097
Microsomal (MIC)	$0.16 \pm 0.02(3)$	$0.146 \pm 0.03(3)$
Plasma membrane (F2)	$0.43 \pm 0.04(3)$	$0.128 \pm 0.01(3)$
Rat myometrium [28]		
Mitochondrial (MIT)	$0.14 \pm 0.03(3)$	$0.138 \pm 0.03(3)$
Microsomal (MIC)	0.42	0.128
Plasma membrane (N1)	$0.72 \pm 0.09(3)$	$0.145 \pm 0.01(3)$

The values are expressed as mean $\pm$ SEM (in n preparations). B_{max} is the density of binding sites per mg membrane protein, and K_d is the dissociation constant for nitrendipine with its binding sites

Results and Discussion

The distribution of high-affinity (Fig. 1, Table 1) [^{3}H]nitrendipine binding was shown to correlate closely (Fig. 2, Table 2) with the distribution of plasma membrane markers in membranes from rat myometrium and rat fundus [20]. Similar detailed studies have not been carried out in vascular smooth muscle membranes, but similar high-affinity binding [32] was observed in microsomal fractions from several vascular smooth muscles (Table 3); B_{max} values (maximum receptor densities expressed in fmol/mg membrane protein), however, were low compared with fundus and myometrium.

Attempts to observe effects of CCA on net efflux of $^{45}Ca^{2+}$ loaded actively (ATP-dependent) or passively into plasma membrane vesicles from rat myometrium, or net uptake into such vesicles, have failed [7] to show changes, except a decrease in ATP-dependent uptake at very high concentrations. A better experimental approach would be to study the effects of CCA on unidirectional efflux of ^{45}Ca from actively or passively loaded plasma membrane vesicles, but this has proved difficult. Part of the problem relates to the complex nature of the efflux curves—whether efflux occurs into Ca^{2+}-containing or Ca^{2+}-free solutions [12]. Presumably, this is due to the efflux of Ca^{2+} from various vesicle compartments (bound to membrane, free-inside vesicles) or to the occurrence of multiple channels by which efflux may occur (Table 4) from vesicles. There may be a leak channel (see above) and Ca^{2+} channels in various states of activation, as well as

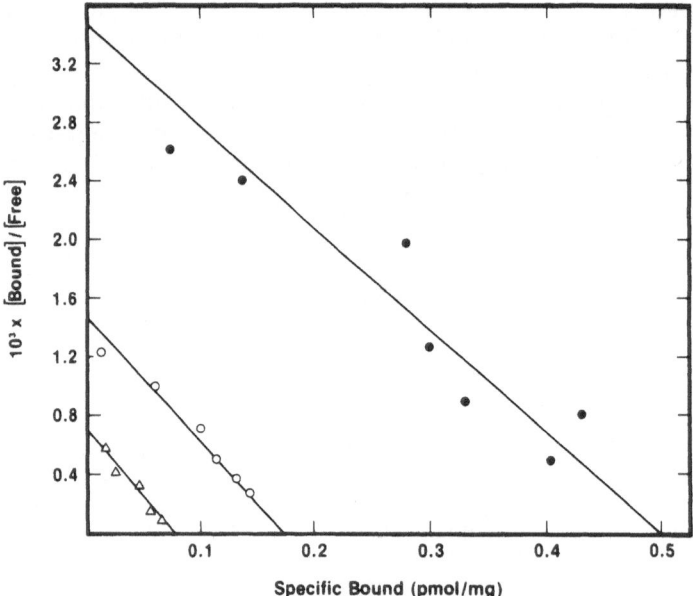

Fig. 1. Scatchard plots for specific [^{3}H]nitrendipine binding to the plasma membrane fraction (●), microsomal fraction (○), and mitochondrial fraction (△) from one rat gastric fundus smooth muscle preparation

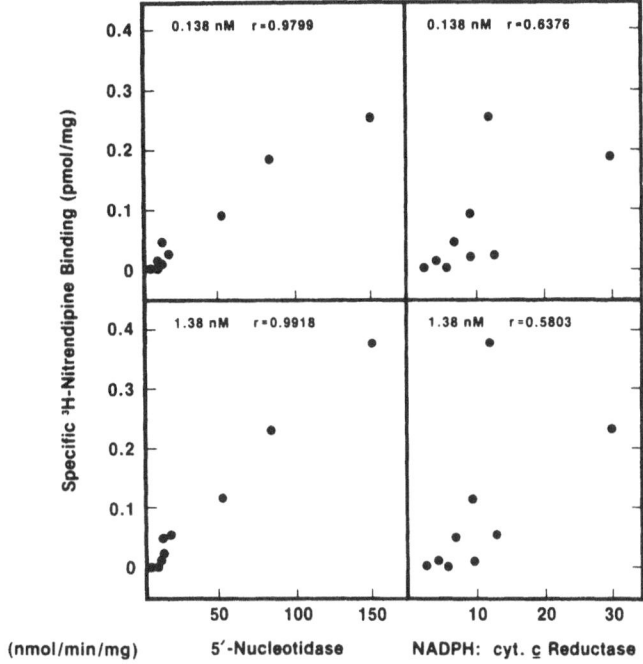

Fig. 2. Correlation between [³H]nitrendipine binding and membrane marker enzyme activities. Binding data were obtained at 0.138 and 1.38 nM [³H]nitrendipine. 5′-nucleotidase and NADPH-cytochrome c reductase activities were expressed in nmol/min/mg. Nine subcellular fractions obtained by differential centrifugation followed by sucrose density gradient centrifugation were prepared from rat gastric fundus smooth muscle. r, linear correlation coefficient

Table 2. Correlation between nitrendipine binding and biochemical markers in subcellular fractions

Nitrendipine	Linear correlation coefficient(r)			
	Rat fundus		Rat myometrium	
	0.138 nM	1.38 nM	0.138 nM	1.38 nM
Biochemical marker				
K⁺-activated ouabain-sensitive				
P-nitrophenylphosphatase	—	—	0.9729	0.9897
5′-nucleotidase	0.9799	0.9918	0.9727	0.9571
Phosphodiesterase I	0.9846	0.9922	—	—
Mg-ATPase	0.9591	0.9777	0.9684	0.9920
Cytochrome c oxidase	0.0643	0.0081	−0.2539	−0.3175
Succinate-dependent cytochrome c reductase	—	—	−0.3503	−0.4099
NADPH-cytochrome c reductase	0.6376	0.5803	−0.2060	−0.1839
Rotenone-insensitive NADH-cytochrome c				
reductase	0.6760	0.5416	—	—

In rat fundus subcellular fractions ($n = 9$), for $P < 0.05$, $r > 0.665$; in rat myometrium ($n = 8$), for $P < 0.05$, $r > 0.700$

Table 3. Binding parameters for nitrendipine at high-affinity sites in vascular muscle membranes

Membrane fraction	K_d (nmol/l)	B_{max} (fmol/mg protein)
Canine mesenteric	0.254	25.0
Canine aorta	0.308	20.3
Rat mesenteric	0.101	18.0

Table 4. Possible modes of Ca efflux from plasma membrane vesicles

Ca leak channels
Ca pump (only outside-out with ATP, Mg^{2+})
Na-Ca exchange (requires Na gradient)
Activated POC or ROC channels (may require vesicle membrane potential)
Inactivated but open POC or ROC channels
Na leak channels
Others

Ca-exchange mechanisms (Na-Ca; Ca pump). Whatever their state, Ca^{2+} channels in vesicles have not yet been demonstrated to be susceptible to CCA, presumably because the channels were inactivated owing to the lack of adequate membrane potential across the vesicle or to the presence of higher than normal $(10^{-7} M)$ Ca^{2+} concentration on both sides (or one side if efflux is into Ca-free solutions) of the vesicle. The ambiguity of the term "inactivated" has to be kept in mind. These membranes clearly had high affinity for Ca^{2+}-channel antagonists, but it is unclear whether they were open or closed, and, if open, susceptible to blockade. Also, occurrence of Na-Ca exchange has been demonstrated to occur in these vesicles [14], and the occurrence of Ca^{2+} loss via Na^+ or other channels cannot be excluded. It is clear that demonstration of the actions of CCA on isolated plasma membrane vesicles will require new protocols, combined with methods of reactivating Ca channels and blocking alternate modes of efflux.

However, if our findings regarding the locus of CCA (nitrendipine)-binding sites to plasma membrane are accepted, the question arises as to whether these are the same sites as involved in the action of CCA in intact cells.

To further establish that CCA acted on plasma membrane sites in intact cells we studied binding of an irreversible antagonist of the dihydropyridine type, diphydropyridine-isothiocyanate (^{3}H-2, 6-dimethyl-3, 5-dicarbomethoxy-4 (2-isothiocyano) phenyl-1, 4-dihydropiridine) (DPSCN) previously studied by Ventner et al. [34]. Microsomal membranes were isolated after strips had been exposed to the ligand in vitro. Some of these membranes were then subjected to digitonin treatment before all were centrifuged on a sucrose gradient. Digitonin forms an insoluble complex with cholesterol and thus associates mainly with membranes such as the cholesterol-containing plasma membrane. This increases the density of such membranes. After digitonin treatment, membranes binding this ligand was found at a higher density, as were membranes containing plasma membrane markers (Fig. 3). This experiment shows clearly that dihydropyridine

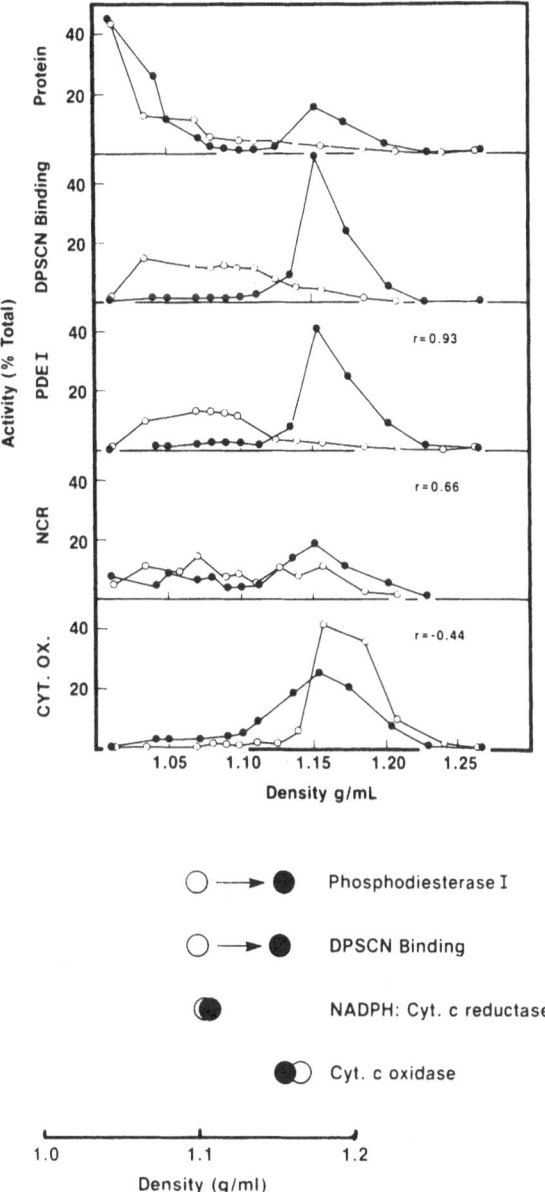

Fig. 3. *Top*: Distribution of activities of digitonin-treated (●) and untreated (○) microsomes on a sucrose density gradient. *PDE I*, phosphodiesterase I; *NCR*, NADPH-cytochrome c reductase; *CYT.OX.*, cytochrome c oxidase; *r*, correlation coefficient. *Bottom*: Summary of weighted mean density shifts of markers upon digitonin treatment. ○, no digitonin; ●, digitonin-treated

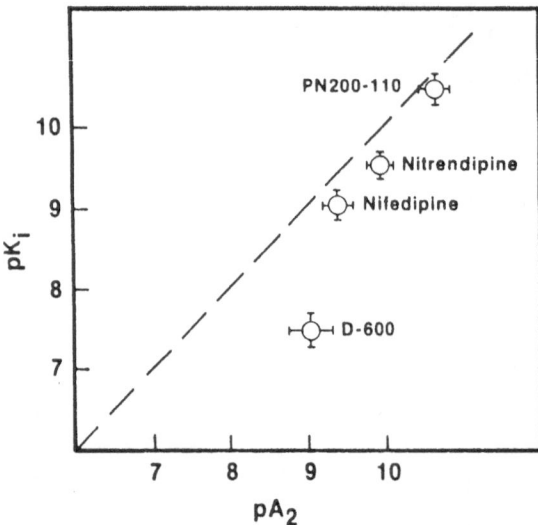

Fig. 4. Correlation between the pK_i for the inhibition of [³H]nitrendipine binding using rat myometrial plasma membranes and the pA_2 for the inhibition of the high K^+ contractions of rat myometrial muscle strips. $r = 0.96$ when the three data points using 1,4-dihydropyridines were analyzed

CCA bind with high affinity to plasma membranes, both in intact cells and after membrane isolation.

A recent study in our laboratory [20] has shown that in rat myometrium, as in guinea pig ileum, longitudinal muscle, and bladder detrusor, there is an excellent correlation (Fig. 4) between Ca-channel antagonism by dihydropyridines (using Ca^{2+} as the agonist in K^+-depolarized membranes) and their competition with ³H-nitrendipine binding. However, as in other smooth muscle tissues (see above), this was not true for D-600, which had a lower dissociation constant (K_i) for competition for binding than predicted from its pA_2 value (negative logarithm of the antagonist concentration required to shift dose-response curves twofold to the right) for Ca-channel antagonism, or for diltiazem, which enhanced binding slightly.

Our findings demonstrate that CCA binding sites in smooth muscle are located mostly, if not exclusively, on plasma membranes in rat myometrium, rat gastric fundus, and guinea pig ileal longitudinal muscle. This appears to be the case whether binding is to intact cells or to isolated membranes. These binding sites may be inactivated Ca channels in isolated membranes; at least, to date, there is no evidence that they are functional or that binding of CCA affects their function. Some evidence exists that Ca^{2+}-channel antagonism can be facilitated by depolarization and that depolarization or accompanying Ca^{2+} entry may lead to inactivation of these channels [4]. If this is so, binding to isolated membranes may provide optimum availability of high-affinity binding sites, i.e., inactivated channels which can bind antagonists but cannot be closed by them. This explanation, if true, would raise questions about the relevance of comparisons between the functional effects of these agents and their membrane binding. However, the studies of the functional effects and binding described above have shown good correlations, at least in the dihydropiridine series. It seems especially important to develop a model, either isolated membrane vesicles or isolated tissues or cells with functional Ca^{2+} channels, in which functional effects can be related directly to binding.

References

1. Agrawal DK, Daniel EE (1985) Two distinct populations of [^{3}H]prazosin and [^{3}H]yohimbine binding sites in the plasma membranes of rat mesenteric artery. J Pharmacol 233:195–203
2. Bolger GT, Gengo P Klockowski R, Luchowski E, Siegel H, Janis RA, Triggle AM, Triggle DN (1983) Characterization of the binding of Ca^{2+}-channel antagonist, [^{3}H]nitrendipene, to guinea pig ileal smooth muscle. J Pharmacol 225:291–309
3. Bolton JB (1979) Mechanisms of action of transmitters and other substances on smooth muscle. Physiol Rev 59:606–718
4. Bolton JB (1985) Calcium exchange in smooth muscle. In: Parratt JR (ed) Control and manipulation of calcium movement. Raven Press, New York, pp 147–168
5. Cauvin C, Loutzenhiser R, Van Breemen C (1983) Mechanism of calcium antagonist-induced vasodilation. Ann Rev Pharmacol Toxicol 23:373–396
6. Crankshaw DJ, Branda LA, Matlib MA, Daniel EE (1978) Localization of the oxytocin receptor in the plasma membrane of rat myometrium. Eur J Biochem 86:481–486
7. Crankshaw DJ, Janis RA, Daniel EE (1977) The effects of Ca^{2+} antagonists on Ca^{2+} accumulation by subcellular fractions of rat myometrium. Can J Physiol Pharmacol 55:1028–1032
8. Daniel EE, Crankshaw D, Kwan CY (1979) Intracellular sources of Ca for activation of smooth muscle. In: Kalsner S (ed) Trends in autonomic pharmacology, vol 1. Urban and Schwarzenberg, Baltimore, pp 443–484
9. Daniel EE, Grover AK, Kwan CY (1982) Isolation and properties of plasma membrane from smooth muscle. Fed Proc 41:2898–2904
10. Daniel EE, Grover AK, Kwan CY (1983) Calcium. In: Stephens NL (ed) Biochemistry of smooth muscle, vol III. CRC Press, Boca Raton, pp 1–88
11. Fosset M, Jarmovich E, Delpont E, Lazdunski M (1983) [^{3}H]nitrendipine receptors in skeletal muscle. Properties and preferential localization in transverse tubules. J Biol Chem 258:6086–6092
12. Grover AK (1984) Analysis of data on efflux of radioactive ions from isolated membrane vesicles. Am J Physiol 247:R445–R448
13. Grover AK, Kwan CY, Crankshaw J, Crankshaw DJ, Garfield RE, Daniel EE (1980) Characteristics of calcium transport and binding by rat myometrium plasma membrane subfractions. Am J Physiol 239:C66–C69.
14. Grover AK, Kwan CY, Daniel EE (1981) Na-Ca exchange in rat myometrium membrane vesicles highly enriched in plasma membranes. Am J Physiol 240:C175–C182
15. Grover AK, Kwan CY, Daniel EE (1982) Ca^{2+}-concentration dependence of Ca uptake by rat myometrium plasma membrane enriched fraction. Am J Physiol 242:C278–C282
16. Grover AK, Kwan CY, Rangachari PK, Daniel EE (1983) Na-Ca exchange in smooth muscle plasma membrane enriched fraction. Am J Physiol 244:C158–C165
17. Grover AK, Kwan CY, Daniel EE, Ahmad S, Ramlal T, Oakes P, Triggle DJ (1985) Subcellular distribution of dihydropyridine isothiocyanate in guinea pig ileal smooth muscle. Arch Int Pharmacodyn Therap 273:74–82
18. Grover AK, Kwan CY, Kostka P, Daniel EE (1985) Binding and degradation of angiotensin II by mesenteric artery subfractions. Eur J Pharmacol 112:137
19. Grover AK, Kwan CY, Luckowski E, Daniel EE, Triggle DJ (1984) Subcellular distribution of [^{3}H]nitrendipine binding in smooth muscle. J Biol Chem 259:2223–2226

20. Grover AK, Oakes PJ (1985) Ca-channel antagonist binding and pharmacology of rat uterine smooth muscle. Life Sciences 37:2187–2192
21. Janis RA, Triggle DJ (1983) New developments in Ca^{2+}-channel antagonists. J Med Chem 26:775–785
22. Kao CY, McCullough JR (1975) Ionic currents in the uterine smooth muscle. J Physiol (Lond) 246:1–36
23. Kitabgi P, Kwan CY, Fox JET, Vincent JP (1984) Characterization of neurotensin binding to rat gastric fundus smooth muscle receptor sties. Peptide 5:917–923
24. Kwan CY, Garfield RE, Daniel EE (1979) An improved method for the isolation of plasma membranes from rat mesenteric arteries. J Mol Cell Cardiol 11:639–659
25. Kwan CY, Sakai Y, Grover AK, Lee RMKW (1982) Isolation and characterization of plasma membrane fraction from gastric fundus smooth muscle of the rat. Mol Physiol 2:107–120
26. Kwan CY, Triggle CR, Grover AK, Lee RMKW, Daniel EE (1983) An analytical approach to the preparation and characterization of subcellular membranes from canine mesenteric arteries. Prep Biochem 13:275–314
27. Kwan CY, Triggle CR, Grover AK, Lee RMKW, Daniel EE (1984) Subcellular fractionation of canine aortic smooth muscle: subcellular distribution of Ca^{2+}-handling properties. J Mol Cell Cardiol 16:747–764
28. Matlib MA, Crankshaw J, Garfield RE, Crankshaw DJ, Kwan CY, Branda LA, Daniel EE (1979) Characterization of membrane fractions and isolation of purified plasma membrane from rat myometrium. J Biol Chem 254:1834–1839
29. Mironneau J (1973) Excitation-contraction coupling in voltage clamped uterine smooth muscle. J Physiol (Lond) 233:127–141
30. Mironneau J (1974) Voltage clamp analysis of the tonic currents in the uterine smooth muscle using the double sucrose gap method. Pfluger Arch 352:197–210
31. Rosenberger LB, Ticku MK, Triggle DK (1979) The effects of Ca^{2+} antagonists on mechanical responses and Ca^{2+} movements in guinea pig ileal longitudinal muscle. Can J Physiol Pharmacol 57:333–347
32. Triggle CR, Agrawal DK, Bolger GT, Daniel EE, Kwan CY, Luchowski EM, Triggle DJ (1982) Calcium-channel antagonist binding to isolated vascular muscle membranes. Can J Physiol Pharmacol 60:1738–1741
33. Triggle DJ, Janis RA (1985) Nitrendipine binding sites and mechanisms of action. In: Seriabine A, Vaniv S, Deck K (eds) Nitrendipine. Urban and Schwarzenberg, Munich, pp 33–52
34. Ventner JC, Fraser CM, Schaber JS, Jung CY, Bolger G, Triggle DJ (1983) Molecular properties of the slow inward Ca channel. J Biol Chem 258:9344–9348
35. Williams LJ, Jones LR (1983) Specific binding of the calcium antagonist [^{3}H]nitrendipine to subcellular fractions isolated from canine myocardium. J Biol Chem 258:5344–5347
36. Yousif FB, Bolger GT, Ruzycky A, Triggle DJ (1984) Ca^{2+}-channel antagonist actions in bladder smooth muscle: comparative pharmacologic and [^{3}H]nitrendipine binding studies. Can J Physiol Pharmacol 63:453–462

Calcium Antagonists
for Essential Hypertension

Therapeutic Role of Calcium Antagonists in Essential Hypertension

A. E. Doyle

Department of Medicine, University of Melbourne, Austin Hospital, Heidelberg, Victoria, 3084, Australia

Summary

This meeting has focussed on a number of issues relevant to the definition of the optimal therapeutic role of calcium antagonists in the treatment of essential hypertension.

A major, and as yet unresolved, question is whether a disturbance of calcium transport mechanisms in vascular smooth muscle represents a fundamental fault in essential hypertension. To demonstrate that this is the case, disturbances of calcium transport and an associated vascular hyper-reactivity must be shown to precede the development of hypertension [1, 2]. The study reported by Mulvany leaves this question unresolved, somewhat since although there was a hint of vascular hypersensitivity to the calcium ion in the young spontaneously hypertensive rats (SHR), his elegant genetic studies rather suggested that this change did not segregate with blood pressure in the F2 SHR-WKY hybrid animals. This finding must cast considerable doubt on the possible pathogenetic role of disturbances in the intravascular calcium ion in hypertension. The alternative is of course that structural change, and in particular hypertrophy of vascular smooth muscle occurring as a consequence of hypertension, might be responsible for the observed hyper-responsiveness to calcium and calcium antagonists in established hypertension both in man and in animals. The presence of such disturbances was clearly demonstrated in many of the papers presented at this meeting.

Even though the pathogenetic role of the calcium ion in essential hypertension is doubtful, there is little doubt that in essential hypertension calcium antagonists, whether dihydropyridine derivates, verapamil or diltiazem, are potent antihypertensive agents [3–5]. It now seems clear that the acute side effects of nifedipine, consisting of reflex tachycardia, headache, facial flushing and ankle oedema, are greatly reduced if a longer acting preparation is used. Nevertheless, the incidence of such side effects may be sufficiently high to limit somewhat the use of these derivates as first-line therapy in mild or moderate hypertension. They remain particularly valuable in combination with beta-blocking drugs [4].

Verapamil and diltiazem are substantially free of the characteristic side effects of the vasodilator dihydropyridines. They seem effective antihypertensive agents, particularly in mild hypertensives, and may be especially useful in patients with concomitant obstructive lung disease and diabetes, in whom beta-blocking drugs may be contraindicated. They are also effective drugs in the relief of angina.

This meeting has underlined the scientific basis of the use of drugs which block calcium transport and has emphasized the potential value of these drugs as therapeutic agents in the treatment of hypertension. There seems no doubt that the development of calcium antagonist drugs represents a major advance in the therapeutics of hypertension.

References

1. Aoki K, Ikeda N, Yamashita K, Tazumi K, Sato I, Hotta K (1974) Cardiovascualr contraction in spontaneously hypertensive rat: Ca^{2+} interaction of myofibrils and subcellular membrane of heart and arterial smooth muscle. Jpn Circ J 38:1115
2. Aoki K, Asano M (1986) Effects of Bay k 8644 and nifedipine on femoral arteries of spontaneously hypertensive rats. Br J Pharmacol 88:221
3. Aoki K, Yoshida T, Kato S, Tazumi K, Sato I, Takikawa K, Hotta K (1976) Hypotensive action and increased plasma renin activity by Ca^{2+} antagonist (nifedipine) in hypertensive patients. Jpn Heart J 17:479
4. Aoki K, Kondo S, Mochizuki A, Yoshida T, Kato S, Kato K, Takikawa K (1978) Antihypertensive effect of cardiovascular effect of cardiovascular Ca^{2+}-antagonist in hypertensive patients in the absence and presence of beta-adrenergic blockade. Am Heart J 96:218
5. Aoki K, Sato K, Kondo S, Yamamoto M (1983) Hypotensive effects of diltiazem to normals and essential hypertensives. Eur J Clin Pharmacol 25:475

Effects of Calcium Antagonists in Essential Hypertension with Special Reference to Renal Function

O. Lederballe Pedersen, L. R. Krusell, C. K. Christensen, L. T. Jespersen, and K. Thomsen

Department of Internal Medicine I, Aarhus Amtssygehus, 8000 Aarhus C, Denmark

Summary. It is difficult to predict the blood pressure response to calcium entry blockers (calcium antagonists) from simple individual factors. The magnitude of the untreated blood pressure and the severity of the disease seem to be major determinants. Regional vascular resistance, age, renin status, and plasma concentrations obtained appear to be factors of limited value in this respect.

In studies on renal function, nifedipine has been found to have significant natriuretic and uricosuric effects without affecting renal hemodynamics. This contrasts with the effect of another vasodilating agent, pinacidil. There is a close relationship between changes in sodium excretion and the changes in uric acid excretion induced by nifedipine. This points to a proximal tubular site of action of nifedipine. Lithium clearance studies confirm this assumption. When higher degrees of vasodilatation in the kidneys are caused by nifedipine, the natriuretic effect may be blunted.

We propose that in addition to the direct vascular effects nifedipine has a specific proximal tubular effect on sodium reabsorption which may play a role in the long-term blood pressure response. Strong vasodilatory effects may counteract or even override the natriuretic effect. Thus, careful titration may be of importance.

Key words: Calcium blocker—Nifedipine—Renal function—Uric acid—Lithium clearance

The idea of using calcium blockers (calcium antagonists) for the treatment of high blood pressure (BP) was conceived by Japanese investigators in the early 1970s [1], but for some reason the introduction of the drugs into routine therapy did not take place until after a considerable delay.

The rationale to using calcium-entry blockade as a more specific vasodilatatory principle in arterial (essential) hypertension is based on research in animal experiments as well as human studies. Four major contributions in this area deserve to be mentioned: *Aoki et al.* (1976) Demonstration of defective Ca^{2+} storage in sarcoplasmic reticulum in the spontaneously hypertensive rat (SHR) [2]. *Lederballe Pedersen et al.* (1978) Evidence of a faster membranal Ca^{2+} turnover in the SHR aorta and enhanced in vitro effects of nifedipine [3]. *Ishii et al.* (1980) Nifedipine causes enhanced vasodilatation in the SHR compared with the normotensive rat [4]. *Hulthén et al.* (1982) Verapamil causes enhanced vasodilatation compared with sodium nitroprusside in the forearm of patients with essential hypertension [5].

Initially, the antihypertensive effect of these drugs was attributed solely to the reduction of vascular resistance [6–9] despite the fact that the natriuretic properties of calcium-entry blockers were reported quite early [10–12].

Individual Factors Influencing the BP Response

As already mentioned, the BP-lowering properties of calcium-entry blockers are not conspicuous in normotensive persons, whereas hypertensives respond with different degrees of BP reduction. A great deal of effort has been devoted to the evaluation of individual factors which may determine the antihypertensive response. Several studies have focused on the following topics: (1) Untreated BP/severity of disease; (2) vascular resistance; (3) dose of the drug/plasma concentration; (4) age of the patient; (5) renin status.

Untreated BP/severity of disease

Guazzi et al. demonstrated the great antihypertensive potency of nifedipine in three cases of hypertensive crisis [7] and Kuwajima et al. confirmed these observations on a greater scale in severe hypertensives [9]. In our own study from 1978, we were able to demonstrate a statistically significant relationship between the magnitude of the untreated BP and the BP reduction obtained after sublingual administration of nifedipine [8]. Similar results were also later reported by other investigators after the administration of verapamil [13]. One might argue that a response pattern of this kind is only what might be expected following a vasodilator, but on the other hand other vasodilators with a different mode of action, e.g., captopril have failed to show this pattern [14].

Vascular resistance

As mentioned above, theoretically, vessel geometry could be expected to cause a greater fall in BP the higher the tone of the vascular smooth muscle cells. However, the smooth muscle of different anatomical regions may show considerable variation in the susceptibility to calcium-entry blockade. In addition, baroreceptor-mediated compensatory reactions and local autoregulatory mechanisms of vital organs may interfere with the effects in the intact organism. Thus, the net outcome may often be different from the effects seen in isolated preparations. Consistent with such considerations, we have not been able to demonstrate a significant relationship between the vascular resistance of two different anatomical regions and the BP reductions obtained. Neither the vascular resistance of the forearm [8] nor the renal vascular resistance seemed to be major determinants of the fall in BP observed (Fig. 1).

Dose of the drug/plasma concentration

Few attempts have been made to construct dose-effect curves in humans but the BP reductions obtained show a definite relationship with dose when normal clinical doses are considered [8]. As far as intra-individual data are concerned, a significant relationship between plasma concentration and decrease in BP has been documented [15]. When *intra*-individual and *inter*-individual data are combined it is evident that the correlation becomes weaker [16, 17]; when only *inter*-individual data are considered, it is no longer possible to demonstrate a significant relationship [8, 18]. The enormous variation among patients in vascular susceptibility to calcium-entry blockade and the differences in

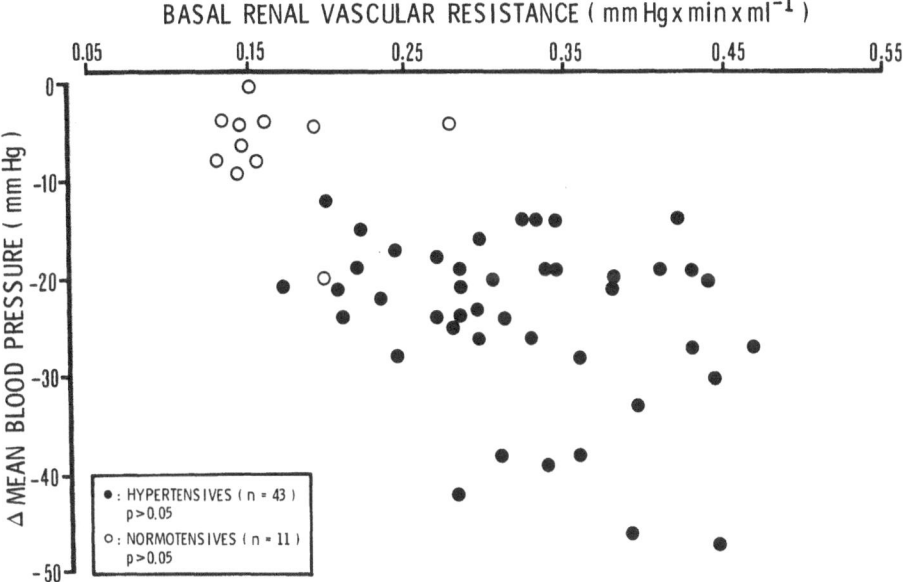

Fig. 1. Relationship between pretreatment renal vascular resistance and the maximal reduction of mean blood pressure following a sublingual dose of 20 mg nifedipine. (Hypertensives in WHO I–III)

baroreceptor-mediated responses caused by age and severity of disease may account for such findings. Thus, it should be borne in mind that the "net" BP reduction only partly reflects the response of the "target organ," which is the vascular bed. This assumption is supported by the fact that despite no significant relationship between plasma concentration and BP decrease a significant relationship between reduction of forearm vascular resistance and plasma concentration may be present [8].

Age of the patient
With increasing age, vascular smooth muscle shows an increasing dependency on extracellular calcium for contractile activation. This has been demonstrated in animal studies in isolated vascular preparations [19]. In addition, baroreceptor sensitivity diminishes with increasing age. Age could, therefore, be expected to be a major determinant of the decrease in BP after calcium blockers. So far, however, only one group of investigators have demonstrated a significant relationship between age and BP fall [13]. The results of our group are shown in Fig. 2. We believe that the lack of correlation is due mainly to the fact that the impact of hypertensive vascular damage is very strong, i.e., hypertensive vessels will show more or less pronounced signs of premature aging [19]. Thus, patient material has to be extremely uniform regarding duration and severity of disease to reveal a correlation between age and BP response.

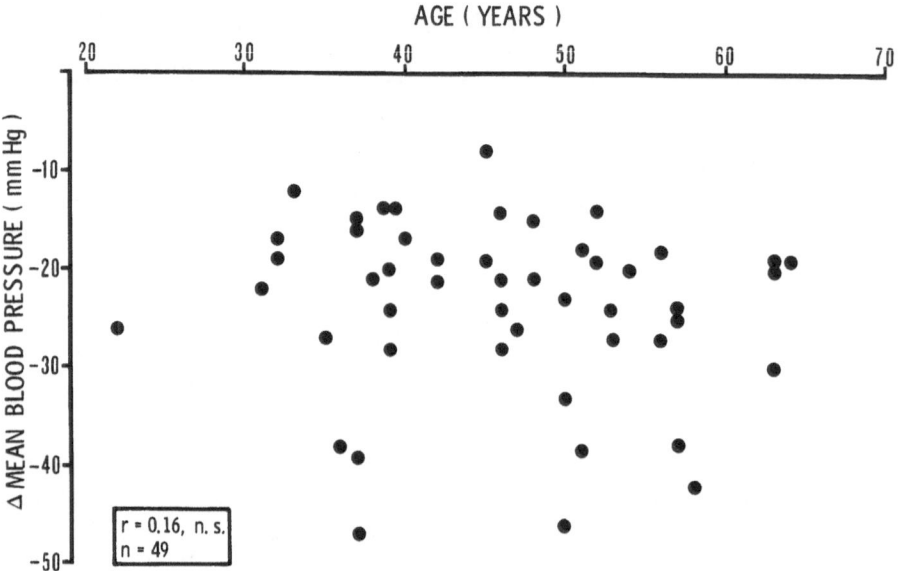

Fig. 2. Relationship between the age of the hypertensive patient (WHO I–III) and the maximal decrease in mean blood pressure following 20 mg nifedipine sublingually.

Renin status

Calcium-entry blockers are effective in reducing the pressor effects of angiotensin II [20]. A relationship between the circulating levels of renin and the BP reductions after calcium blockade could, therefore, be expected. We have seen a significant correlation of this kind only in a small group of 13 patients who received nifedipine acutely; during chronic therapy, the relationship was non-significant [21]. In accordance with these findings, most investigators have reported the renin levels to be of no clinical importance—except for one group who surprisingly found the plasma renin levels to be inversely correlated with BP reduction [13]. They explain their finding by the greater intracellular sodium concentration in low-renin patients and subsequent accumulation of calcium, which enhances arteriolar tone. The blunted reflex response in renin in low-renin patients following the administration of calcium blockers may also help to explain the response pattern [21]. Finally, it should be mentioned that well-performed animal experiments do not point to renin as a determinant factor for the BP reductions obtained by calcium blockade [22].

Effects of Calcium-Entry Blockers on Renal Function

Effects on renal hemodynamics

Population sample studies have shown that there is a decrease in renal blood flow (RBF) with increasing BP, whereas the glomerular filtration rate (GFR) is not altered [23]. This means that renal vascular resistance (RVR) increases when BP

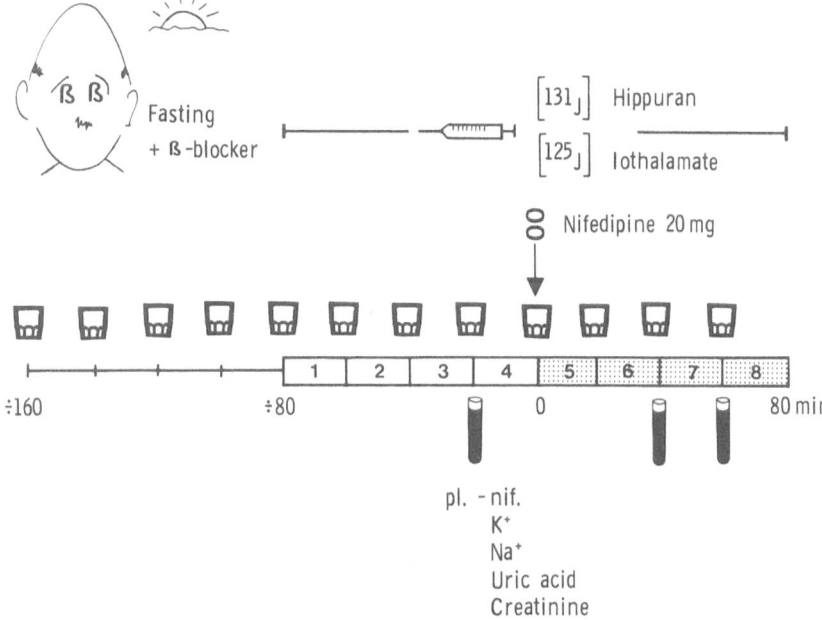

Fig. 3. Schematic presentation of our setup for studies of renal hemodynamics and clearance of electrolytes, creatinine, and uric acid. [For details—27]

rises, but autoregulatory mechanisms keep the GFR at normal levels. Like other vasodilating principles, calcium blockade will affect RVR but the reports on the effects on GFR and RPF have been somewhat contradictory. In experiments in dogs, verapamil, but not nifedipine, was shown to increase RBF, whereas neither drug affected GFR [24]. Klütsch et al. [10] demonstrated a transient increase in RPF and GFR after i.v. nifedipine in essential hypertensives, and similar findings have been reported by Yokoyama and Kaburagi [25]. In our own experiments (methodology given in Fig. 3), we found no significant effect of sublingual nifedipine on GFR and RPF in normotensive subjects and in untreated hypertensive patients [26]. Previous studies in hypertensive patients on beta-receptor blockade showed the same response pattern [27]. Thus, autoregulatory mechanisms may ensure constant GFR and RPF when the drugs are given by the oral route.

Effects on sodium excretion and diuresis
According to the theories of "pressure natriuresis," a fall in BP should invariably cause sodium retention to ensure pressure/volume homeostasis [28]. However, natriuretic properties were early recognized features of calcium-entry blockers and in this respect they differ distinctly from other types of vasodilators (Fig. 4) [29]. Thus, the natriuretic effects seem to be primarily separated from the effects on renal hemodynamics. This assumption gains support from animal studies in

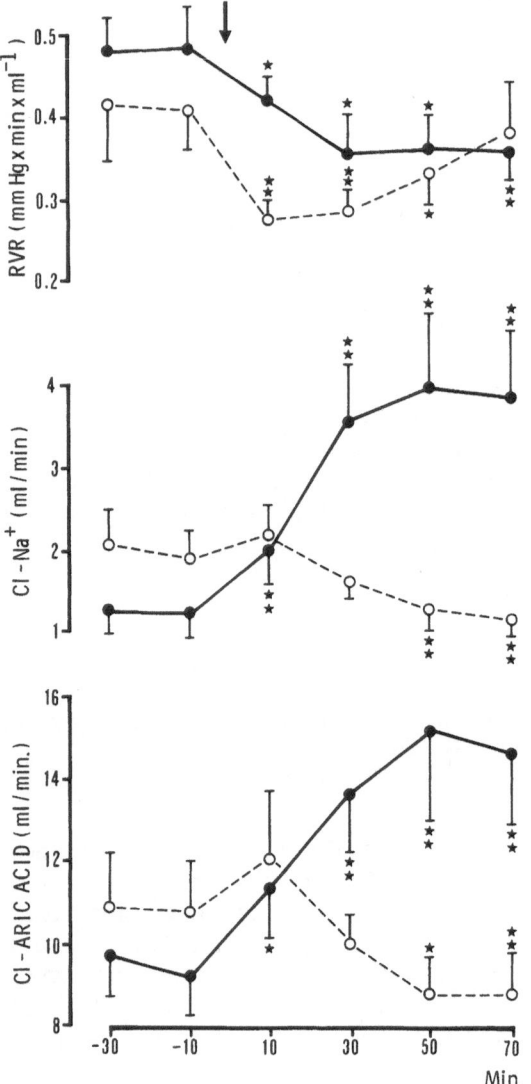

● NIFEDIPINE 20 mg subl.   (n = 10)
○ PINACIDIL   0.1 mg / kg i. v. (n = 10)

Fig. 4. Renal vascular resistance (*RVR*), clearance of sodium (*Cl-Na$^+$*), and clearance of uric acid following the sublingual administration (↓) of 20 mg nifedipine or 0.1 mg/kg i.v. pinacidil in hypertensive patients on chronic beta blockade. [For details—27, 29]

which an effect on reabsorption of sodium and water in the distal tubules was found [30]. Further support was gained from human studies where nonhypotensive doses of felodipine were administered [31]. Interestingly, a negative correlation between the change in diastolic BP and the percentage change in diuresis was demonstrated by Edgar et al. [31]. This means that with higher degrees of vasodilatation there is a definite impact of "pressure natriuresis," which will cause sodium retention. The natriuretic effect is therefore counterbalanced to varying degrees by the vasodilatation per se—and possibly may even be overrid-

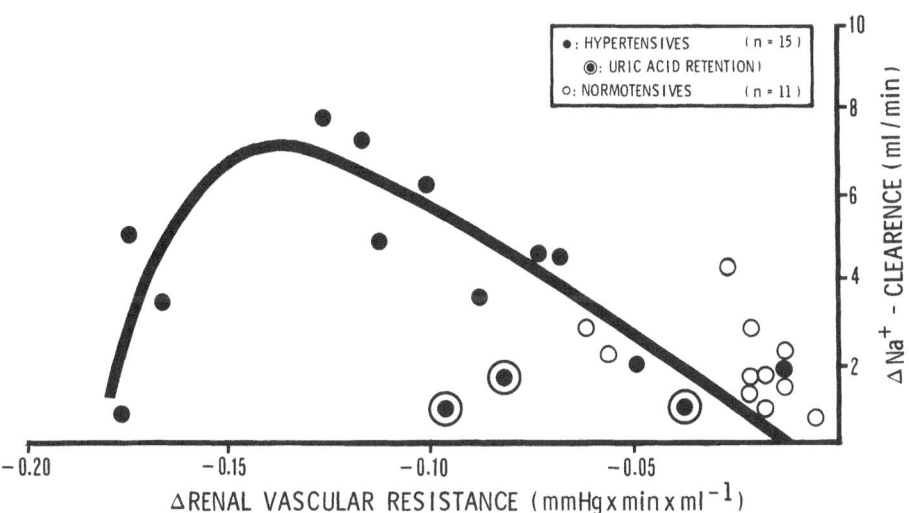

Fig. 5. Relationship between the change in renal vascular resistance and the change in sodium clearance induced by the acute administration of 20 mg nifedipine. [For details—26]

den. Recent experiments in our department (Fig. 5) also suggest that when critical levels of vasodilatation are reached sodium excretion will drop dramatically [26].

The acute natriuretic effects of calcium-entry blockers seem to be withheld during maintained therapy [12] and small but statistically significant body weight reductions have been reported in short-term studies [8, 12]. Whether long-term studies will reveal another pattern has not yet been clarified as volume studies of longer duration are still lacking.

Effects on uric acid excretion

The acute uricosuric effect of nifedipine was first noted in a study in hypertensive patients on chronic betablockade (Figs. 4, 6) [27]. This is a desirable ability for an antihypertensive agent since most drugs, especially those with natriuretic properties, seem to cause retention of uric acid [29, 32]. Uric acid is freely filtered in the glomerulus and undergoes secretion as well as reabsorption in the proximal tubule, whereas no handling by the tubular cells takes place in the distal part of the nephron (Fig. 7). Thus, the uricosuric action of calcium-entry blockers is bound to be a proximal tubular effect. The close correlation between the changes in uric acid excretion and sodium excretion suggest that the natriuretic effect is also a proximal tubular event. This would contrast sharply with the findings in animal studies [30].

The significance of the uricosuric effect during chronic therapy is not known. After 6 weeks of treatment with nifedipine, no change in serum uric acid was found [8].

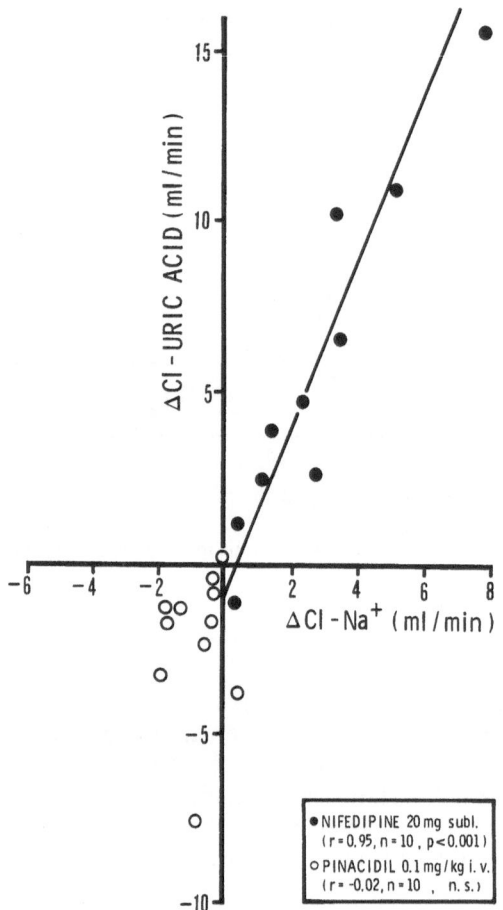

Fig. 6. Relationship between the change in renal sodium and uric acid clearance after 20 mg nifedipine sublingually or 0.1 mg/kg i.v. pinacidil in hypertensive patients receiving a beta blocker. [For details—27, 29]

Effects on lithium clearance

Renal lithium clearance has recently been introduced as a fairly specific tool for the measurement of proximal tubular sodium reabsorption (Fig. 8) [33]. In the experimental setup, 75% of the filtered amount of lithium ions are reabsorbed in the proximal tubule and the rest are delivered in the urine. Few drugs are known to affect the clearance of lithium but clinical reports have emerged in which decreases of serum lithium values in psychiatric patients have been noted following verapamil treatment [34]. Recently, we have applied the lithium clearance methodology in studies of the acute renal effects of nifedipine, and, as can be seen from Fig. 9, there seems to be a close relationship between the changes in sodium clearance and lithium clearance [35]. Thus, these results support the above-mentioned findings of increased uric acid excretion and point to a proximal tubular site of action of nifedipine.

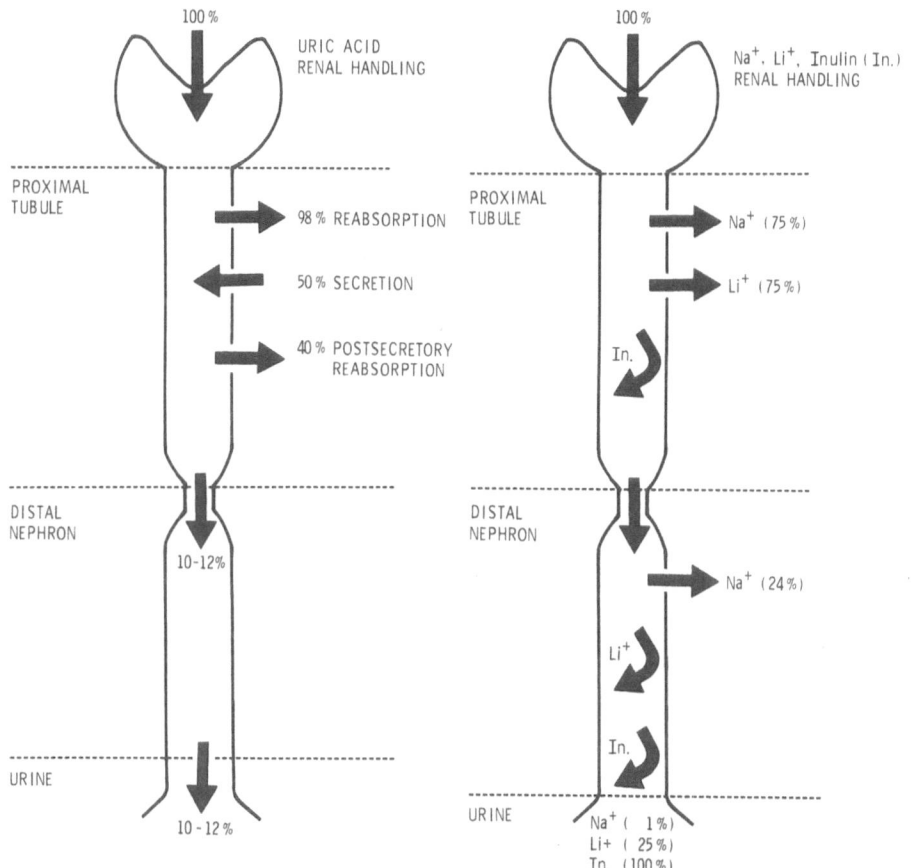

Fig. 7. Schematic presentation of the renal handling of uric acid in humans

Fig. 8. Schematic presentation of the renal handling of sodium, lithium, and inulin

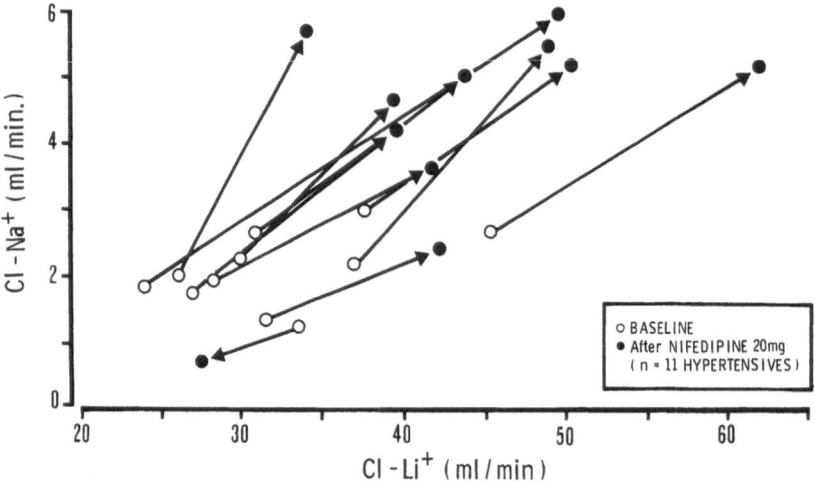

Fig. 9. Relationship between lithium and sodium clearance values before (○) and after (●) the sublingual administration of 20 mg nifedipine in 11 hypertensive patients [For details—35]

References

1. Murakami M, Murakami E, Takekoshi N, Tsuchiya M, Kin T, Onoe T, Takeuchi N, Funatsu T, Hara S, Ishise S, Mifune J, Maeda M (1972) Antihypertensive effect of 4(-2′-nitrophenyl)-2,6-dimethyl-1,4-dihydropyridine-3,5-dicarbonic acid dimethylester (Nifedipine, Bay-a 1040), a new coronary dilator. Jpn Heart J 13:128–135

2. Aoki K, Yamashita K, Suzuki A, Takikawa K, Hotta K (1976) Uptake of calcium ions by sarcoplasmic reticulum from heart and arterial smooth muscle in the spontaneously hypertensive rat (SHR). Clin Exp Pharmacol Physiol Suppl 3:27–30

3. Lederballe Pedersen O, Mikkelsen E, Andersson K-E (1978) Effects of extracellular calcium on potassium and noradrenaline induced contractions in the aorta of spontaneously hypertensive rats—Increased sensitivity to nifedipine. Acta Pharmacol Toxicol 43:137–144

4. Ishii H, Itoh K, Nose T (1980) Different antihypertensive effects of nifedipine in conscious experimental hypertensive and normotensive rats. Eur J Pharmacol 64:21–29

5. Hulthén UL, Bolli P, Amann FW, Kiowski W, Bühler FR (1982) Enhanced vasodilatation in essential hypertension by calcium channel blockade with verapamil. Hypertension 4, suppl. II:II-26–II-31

6. Aoki K, Yoshida T, Kato S, Tazumi K, Sato I, Takikawa K, Hotta K (1976) Hypotensive action and increased plasma renin activity by Ca²⁺ antagonist (nifedipine) in hypertensive patients. Jpn Heart J 17:479–484

7. Guazzi M, Olivari MT, Polese A, Fiorentini C, Magrini F, Moruzzi P (1977) Nifedipine, a new antihypertensive with rapid action. Clin Pharmacol Therap 22:528–532

8. Lederballe Pedersen O, Mikkelsen E (1978) Acute and chronic effects of nifedipine in arterial hypertension. Eur J Clin Pharmacol 14:375–381

9. Kuwajima I, Ueda K, Kamata C, Matsushita S, Kuramoto K, Murakami M, Hada Y (1978) A study of the effects of nifedipine in hypertensive crises and severe hypertension. Jpn Heart J 19:455–467

10. Klütsch K, Schmidt P, Grosswendt J (1972) Der Einfluß von BAY a 1040 auf die Nierenfunktion des Hypertonikers. Arzneim-Forsch 22:377–380

11. Kinoshita M, Kusukawa R, Shimono Y, Motomura M, Tomonaga G, Hoshino T (1978) Effects of diltiazem hydrochloride on renal hemodynamics and urinary electrolyte excretion. Jpn Circ J 42:553–560

12. Leonetti G, Sala C, Bianchini C, Terzoli L, Zanchetti A (1980) Antihypertensive and renal effects of orally administered verapamil. Eur J Clin Pharmacol 18:375–382

13. Erne P, Bolli P, Bertel O, Hulthén UL, Kiowski W, Müller FB, Bühler F (1983) Factors influencing the hypotensive effects of calcium antagonists. Hypertension 5 (Suppl II): II-97–II-102

14. MacGregor G (1982) Contrasting effects of calcium antagonist, captopril and propranolol in normotensive and hypertensive subjects—a functional abnormality of arteriolar smooth muscle in essential hypertension. J Cardiovase Pharmacol 4, Suppl 3:S-538–S362

15. Pasanisi F, Reid JL (1983) Plasma nifedipine levels and fall in blood pressure in a 53 year old woman. Europ J Clin Pharmacol 25:143–144

16. Aoki K, Sato K, Kawaguchi Y, Yamamoto M (1982) Acute and long-term hypotensive effects and plasma concentrations of nifedipine in patients with essential hypertension. Eur J Clin Pharmacol 23:197–201

17. Taburet AM, Singlas E, Colin J-N, Banzet O, Thibonnier M, Corvol P (1983) Pharmacokinetic studies of nifedipine tablet. Correlation with antihypertensive effects. Hypertension 5 (Suppl II): II-29–II-33

18. Lederballe Pedersen O, Christensen CK, Mikkelsen E, Rämsch KD (1980) Relationship between the antihypertensive effect and steady-state plasma concentration of nifedipine given alone or in combination with a beta-adrenoceptor blocking agent. Eur J Clin Pharmacol 18:287–293

19. Lederballe Pedersen O (1979) Role of extracellular calcium in isometric contractions of the SHR aorta. Influence of age and antihypertensive treatment. Arch Int Pharmacodyn Thérap 239:208–220

20. Vierhapper H, Waldhäusl (1982) Reduced pressor effect of angiotensin II and of noradrenaline in normal man following the oral administration of the calcium-antagonist nifedipine. Eur J Clin Med 12:263–267

21. Lederballe Pedersen O, Mikkelsen E, Christensen NJ, Kornerup HJ, Pedersen EB (1979) Effect of nifedipine on plasma renin, aldosterone and catecholamines in arterial hypertension. Eur J Clin Pharmacol 15:235–240

22. Waeber B, Nussberger J, Brunner HR (1985) Does renin determine the blood pressure response to calcium entry blockers? Hypertension 7:223–227

23. Ljungman S, Aurell M, Hartford M, Wikstrand J, Wilhelmsen L, Berglund G (1980) Blood pressure and renal function. Acta Med Scand 208:17–25

24. Dietz JR, Davis JO, Freeman RH, Villarreal D, Echtenkamp SF (1983) Effects of intrarenal infusion of calcium entry blockers in anesthetized dogs. Hypertension 5:482–488

25. Yokoyama S, Kaburagi T (1983) Clinical effects of intravenous nifedipine on renal function. J Cardiovasc Pharmacol 5:67–71

26. Krusell LR, Christensen CK, Lederballe Pedersen O (1985) Acute natriuretic effects of nifedipine in hypertensive patients and normotensive controls—a proximal tubular effect? (to be published)

27. Christensen CK, Lederballe Pedersen O, Mikkelsen E (1982) Renal effects of acute calcium blockade with nifedipine in hypertensive patients receiving beta-adrenoceptor blocking drugs. Clin Pharmacol Therap 32:572–576

28. Omvik P, Tarazi RC, Bravo EL (1980) Regulation of sodium balance in hypertension. Hypertension 2:515–523

29. Krusell LR, Christensen CK, Lederballe Pedersen O (1985) Renal effects of pinacidil in hypertensive patients on chronic beta-blockade. Eur J Clin Pharmacol (in press)

30. DiBona GF (1985) Effects of felodipine on renal function in animals. Drugs 29, Suppl 2:168–175

31. Edgar B, Bengtsson B, Elmfeldt D, Lundborge P, Nyberg G, Raner S, Rönn O (1985) Acute diuretic/natriuretic properties of felodipine in man. Drugs 29 (Suppl 2): 176–184

32. Lederballe Pedersen O, Mikkelsen E (1979) Serum potassium and uric acid changes during treatment with timolol alone and in combination with a diuretic. Clin Pharmacol Therap 26:339–343

33. Thomsen K (1984) Lithium clearence: A new method for determining proximal and distal tubular reabsorption of sodium and water. Nephron 37:217–223

34. Weinrauch LA, Belok S, D'Elia JA (1984) Decreased serum lithium during verapamil therapy. Am Heart J 108:1378–1380
35. Krusell LR, Thomsen K, Christensen CK, Lederballe Pedersen O (to be published) Inhibition of proximal tubular sodium reabsorption by nifedipine

Dihydropyridines As Antihypertensive Agents

C. Rosendorff and C. Goodman

MRC/University Criculation Research Unit and Departments of Physiology and Medicine, University of the Witwatersrand Medical School, Parktown 2193, Johannesburg, South Africa

Summary. Vascular smooth muscle tone is increased by inward transmembrane flux of Ca^{2+} through voltage-dependent and receptor-operated channels, as well as from intracellular stores. Calcium entry blockers selectively and reversibly reduce the influx of Ca^{2+} into the cell through the cell membrane and from bound sites within the cell. The ability of Ca^{2+} channel blockers to relax vascular smooth muscle and, therefore, to decrease peripheral vascular resistance makes them useful antihypertensive drugs. Nifedipine is the best known example of the 1,4-dihydropyridine group of Ca^{2+} channel blockers, which also includes nitrendipine, nisoldipine, and nimodipine. Nifedipine is effective in lowering blood pressure in patients with arterial hypertension and has a rapid onset of action, which makes nifedipine eminently suitable for the emergency treatment of hypertension. In chronic therapy, nifedipine is an effective antihypertensive drug with few contraindications and side effects.

Nisoldipine at 10 mg once a day was compared with nifedipine at 20 mg twice a day in a randomized double-blind double-dummy crossover study of efficacy and safety in 30 patients with mild to moderate essential hypertension (untreated supine phase V diastolic blood pressure of 95–120 mmHg) treated with each drug for 8 weeks. The two agents were equally effective in reducing supine and standing blood pressures. Heart rates increased significantly on nisoldipine but not on nifedipine. The side-effect profile was similar, except that ankle edema was significantly more common with nifedipine.

Nisoldipine is a new dihydropyridine calcium channel blocking drug that is potent, effective, and relatively safe in once-daily monotherapy for mild to moderate essential hypertension.

Key words: Calcium channel blockers—Dihydropyridines—Nifedipine—Nisoldipine—Nitrendipine—Hypertension

Essential hypertension is characterized by an increased peripheral vascular resistance. The elevated arteriolar tone may be due to adaptive structural changes [1], to increased autonomic activity [2], to activation of the renin-angiotensin system [3], to changes in the vascular smooth muscle sodium [4] and calcium content [5], or any combination of these. In recent years, there has been increasing interest in the changes in the transmembrane flux of Ca^{2+}, which may affect vascular smooth muscle contractility, and in the calcium channel blocking agents, of which the dihydropyridines are a major subgroup, as antihypertensive drugs.

Role of Calcium Ions in Vascular Tone

There are two major stimuli to the movement of Ca^{2+} ions from the outside to the inside of vascular smooth muscle cells [6, 7]. One is related to depolarization of the membrane and depends on raised extracellular K^+ concentration ("voltage-dependent channels"). The second mechanism for increasing intracellular Ca^{2+} is an activation of "receptor-operated channels", particularly by norepinephrine [8, 9] and, perhaps quantitatively less important, the norepinephrine-induced release of Ca^{2+} from intracellular stores. A third mechanism [10] for increasing vascular smooth muscle tone relates to another linked transport mechanism, namely the transport of Na^+ (inward) and Ca^{2+} (outward). Any reduction in the Na^+ gradient (due to a rise in the internal Na^+ concentration following decreased activity of the Na^+-K^+ pump) would hinder the outward transport of Ca^{2+} through this carrier mechanism, thus increasing the intracellular Ca^{2+} concentration.

Any or all of these three mechanisms may operate to increase intracellular Ca^{2+} and cause an increase in vascular tone, in peripheral resistance, and hence in arterial pressure. Inhibition of Na^+,K^+-ATPase lowers the efficiency of the Na^+-K^+ pump, allows the extracellular accumulation of K^+, with an increase in membrane excitability, and an activation of voltage-dependent Ca^{2+} channels. Sympathetic overactivity will activate smooth muscle, at least partly through receptor-operated Ca^{2+} channels. Lastly, Na^+-K^+ pump failure will allow the intracellular accumulation of Na^+, a slowing of Na^+-Ca^{2+} countertransport, and a rise in intracellular Ca^{2+}. The mechanisms by which intracellular Ca^{2+} activates smooth muscle contraction are still controversial [11]. One postulated sequence of events is that Ca^{2+} in the cell binds with a 16 500-dalton Ca^{2+}-binding protein (calmodulin) and the Ca^{2+}-calmodulin complex activates myosin light-chain kinase. This activated enzyme phosphorylates myosin, which results in contraction. Relaxation depends on the inactivation of myosin light-chain kinase. This may be produced by protein kinase, which is activated by cyclic AMP. An important trigger to cyclic AMP formation is the β_2-adrenoreceptor in the vascular smooth muscle cell membrane.

There are some experimental findings which are not in accord with this theory. For example, de Mendonca et al. [12] have found a decrease in another Na^+-K^+ transport system in red blood cells from hypertensive patients. This is not the Na^+-K^+ pump, because this system cannot be inhibited by ouabain, which is specific to Na^+-K^+-ATPase. Also, there is no direct evidence that the vascular smooth muscle membrane of hypertensive patients shares the electrolyte abnormality which has been demonstrated in their red blood cells, nor that such smooth muscle contains a higher concentration of free intracellular Ca^{2+} than that of normotensive subjects. However, rats with experimental hypertension have increased arteriolar smooth muscle Ca^{2+} transport [13], and drugs which specifically reduce the influx of Ca^{2+} into the cell through the cell membrane and form bound sites within the cell have a vasodilator antihypertensive action. It might also be predicted that the degree of blood pressure reduction brought about by Ca^{2+} antagonists is directly related to the magnitude of the pretreatment blood pressure, and, generally, this has been found to be the case.

What has not been established with certainty in vascular smooth muscle is the relative contribution of Ca^{2+}-channels, which are opened by a rise in the extracellular K^+ and, by implication, by action potentials (voltage-dependent channels), and those which are switched on by norepinephrine, acetylcholine, 5-

hydroxytryptamine, histamine, ergotamine, and angiotensin II (neurotransmitter or receptor-operated channels). Also, what is not clear is the interrelationship between the two types of channel or the role of the release of Ca^{2+} from intracellular organelles such as the sarcoplasmic reticulum and mitochondria.

Lastly, there is controversy over the intracellular action of Ca^{2+} in initiating interactions between the contractile proteins of vascular smooth muscle. The Ca^{2+}-calmodulin, myosin light-chain kinase, myosin-phosphate sequence [14, 15], calcium-leiotonin regulation of contraction [16], and the concept of myosin phosphorylation being necessary for cross-bridge cycling but not for actin-myosin "latch" cross-bridging [17] are all different models of Ca^{2+} interactions with smooth muscle contractile proteins. Regardless of which of these Ca^{2+}-activated mechanisms proves important in vascular smooth muscle, it is agreed that an increase in cytostolic Ca^{2+} concentration represents the signal that initiates the contractile process in vascular smooth muscle.

Dihydropyridine Calcium Channel Blockers in Hypertension

The ability of Ca^{2+} channel blockers to relax vascular smooth muscle and, therefore, to decrease peripheral vascular resistance makes them useful antihypertensive drugs [5]. However, the number of good clinical trials of these agents in the treatment of arterial hypertension is quite small. Most studies have been performed on nifedipine and verapamil, with a few on diltiazem and tiapamil.

Nifedipine is the best known example of the 1,4-dihydropyridine group of Ca^{2+} channel blockers (Fig. 1). Nifedipine is an effective antihypertensive drug at total daily doses of 15–60 mg. The acute effect, which comes on within 15–20 min, is dose-related and the higher the blood pressure or the total peripheral resistance before treatment, the greater the fall in blood pressure [18]. Normotensive patients do not show a drop in blood pressure in response to nifedipine. Treatment of hypertension with 10–20 mg orally or sublingually lowers blood pressure within 15–20 min [18, 19]. This rapid onset of action makes nifedipine a drug which is eminently suitable for the emergency treatment of hypertension [18–20]. The extent of the blood pressure fall in these patients was 21%–35% [18, 21] and was seen 30 min after the oral administration of the 10-mg capsule. This acute reduction in blood pressure was often [22–24] but not always [18, 25] accompanied by an increase in heart rate, probably mediated by a baroreceptor reflex stimulation.

Nifedipine increases urinary volume and urinary Na^+ secretion [26], in contrast to many other types of vasodilator drugs [27]. Plasma renin activity and plasma norepinephrine concentration usually increase in response to 10 mg or more of nifedipine [22, 25, 28]. However, plasma aldosterone does not change [24, 29]. In one study, nifedipine was shown to be an inhibitor of the angiotensin II-mediated release of aldosterone [30].

As chronic therapy, nifedipine is an effective drug [31–36] at total daily doses of 15–60 mg. In most studies, the heart rate tended to remain unchanged or decreased, which may be explained on the basis of resetting of the baroreflex mechanism. Nifedipine did not produce postural hypotension and tolerance

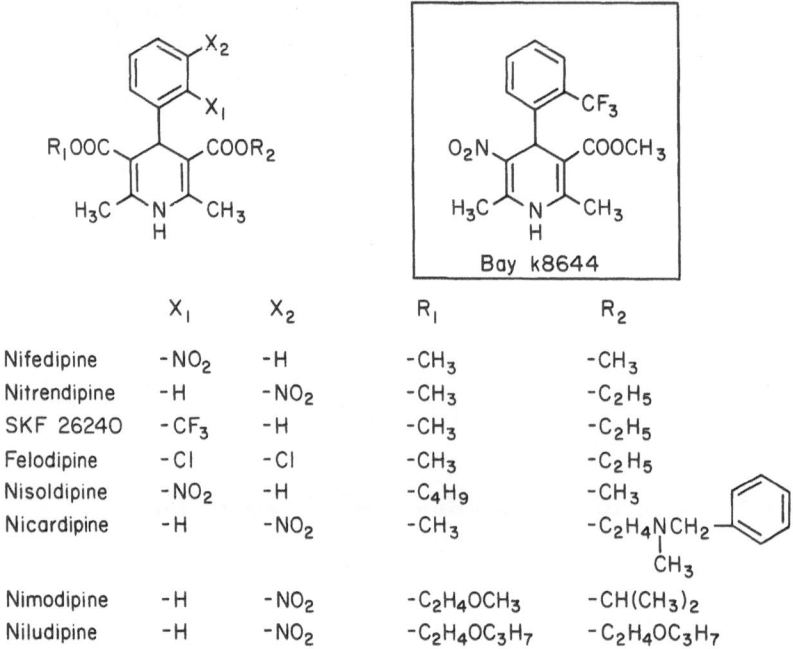

	X_1	X_2	R_1	R_2
Nifedipine	$-NO_2$	$-H$	$-CH_3$	$-CH_3$
Nitrendipine	$-H$	$-NO_2$	$-CH_3$	$-C_2H_5$
SKF 26240	$-CF_3$	$-H$	$-CH_3$	$-C_2H_5$
Felodipine	$-Cl$	$-Cl$	$-CH_3$	$-C_2H_5$
Nisoldipine	$-NO_2$	$-H$	$-C_4H_9$	$-CH_3$
Nicardipine	$-H$	$-NO_2$	$-CH_3$	$-C_2H_4NCH_2-\bigcirc$ / CH_3
Nimodipine	$-H$	$-NO_2$	$-C_2H_4OCH_3$	$-CH(CH_3)_2$
Niludipine	$-H$	$-NO_2$	$-C_2H_4OC_3H_7$	$-C_2H_4OC_3H_7$

Fig. 1. The molecular structure of some dihydropyridine calcium channel blockers and BAY K8644 (*in box*), a calcium agonist

did not develop [33, 34]. There was no change in body weight, suggesting the absence of Na^+ and fluid retention [19, 35, 38]. Plasma volume was measured in one study on 18 patients treated with nifedipine and found to be unchanged after a year [19]. Also, in contrast to other vasodilators, long-term treatment with nifedipine did not result in any consistent increase in plasma renin activity [25, 29]. However, plasma renin was increased by nifedipine in one study [37] in which nifedipine was found to be as effective an antihypertensive drug as prazosin in a double-blind crossover trial. Recently Bühler and his colleagues [38] have suggested that calcium channel blockers are particularly indicated in older patients and in those with low renin hypertension, in whom betablockers and angiotensin converting enzyme inhibitors would probably be less effective.

Antihypertensive Efficacy of Nisoldipine

Clinical experience of calcium channel blockers in hypertension was, until recently, confined to nifedipine and the phenylalkylamine, verapamil. We investigated [39] the antihypertensive efficacy and safety of nisoldipine in a double-blind double-dummy crossover study versus nifedipine. Nisoldipine is four to ten times more potent than nifedipine as an antagonist of vascular contractions in vitro, and is, therefore, probably the most potent vasodilator and

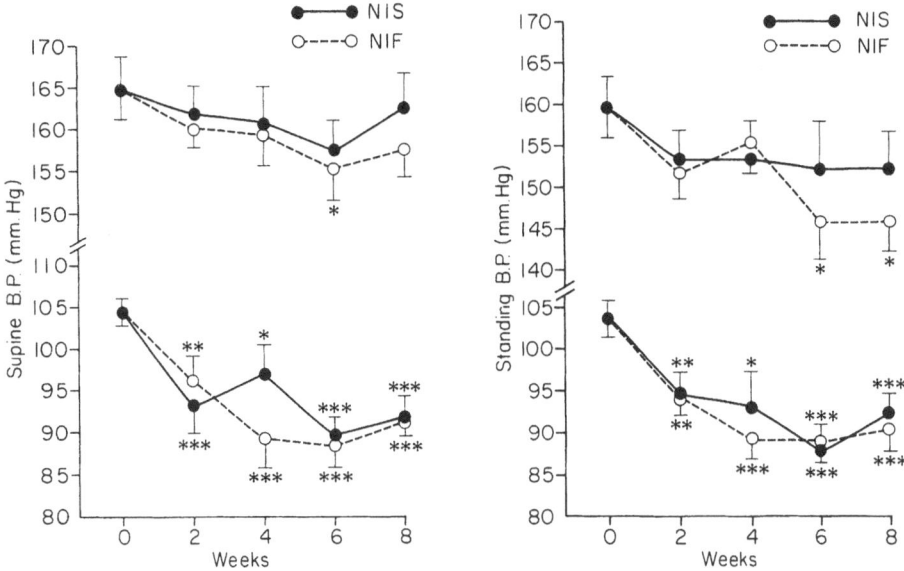

Fig. 2. Nisoldipine vs. nifedipine. Mean supine (*left*) and standing (*right*) systolic and diastolic blood pressure ($\pm$ SEM) with time. *$P < 0.05$, **$P < 0.005$, ***$P < 0.0005$. *NIS* nisoldipine, *NIF* nifedipine. Reproduced by permission from Rosendorff and Goodman [39]

Ca^{2+} antagonist known. However, as a negative inotropic agent nisoldipine is only equipotent to or even less potent than nifedipine. Since the underlying hemodynamic alteration in most forms of established hypertension is an increase in total peripheral resistance [40], an increase in the vasodilator potency without any increase in negative inotropy could be of great therapeutic advantage.

Thirty patients with mild to moderate essential hypertension, defined as un-treated supine diastolic blood pressure (Phase V) of 95–120 mmHg, were treated with each drug as monotherapy for 8 weeks, with a 2-week washout between treatment periods. Doses were 20 mg nifedipine retard b.i.d. and 10 mg nisoldi-pine in the morning. Results are shown in Fig. 2. There were no statistically significant differences in the blood pressure responses of the two groups based on the order of administration of the drugs, so the two groups were pooled to simplify the comparison of the effects of the two drugs.

The mean supine blood pressure at the end of the baseline period was 165.0 ± 3.5 mmHg (systolic) and 104.5 ± 1.8 mmHg (diastolic). On nisoldipine, the systolic pressure fell over 6 weeks to a low of 157.5 ± 3.5 mmHg, but rose again, slightly, to 162.7 ± 4.0 at week 8. None of the values were significantly different from the baseline pressure. Nifedipine caused a significant decrease in supine systolic pressure only at week 6 (155.3 ± 3.6 mmHg), also with a small rebound at week 8. Both nisoldipine and nifedipine caused a significant decrease in supine diastolic pressure throughout the active treatment periods to the lowest values of 89.6 ± 2.3 mmHg and 88.2 ± 2.2 mmHg, respectively, both at week 6.

Standing systolic, but not diastolic, pressures were significantly lower than supine pressures. The mean standing blood pressure at the end of the baseline period was 159.6 ± 3.7 mmHg (systolic) and 103.6 ± 2.1 mmHg (diastolic). On nisoldipine, the systolic pressure fell to 152.0 ± 5.6 mmHg and 151.6 ± 4.7 mmHg at 6 and 8 weeks, respectively; neither was significantly lower than baseline values. Corresponding values for nifedipine were 145.7 ± 4.2 mmHg and 145.9 ± 3.5 mmHg, both of which were significantly ($P < 0.05$) lower than baseline values. As with the supine pressures, the changes in the standing diastolic pressures were more impressive than the systolic pressures; lowest mean values, both at 6 weeks, were 87.5 ± 3.1 mmHg (nisoldipine) and 88.8 ± 2.4 mmHg (nifedipine). All mean standing diastolic pressures, from weeks 2 to 8 inclusive, were significantly lower than baseline values.

There were no significant differences in mean blood pressures, supine or standing, systolic or diastolic, between the nisoldipine and the nifedipine periods.

The mean pulse rate tended to increase with treatment with nisoldipine but not nifedipine. On nisoldipine, mean supine pulse rate increased from 80.2 ± 3.1/min to 87.9 ± 2.6/min ($P < 0.05$) at week 4 and mean standing pulse rate rose from 92.5 ± 2.3/min to 99.2 ± 3.0/min ($P < 0.05$) at week 4. Mean standing pulse rate was significantly higher in the nisoldipine than in the nifedipine group at weeks 2–4.

On nisoldipine, eight patients were withdrawn from therapy ("treatment failures"), four because of inadequate control (diastolic pressure over 95 mmHg), three at week 2 and one at week 4. Another four patients were withdrawn because of severe headaches. On nifedipine, four patients were treatment failures, two due to inadequate control (at weeks 2 and 4) and one each due to headache/flushing and palpitations, both at week 2. The side-effect profiles were similar, particularly for the incidence of headache and hot flushes, but ankle edema was more common during nifedipine (five patients) than during nisoldipine (one patient) treatment. There were no significant effects of either nisoldipine or nifedipine on any of the hematological or biochemical parameters measured, nor was there any difference between them.

The trial showed that nisoldipine, a dihydropyridine analogue of nifedipine, at a dose of 10 mg once a day is as effective as nifedipine at 20 mg twice a day as monotherapy for mild to moderate essential hypertension. Like nifedipine, it is more effective in reducing diastolic than systolic blood pressure, but it produced a slightly though significantly greater degree of reflex tachycardia than nifedipine. The side-effect profile was similar with respect to the incidence of headache and hot flushes, but ankle edema was significantly less common in the nisoldipine group.

From the point of view of convenience and compliance, monotherapy is an ideal for antihypertensive therapy. Diuretics and betablockers, as the traditional "first-step" monotherapy drugs, are effective and well tolerated but have metabolic side effects which, over some years, may produce adverse cardiovascular effects that could partially negate any benefit achieved from blood pressure reduction. This has led to a search for alternative "first-step" drugs, of which at present the most likely candidates are alpha adrenoreceptor blocking drugs, angiotensin converting enzyme inhibitors, and calcium antagonists.

Calcium channel blockers inhibit smooth muscle contraction, reducing vascular resistance, thus counteracting the basic hemodynamic abnormality in essential hypertension. Calcium antagonists have the advantage of dilating coronary vessels, they do not evoke tolerance during long-term treatment, in contrast to other directly acting dilator drugs, and they do not consistently lead to a rise in plasma renin activity. In in vitro experiments, they have a negatively inotropic action on the heart; in patients, they sometimes produce slight dependent edema [41].

Nifedipine is reasonably well established as an antihypertensive agent [5], either alone or in combination with other drugs, including propranolol [12, 22, 42], atenolol, and bendrofluazide [43]. This paper reports the first controlled clinical study of nisoldipine in hypertension. Nisoldipine acts preferentially on vascular smooth muscle; in vitro it inhibits Ca^{2+}-, Ba^{2+}-, or K^+-induced contraction of smooth muscle preparations in substantially lower concentrations than the spontaneous or electrically stimulated contractility of heart muscle preparations [44]. It thus differs from nifedipine, which inhibits vascular and myocardial preparations equipotentially. It is also four to ten times more potent in terms of inhibition of vascular smooth muscle contraction than nifedipine, previously described as the most potent known calcium antagonist compound [45].

In the present study, the similarity of blood pressure responses to doses of nisoldipine, 10 mg once a day, and nifedipine, 20 mg twice a day, suggests a clinical potency ratio of about 4:1. Both drugs are moderately effective at 24 and 12 h, respectively, after the previous dose; it is possible, even probable, that blood pressure responses would have been even more impressive if they had been measured less than 24 and 12 h, respectively, after the previous dose and if dose titration to higher doses had been incorporated into the trial design. The significantly higher pulse rate in the nisoldipine group is likely to be a function of the lower specificity of nisoldipine for the heart than for vascular smooth muscle, allowing an unblocked reflex increase in heart rate. In a therapeutic situation, this could be a disadvantage when the hypertension is associated with a hyperkinetic circulation, a raised cardiac output, a rapid heart rate, or angina, or an advantage, in hypertension is associated with bradyarrhythmias, a low cardiac output, or as concomitant therapy with beta adrenoreceptor blockers.

There was a significant difference between nisoldipine and nifedipine in the incidence of ankle edema; only one patient on nisoldipine had ankle edema compared with five on nifedipine. Almost 0.6% of 4863 patients treated with nifedipine had edema of the legs [46]. There is no clear explanation of this effect; it may be related to a local change in capillary permeability [47]. The much lower incidence of ankle edema during the nisoldipine period is clearly an advantage.

Nitrendipine

Nitrendipine (Fig.1) is a dihydropyridine derivative with a chemical structure and mechanism of action similar to that of nifedipine, but with a duration of action longer than that of nifedipine [48]. The maximum blood pressure effect of oral nitrendipine is achieved in 60–90 min and the blood pressure remains at this level for 6–8 h [49]. In chronic studies, it has been shown to have significant antihypertensive effects at a dose of 20 or 40 mg once a day [50], twice a day alone or in combination with propranolol and/or hydrochlorothiazide [51], or as third-step therapy with a variety of other antihypertensive drugs [52]. As with nisoldipine, reflex tachycardia does occur [53, 54].

References

1. Folkow B (1971) The haemodynamic consequences of adaptive structural changes of the resistance vessels in hypertension. Clin Sci Mol Med 41:1–12
2. Hurwitz ML, Rosendorff C (1985) Cardiovascular adrenoreceptor number and function in experimental hypertension in the baboon. J Cardiovasc Pharmacol 7 (56): S172–S177
3. Laragh JH (1981) Position paper: The renin-angiotensin-aldosterone system for blood pressure regulation and for subdividing patients to reveal and analyze different forms of hypertension. In: Laragh JH, Bühler FR, Seldin DW (eds) Frontiers in hypertension research. Springer Berlin, Heidelberg New York, pp 183–194
4. Blaustein MP (1984) Sodium transport and hypertension. Hypertension 6(4): 445–453
5. Rosendorff C (1984) Calcium channel blockers and hypertension. In: Opie LH (ed) Calcium antagonists and cardiovascular disease. Raven, New York, pp 323–331
6. Meisheri KD, Hwang O, van Breemen C (1981) Evidence for two separate Ca^{2+} pathways in smooth muscle plasmalemma. J Memb Biol 59:10–25
7. van Breemen C, Mangel A, Fahim M, Meisheri K (1982) Selectivity of calcium antagonistic action in vascular smooth muscle. Am J Cardiol 49:507–510
8. Godfraind T (1981) Calcium influx and receptor-response coupling. In: Weis GB (ed) New perspective on calcium antagonists. American Physiol Soc, Bethesda, pp 95–107
9. Godfraid T (1981) Mechanisms of action of calcium entry blockers. Federation Proc 40: 2866–2871
10. Blaustein MP (1977) Sodium ions, calcium ions, blood pressure regulation, and hypertension: A reassessment and a hypothesis. Am J Physiol 232:C165–C173
11. Gevers W (1984) Calcium and the contractile mechanisms in heart and smooth muscle. In: Opie LH (ed) Calcium antagonists and cardiovascular disease. Raven, New York, pp 67–74
12. De Mendonca M, Grichois ML, Garay RP, Sassrd J, Ben-Ishay D, Meyers P (1980) Abnormal net Na^+ and K^+ fluxes in erythrocytes of three varieties of genetically hypertensive rats. Proc Nat Acad Sci USA 77:4283–4286
13. Wei JW, Janis RA, Daniel EE (1977) Alterations in calcium transport and binding by the plasma membrane of mesenteric arteries from spontaneously hypertensive rats. Blood Vessels 14:55–64
14. Aldestein RS, Hathaway DR (1979) Role of calcium and cyclic adenosine 3:5'-monophosphate in regulating smooth muscle contraction. Mechanisms of excitation-contraction coupling in smooth muscle. Am J Cardiol 44:783–787
15. Hartshorne DJ (1980) Biochemical basis for contraction of vascular smooth muscle. Chest 78:140–149
16. Ebashi S (1980) Regulation of muscle contraction. Proc R Soc Lond B207:259–286
17. Aksoy MO, Murphy RA, Kamm KE (1982) Role of Ca^{2+} and myosin light chain phosphorylation in regulation of smooth muscle. Am J Physiol 242:C109–116
18. Guazzi MD, Fiorentine C, Olivari MT, Bartorelli A, Necchi G, Polese A (1980) Short- and long-term efficacy of a calcium-antagonistic agent (nifedipine) combined with methyldopa in the treatment of severe hypertension. Circulation 61:913–919
19. Guazzi MD, Olivari MT, Polese A, Fiorentini C, Magrini F, Morizzi P (1977) Nifedipine, a new antihypertensive with rapid action. Clin Pharmacol Ther 22:528–532
20. Bartorelli C, Magrini F, Moruzzi P, Olivari MT, Polese A, Fiorentini C, Guazzi M (1978) Haemodynamic effects of a calcium antagonistic agent (nifedipine) in hypertension: therapeutic implications. Clin Sci Mol Med 55:291S–292S
21. Kuwajima I, Ueda K, Kamata C, Matsushita S, Kuramoto K, Murakami M, Hata Y (1978) A

study on the effects of nifedipine in hypertensive crises and severe hypertension. Jpn Heart J 19:455–467

22. Aoki K, Kondo S, Mochizuki A, Yoshida T, Kato S, Kato K, Takikawa K (1978) Antihypertensive effect of cardiovascular Ca^{2+}-antagonist in hypertensive patients in the absence and presence of beta-adrenergic blockade. Am Heart J 96:218–226

23. Lederballe Pedersen O, Christensen NJ, Rämsch KD (1980) Comparison of acute effects of nifedipine in normotensive and hypertensive man. J Cardiovasc Pharmacol 2:357–366

24. Thibonnier M, Bonnet F, Corvol P (1980) Antihypertensive effect of fractionated sublingual administration of nifedipine in moderate essential hypertension. Eur J Clin Pharmacol 17:161–164

25. Corea L, Alunni G, Bentivoglio M, Boschetti E, Cosmi F, Giaimo MD, Miele N, Motolese M (1980) Acute and long-term effects of nifedipine on plasma renin activity and plasma catecholamines in controls and hypertensive patients before and after metoprolol. Acta Therap 6:177–182

26. Klütsch K, Schmidt P, Grosswendt J (1972) Der Einfluss von Bay a 1040 auf die Nierenfunktion des Hypertonikers. Drug Res 22:377–380

27. Koch-Weser J (1974) Vasodilator drugs in the treatment of hypertension. Arch Intern Med 133:1017–1027

28. Corea L, Miele N, Bentivoglio M, Boschett E, Agabiti-Rosei E, Muresan G (1979) Acute and chronic effects of nifedipine on plasma renin activity and plasma adrenaline and noradrenaline in controls and hypertensive patients. Clin Sci: 115S–117S

29. Lederballe Pedersen O, Mikkelsen E, Christensen NJ, Kornerup HJ, Pedersen EB (1979) Effect of nifedipine on plasma renin, aldosterone and catecholamines in arterial hypertension. Europ J Clin Pharmacol 15:235–239

30. Millar JA, McLean K, Reid JL (1981) Calcium antagonists decrease adrenal and vascular responsiveness to angiotensin II in normal man. Clin Sci 61:65S–68S

31. Massie BM, Hirsch AT, Inouye IK, Tubau JF (1984) Calcium channel blockers as antihypertensive agents. Am J Med 77:135–142

32. Klein WW (1984) Treatment of hypertension with calcium channel blockers: European data. Am J Med 77:143–146

33. Murakami M, Murakami F, Takekoshi N, Tsuchiya M, Kin T, Onoe T, Takeuchi N, Funatsu T, Hara S, Ishise S, Mifune J, Maeda M (1972) Antihypertensive effect of 4-(2'-Nitrophenyl)-2-6-dimethyl-1, 4-dihydropyridine-3, 5-dicarbonic acid dimethylester (nifedipine, BAY a1040), a new coronary dilator. Jpn Heart J 13:128–135

34. Ekelund L-G, Orö L (1979) Antianginal efficiency of nifedipine (Adalat) with and without a beta-blocker, studied with exercise test. A double-blind, randomised subacute study. Clin Cardiol 2:203–211

35. Lederballe Pedersen O, Mikkelsen E (1978) Acute and chronic effects of nifedipine in arterial hypertension. Eur J Clin Pharmacol 14:375–381

36. Olivari MT, Bartorelli C, Polese A, Fiorentine C, Moruzzi P, Guazzi MD (1979) Treatment of hypertension with nifedipine, a calcium antagonistic agent. Circulation 59:1056–1062

37. Corea L, Bentivoglio M, Cosmi F, Alunni G, Carnovali M (1981b) Nifedipine versus prazosin in essential hypertension: A double-blind study. Curr Ther Res 30:708–717

38. Müller FB, Bolli P, Erne P, Kiowski W, Bühler FR (1984) Use of calcium antagonists as monotherapy in the management of hypertension 77:11–15

39. Rosendorff C, Goodman C (1985) Double-blind double-dummy crossover study of the efficacy and safety of nisoldipine (BAY k5552) versus nifedipine. Curr Ther Res 37:912–920

40. Freis ED (1960) Hemodynamics in hypertension. Physiol Rev 40:27–54

41. Robinson BF, Bayley S, Dobbs RJ (1983) Long term efficacy of calcium antagonists in resistant hypertension. Hypertension 5:II 122–II 124

42. Yagil Y, Kobrin I, Stessman J, Ghanem J, Leibel B, Ben-Ishay D (1983) Effectiveness of combined nifedipine and propranolol treatment in hypertension. Hypertension 5:II 113–II 117

43. Murphy MB, Scriven AJI, Dollery CT (1983) Efficacy of nifedipine as step 3 antihypertensive drug. Hypertension 5:II 118–II 121

44. Kazda S, Garthoff B, Meyer H, Schlossman K, Stoepel K, Towart R, Vater W, Wehinger E

(1980) Pharmacology of a new calcium antagonistic compound, isobutyl methyl 1,4-dihydro-2,6-dimethyl-4(2-nitrophenyl)-3,5-pyridinedicar boxylate (nisoldipine, BAY k5552). Arzeneim-Forch Drug Res 39(II), 12:2144–2162

45. Fleckenstein A (1984) Calcium antagonism: History and prospects for a multifaceted, phamacodynamic principle. In: Opie LH (ed) Calcium antagonists and cardiovascular disease. Raven, New York, pp 9–28
46. Ebner F, Donath M (1980) Mode of action and efficacy of nifedipine. In Puech P, Krebs L (eds) Proc 4th Intern Adalat Symposium. Exerpta Medica, Amsterdam, pp 25–34
47. Krebs R (1983) Adverse reactions with calcium antagonists. Hypertension 5:II 125–II 129
48. Deck K, Stoepel K, Leibowitz D, Taylor R, Vanov S (1984) Some aspects of the clinical pharmacology of nitrendipine. In: Scriabine A, Vanov S, Deck K (eds) Nitrendipine. Urbant and Schwarzenberg, Baltimore, pp 397–407
49. Burris JF, Notargiacomo AV, Papademetriou V, Freis ED (1982) Acute and short-term effects of a new calcium antagonist in hypertension. Hypertension 4 (Suppl II):II 32–35
50. Andren L, Hansson L, Oro L, Ryman T (1982) Experience with nitrendipine—a new calcium antagonist—in hypertension. J Cardiovasc Pharmacol 4:S387–391
51. Jain AK, McMahon FG, Ryan JR, Maronde R, Vlachis N, Mroczek W (1984) Efficacy and safety of nitrendipine in patients with severe hypertension: A multiclinic study. J Cardiovasc Pharmacol 6:S1053–S1059
52. Höffler D, Stoepel K (1984) Nitrendipine in hypertension that is difficult to control. J Cardiovasc Pharmacol 6:S1060–S1062
53. Ventura HO, Messerli FH, Oigman W, Dunn FG, Reisin E, Frohlich ED (1983) Immediate hemodynamic effects of a new calcium-channel blocking agent (nitrendipine) in essential hypertension. Am J Cardiol 51:783–786
54. Fouad FM, Pedrinelli R, Bravo EL, Abi-Samra F, Textor SC, Tarazi RC (1984) Clinical and systemic hemodynamic effects of nitrendipine. Clin Pharmacol Ther 35:768–775

Calcium Antagonists in Patients with Hypertension and Diabetes Mellitus

Effects of Calcium Antagonist Nitrendipine on Glucose Homeostasis*

B. N. Trost and P. Weidmann `

Medizinische Poliklinik, University of Berne, Switzerland

Summary. In ten elderly patients with diabetes mellitus type II and mild to moderate hypertension, both of which had been present for several years, it was demonstrated by means of fasting blood sugar levels, urinary glucose excretion, and behavior of plasma glucose and insulin concentrations after a standard breakfast as well as by measurements of the glycosylated hemoglobin A_1 that antihypertensive long-term monotherapy with about 30 mg nitrendipine every morning for 12 months was able to lower blood pressure reproducibly compared with placebo. Despite some apprehension derived mostly from in vitro experiments, nitrendipine did not impair overall glucose homeostasis.

Key words: Calcium antagonists—Diabetes mellitus—Glucose homeostasis—Hypertension—Nitrendipine

Cardiovascular complications are the main cause of disability and premature death among patients with diabetes mellitus [1–3]. These complications are due to the known sequelae of the altered carbohydrate metabolism itself but, equally, to additional cardiovascular risk factors, particularly hypertension [1]. Furthermore, because of the increased prevalence of hypertension in patients with diabetes mellitus compared with the nondiabetic population [2–5] (at present it is uncertain if the two problems are merely associated, e.g., by the link of obesity [2], or if they are causally connected by common pathophysiological factors) blood pressure in diabetics deserves special attention. If the blood pressure is abnormal it needs to be carefully integrated into overall diagnostic and therapeutic considerations.

If general measures, like reducing overweight, salt intake, smoking, and stress as well as omitting medication that might elevate blood pressure, fail or are unrealistic, hypertension has to be treated with appropriate drugs [6]. In this context, "*appropriate*" means: (a) lowering the elevated blood pressure effectively; (b) not deteriorating the glucose metabolism already altered; (c) no unfavorable influence on associated cardiovascular risk factors, e.g., hyperlipoproteinemia; (d) not aggravating the complications of diabetes mellitus (besides the classic ones, especially sexual impotence and orthostatic hypotension); (e) not interacting

* This study was supported in part by the Swiss National Science Foundation and Bayer AG, Leverkusen, Federal Republic of Germany

adversely with the current antidiabetic therapy; (f) having as few other side effects as possible; (g) to be taken once a day; (h) being economically sound.

In the following, we shall focus our attention to items a and b, namely whether the calcium antagonist nitrendipine lowers high blood pressure adequately and deteriorates the impaired glucose homeostasis.

Patients and Methods

In a still ongoing placebo-controlled single-blind long-term study, ten patients (six women, four men) with a mean age of 57 ± 2 (SEM) years (range, 48–67 years), who had suffered from diabetes mellitus type II for 11 ± 3 years and from mild to moderate hypertension for 13 ± 2 years, underwent an identical test protocol 1 month after daily intake of placebo as well as $1\frac{1}{2}$, 6, and 12 months after an antihypertensive monotherapy with 35 ± 6, 30 ± 4, and 30 ± 3 mg nitrendipine p.o. every morning (Fig. 1). The antidiabetic regimen (diet alone—two patients; oral hypoglycemic drugs—four; insulin—four) remained unchanged during this period (for nonspecific alterations, see Discussion).

Blood pressure was monitored with a Physiometrics SR 2 automatic recorder (Physiometrics International, Malibu, CA, USA) 90 min after intake of placebo or verum. The monitoring was carried out after 1 h of recumbency in a warm, quiet room and after 5 min in the upright position. The values are the means of three determinations.

A standard breakfast for dynamic testing of glucose homeostasis, which was taken about 1 h after placebo or nitrendipine, was intraindividually identical; the

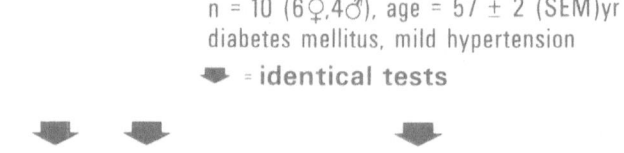

n = 10 (6♀,4♂), age = 57 ± 2 (SEM)yr
diabetes mellitus, mild hypertension

➥ = identical tests

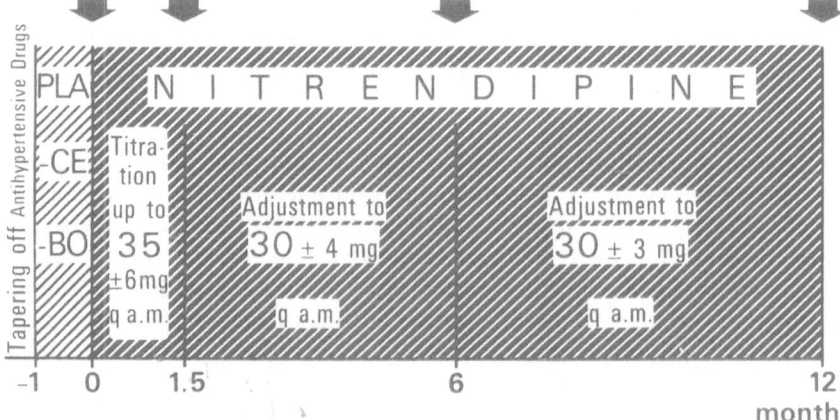

Fig. 1. Study design. For explanation see text. *q a.m.* every morning

main carbohydrate load usually consisted of 90 g rye bread. Before and 1 h and 2 h after breakfast, blood was obtained for determination of glucose and insulin.

All patients, wearing only underwear, were weighed on the same mechanical balance.

Measurements of plasma and urine glucose levels (hexokinase method, Greiner-G 400 Autoanalyzer), determinations of plasma immunoreactive insulin [7], and calculations of the glycosylated hemoglobin A_1 (HbA$_1$) (Bio-Rad column test in whole blood; Bio-Rad Clinical Division, Richmond, CA, USA) were performed with the usual routine methods in the Zentrallabor Department of the Inselspital, Berne (Director—Prof. J. P. Colombo, MD).

Student's two-sided paired t-test was used for statistical analysis.

Results

Blood pressure, systolic and diastolic, was lowered by nitrendipine versus placebo, mostly in a highly significant manner (Fig. 2). Mean supine blood pressure fell by 15% on average, whereas mean upright pressure was decreased by 26%. After 6 weeks of verum treatment, this occurred to about the same degree as 6 and 12 months after initiation of therapy.

Fasting blood sugar, i.e., the means of three samples each measured on 3 consecutive mornings, remained statistically unchanged by the calcium antagonist (Fig. 3). This was somewhat corroborated by significant pair-correlations

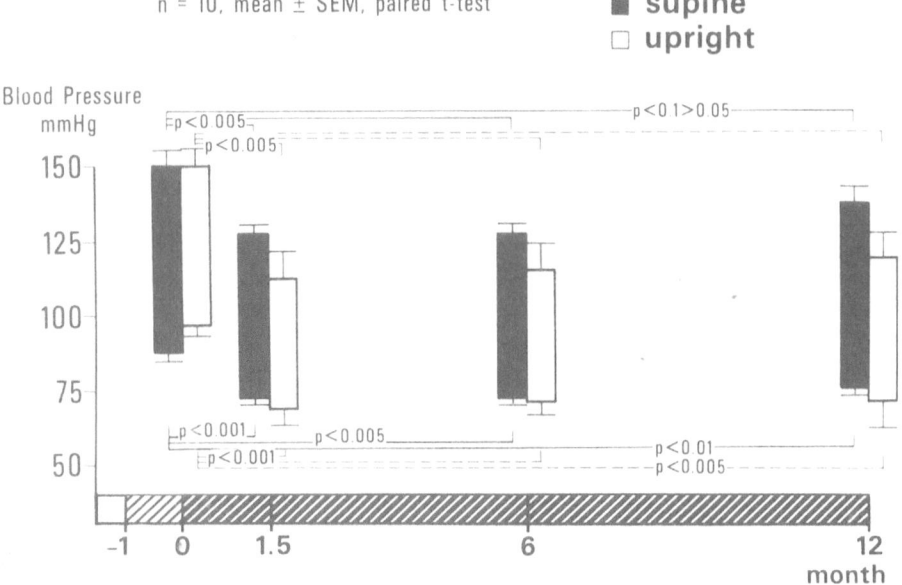

Fig. 2. Blood pressure in nitrendipine-treated diabetic patients. *Hatched areas* symbolize treatment and correspond to those in Fig. 1

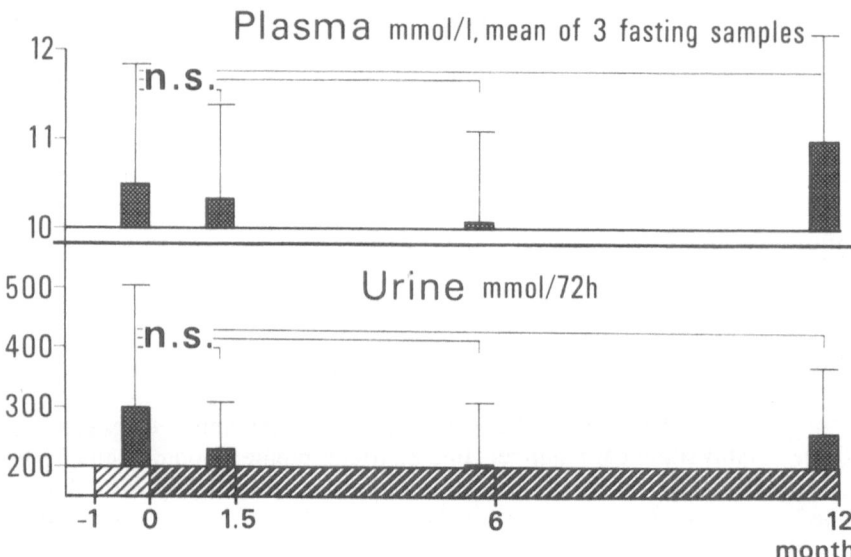

Fig. 3. Glucose levels in plasma and urine in nitrendipine-treated diabetics. *Hatched areas* symbolize treatment and correspond to those in Fig. 1

between each of the different times of determination (r 0.66–0.92; $P < 0.05$– < 0.001).

The *excretion of glucose in 72-h urine* collected over 3 consecutive days was unaltered by the treatment with nitrendipine (Fig. 3). However, the creatinine concentration 1 year after beginning therapy was significantly increased (33 ± 3 versus 38 ± 3 mmol/72h, $P < 0.005$), which was not observed after $1\frac{1}{2}$ and 6 months. Pair-correlations concerning sugar excretion were in part, and those relating to the concentration of creatinine (r 0.90–0.98) were always, highly significant between all periods of analysis.

A *standard breakfast* did not statistically affect the incremental area under the curve of plasma glucose over a period of 120 min after 6 weeks of therapy with nitrendipine, whereas after 6 and 12 months of treatment the areas were significantly larger in spite of the smaller dose of the calcium antagonist prescribed (Fig. 4). Statistically, no corresponding changes were manifest under the analogous curve of plasma insulin levels. However, there was a slight tendency to increased areas after 6 and 12 months of nitrendipine therapy under the insulin curves (Fig. 4).

The course of *HbA₁ percentages* (Fig. 5) showed the following. The average blood sugar levels for several weeks before the trial must have been significantly higher than during the placebo period of 4 weeks and the first 6 weeks on calcium antagonist treatment ($P < 0.01$ for both differences). The difference between HbA_1 levels after the placebo phase and the first 6 weeks of verum therapy was statistically suggestive of a decrease ($P < 0.1 > 0.05$). The values after 6 and 12

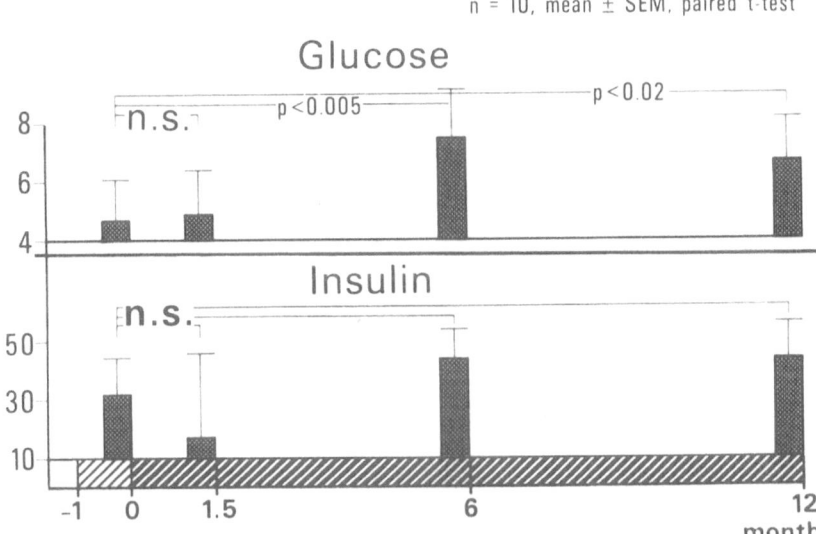

Fig. 4. Standard breakfast in nitrendipine-treated diabetic patients. Incremental areas under the curve (arbitrary units) of plasma glucose and insulin concentrations for 120 min after a standard breakfast. *Hatched areas* symbolize treatment and correspond to those in Fig. 1

months of nitrendipine treatment were not statistically distinguishable from each other nor from each of the three earlier determinations. Furthermore, every single pair-correlation of HbA$_1$ percentages at each point in time compared with every other point was statistically significant (r 0.65–0.97, P mostly < 0.001).

Body weight showed a striking parallelism with HbA$_1$ levels: A significant fall was noted from the prestudy value to that after placebo treatment (86 $\pm$ 8 versus 84 $\pm$ 8 kg, $P < 0.02$) and to the value after 6 weeks of calcium antagonist therapy (86 $\pm$ 8 versus 83 $\pm$ 8 kg, $P < 0.005$). However, a comparison of weights after 6 and 12 months of intake of nitrendipine (83 $\pm$ 8 and 84 $\pm$ 7 kg, respectively) did not result in a statistical distinction either between each other or between each of the earlier measurements mentioned above.

Discussion

From blood pressure studies, we can conclude that mild to moderate hypertension in elderly patients with diabetes mellitus type II can reproducibly be brought into normal limits by an antihypertensive monotherapy of about 30 mg nitrendipine daily for a period of several weeks or months. These results were obtained after 90 min of drug ingestion; the previous dose had been swallowed about 24 h earlier. Thus, there are no indications of tachyphylaxis. On the other hand, the present data are unable to provide information on the duration of action of a single dose of the calcium antagonist. If the results obtained by Deck et al. [8], Hansson et al. [9], Vlachakis et al. [10], and Esper et al. [11] in nondiabetic subjects

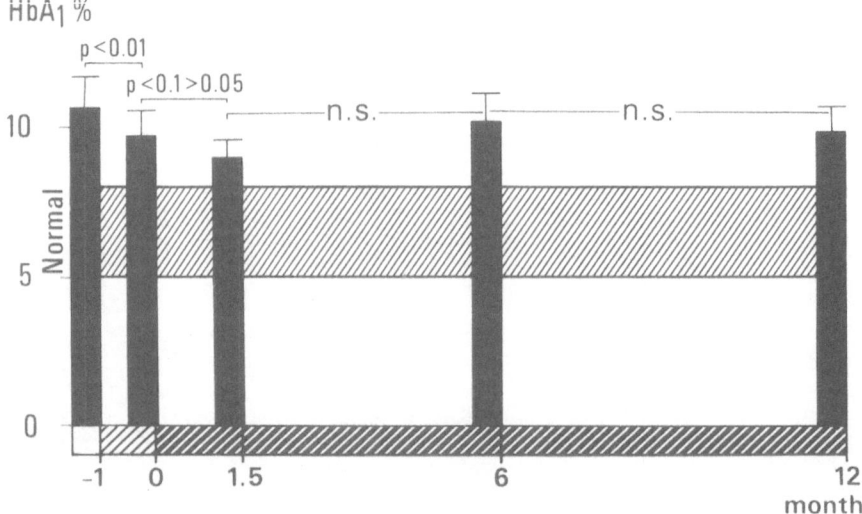

Fig. 5. Blood levels of the glycosylated HbA$_1$ in nitrendipine-treated diabetics. The *first column on the left* corresponds to the values obtained just before patients entered the study, i.e., before tapering off the antihypertensive regimen and beginning with the placebo phase. *Hatched areas* symbolize treatment and correspond to those in Fig. 1

with essential hypertension treated with nitrendipine may be extended to our patients with diabetes mellitus (the decrease in blood pressure 90 min after drug intake is in perfect agreement), it may be assumed that the hypotensive effect lasts for a minimum of 8 h and that the patients do become normotensive.

The finding of a dependence of the second phase of insulin release after a glucose challenge on a normal influx of calcium ions into the pancreatic beta cells [12] has led to some apprehension concerning the use of calcium antagonists in patients with diabetes mellitus type II, since a deterioration of their glucose homeostasis was anticipated. As we have shown in a detailed review article [13], this fear—derived mostly from in vitro experiments—could not be substantiated in man, and diabetic patients in particular, from a clinical point of view. However, with higher dosages and after a glucose tolerance test (a debatable method, at least in diabetics), a transient rise in blood glucose and a *relative* decrease in insulin stimulation may occur after administration of a calcium antagonist.

In the present paper, we demonstrate for the first time that an antihypertensive monotherapy with nitrendipine *for 12 months* essentially does not alter carbohydrate metabolism in type II diabetics. The small increase of areas under the plasma glucose curve after a standard breakfast together with the slight *relative* decrease of areas under the plasma insulin curve point to the pathophysiological background cited above. Nevertheless, the possibilities of a diminished sensitivity of insulin receptors and calcium antagonist-provoked changes in other hormones should not be excluded a priori. Furthermore, three particular circumstances need to be kept in mind. First, after a standard breakfast, carbohydrate metabolism parameters were obtained at a time when nitrendipine plasma levels are the highest [14] and therefore, in this respect, during the most unfavorable period of the day. Second, 30 mg nitrendipine is a relatively high dose in elderly patients. Third, the carbohydrate load of about 90 g bread was about twice as much as these patients normally had for breakfast.

The time-course of HbA$_1$ levels, which are at present considered to be the most solid and representative parameter of glucose homeostasis [15–17], proves that possible calcium antagonist-induced small postprandial changes are most likely negligible. At first glance (Fig. 5), one might even believe that carbohydrate metabolism becomes *ameliorated* by nitrendipine. We do not think this is the case for several reasons. To begin with, something happened unintentionally which we consider a nonspecific effect of the trial and the investigator: Patients did reduce their body weight, which in practical terms most likely means that they stuck to their diet more precisely. This explanation is obvious for the time-courses of body weight as well as of HbA$_1$ percentage, since during the two early periods (4 weeks on placebo and the first 6 weeks on verum) all patients were examined extensively by the investigator (B.N.T.) every 2 weeks for 2 h following a standard protocol; later, short controls were made at the outpatient clinic at best every month, as had been the case before they entered the study. A second possibility to explain the decrease in HbA$_1$ levels especially after the placebo phase could be the favorable effect of being taken off the antihypertensive regimen, which in all ten patients included a diuretic drug [18, 19]. Finally, it is almost certain that an overall bloodletting of about 400 ml due to many other items of investigation at the end of the placebo period must have had some influence on the lowering of HbA$_1$ at the end of the first verum phase of 6 weeks [15, 20, 21]. In spite of the three objections just raised against an amelioration of glucose homeostasis caused by calcium antagonist therapy, we do not have any evidence for a deterioration of overall carbohydrate metabolism due to nitrendipine.

In conclusion, we were able to demonstrate that an antihypertensive monotherapy with about 30 mg nitrendipine every morning in elderly type II diabetics with mild to moderate hypertension over a period of 12 months is effective in lowering blood pressure adequately and does not impair overall glucose homeostasis. Therefore, it is not justified to withhold the benefit of calcium antagonist therapy from these patients based on the apprehension of deteriorating their diabetes mellitus, especially in view of their frequent cardiovascular problems.

References

1. Kannel WB, McGee DL (1979) Diabetes and cardiovascular disease (the Framingham study). JAMA 241:2035–2038
2. Barrett-Connor E, Criqui MH, Klauber MR, Holdbrook M (1981) Diabetes and hypertension in a community of older adults. Am J Epidemiol 113:276–284
3. Christlieb AR (1982) Treating hypertension in the patient with diabetes mellitus. Med Clin North Am 66:1373–1388
4. Passa P, Lombrail P, Eschwege E, Canivet J (1983) Prévalence de l'hypertension artérielle chez

le diabétique, influence des traitements antihypertenseurs sur le contrôle métabolique. Arch Mal Coeur 76: 169–171

5. Uusitupa M, Siitonen O, Aro A, Pyörälä K (1985) Prevalence of coronary heart disease, left ventricular failure and hypertension in middle-aged, newly diagnosed type 2 (non-insulin-dependent) diabetic subjects. Diabetologia 28: 22–27

6. Trost BN, Weidmann P, Beretta-Piccoli C (1985) Antihypertensive therapy in diabetic patients. Hypertension 7 (Suppl II): II-102–II-108

7. Löffler G, Weiss L (1975) Radioimmunologische Bestimmung von Insulin im Serum. In: Breuer H, Hamel D, Krüskemper HL (eds) Methoden der Hormonbestimmung. Thieme, Stuttgart, pp 75–88

8. Deck K, Stoepel K, Leibowitz D, Taylor R, Vanov S (1984) Some aspects of the clinical pharmacology of nitrendipine. In: Scriabine A, Vanov S, Deck K (eds) Nitrendipine. Urban and Schwarzenberg, Baltimore, pp 397–407

9. Hansson L, Andrén L, Orö L, Ryman T (1984) The antihypertensive effects and pharmacokinetics of nitrendipine in patients with essential hypertension. In: Scriabine A, Vanov S, Deck K (eds) Nitrendipine. Urban and Schwarzenberg, Baltimore, pp 423–433

10. Vlachakis ND, Vanov SK, Taylor RJ, Pun EFC (1984) Controlled comparison of nitrendipine and placebo in the treatment of hypertension. In: Scriabine A, Vanov S, Deck K (eds) Nitrendipine. Urban and Schwarzenberg, Baltimore, pp 443–449

11. Esper RJ, Esper RC, Cassola D, Spiritoso RA, Mosca H, Sami HH, Castro JM, Rohwedder RW (1984) Effectiveness of nitrendipine in the treatment of essential hypertension: a multicenter trial. In: Scriabine A, Vanov S, Deck K (eds) Nitrendipine. Urban and Schwarzenberg, Baltimore, pp 477–489

12. Wollheim CB, Sharp GWG (1981) Regulation of insulin release by calcium. Physiol Rev 61: 914–973

13. Trost BN, Weidmann P (1984) Effects of nitrendipine and other calcium antagonists on glucose metabolism in man. J Cardiovasc Pharmacol 6: S 986–995

14. Raemsch KD, Sommer J (1984) Pharmacokinetics and metabolism of nitrendipine. In: Scriabine A, Vanov S, Deck K (eds) Nitrendipine. Urban and Schwarzenberg, Baltimore, pp 409–421

15. Gabbay KH (1982) Glycosylated hemoglobin and diabetes mellitus. Med Clin North Am 66: 1309–1315

16. Kennedy L, Baynes JW (1984) Non-enzymatic glycosylation and the chronic complications of diabetes: an overview. Diabetologia 26: 93–98

17. Nathan DM, Singer DE, Hurxthal K, Goodson JD (1984) The clinical information value of the glycosylated hemoglobin assay. N Eng J Med 310: 341–346

18. Ames RP, Hill P (1982) Improvement of glucose tolerance and lowering of glycohemoglobin and serum lipid concentrations after discontinuation of antihypertensive drug therapy. Circulation 65: 899–904

19. Bloomgarden ZT, Ginsberg-Fellner F, Rayfield EJ, Bookman J, Brown WV (1984) Elevated hemoglobin A_{1c} and low-density lipoprotein cholesterol levels in thiazide-treated diabetic patients. Am J med 77: 823–827

20. Bunn HF, Haney DN, Kamin S, Gabbay KH, Gallop PM (1976) The biosynthesis of human hemoglobin A_{1c}: Slow glycosylation of hemoglobin in vivo. J Clin Invest 57: 1652–1659

21. Fitzgibbons JF, Koler RD, Jones RT (1976) Red cell age-related changes of hemoglobins A_{1a+b} and A_{1c} in normal and diabetic subjects. J Clin Invest 58: 820–824

Epidemiological Studies on the Role of Sodium, Potassium, Calcium, and Magnesium in Hypertension

H. Kesteloot[1], J. Geboers[1], and D.X. Huang[2]

[1]Department of Epidemiology, St. Rafaël University Hospital, Gasthuisberg, 3000 Leuven, Belgium
[2]Department of Cardiology, Chinese PLA General Hospital, Beijing, People's Republic of China

Summary. The relationship between cations and blood pressure is complex. In countries with a high sodium intake (more than 200 mmol/24 h) a significant positive relationship is found between sodium intake and the urinary 24-h Na/K ratio and blood pressure, and a significant negative relationship is found for potassium intake. Such a positive relationship, however, cannot be demonstrated in Western countries. The serum calcium level correlates positively with blood pressure, but is influenced by sodium and potassium intake and correlates negatively with the 24-h urinary Na/K ratio. The relationship between 24-h urinary calcium and magnesium and blood pressure is also complex, and varying results have been obtained in different populations. The 24-h urinary magnesium excretion correlates negatively with blood pressure in a Western population, but not in the People's Republic of China. Presently, no general conclusions can be drawn on the role of cations in blood pressure regulation at the population level.

Key words: Blood pressure regulation—24 hour urinary excretion of sodium, potassium, calcium, and magnesium—serum calcium

Epidemiological studies have for many years shown that important differences in cerebrovascular mortality and morbidity exist among different populations. Although hypertension is a worldwide problem, its prevalence is particularly high in Northeast Asia, as is the prevalence of cerebrovascular disease. For a long time, differences in the prevalence of cerebrovascular disease have been ascribed to differences in dietary habits, and in particular, the role of sodium has been examined in this respect. Only recently has the role of other cations in blood pressure regulation at the population level become a focus of attention. The purpose of this study is to present data on the possible role of several cations as determinants of blood pressure in the population. Use will be made of several large epidemiological studies performed by our department in which sodium, potassium, calcium (urinary or seral), and magnesium were measured together with blood pressure and other cardiovascular risk factors.

Sodium, Potassium, and Blood Pressure

In Korea, we were able to demonstrate a significant independent positive correlation between sodium and blood pressure and a significant independent negative correlation between potassium and blood pressure [1, 2]. The characteristics of

Table 1. Anthropometric data, urinary electrolyte excretion, and blood pressure in Korean and Belgian populations (mean ± SD)

| | Korea | | Belgium | |
	M (n = 200)	F (n = 258)	M (n = 133)	F (n = 167)
Age (years)	37.5 ± 14.3	39.7 ± 13.7	39.3 ± 11.0	40.0 ± 12.2
H (cm)	166.6 ± 6.6	155.4 ± 5.2	174.0 ± 6.4	161.3 ± 6.4
W (kg)	60.2 ± 8.2	50.4 ± 7.3	75.4 ± 10.8	60.7 ± 8.2
W/H² (kg/m²)	0.22 ± 0.024	0.21 ± 0.029	0.25 ± 0.033	0.23 ± 0.031
Na (mmol/24 h)	294.2 ± 133.4	266.5 ± 107.6	183.9 ± 44.6	152.6 ± 43.8
K (mmol/24 h)	57.1 ± 43.8	54.7 ± 27.5	76.7 ± 15.4	65.3 ± 12.5
SBP (mmHg)	125.2 ± 14.2	120.5 ± 18.6	121.4 ± 12.6	114.6 ± 13.9
DBP (mmHg)	81.2 ± 10.6	77.9 ± 12.0	78.5 ± 8.6	73.0 ± 8.4

M males, *F* females, *H* height, *W* weight

Table 2. Significance of independent relationships[a] of sodium and potassium with blood pressure (*t*-values)

| | | n | SBP | | DBP | | R^b | |
			Na	K	Na	K	SBP	DBP
Belgium	M	133	—	—	—	—	0.51	0.53
	F	167	—	—	+2.0*	—	0.55	0.59
	M+F	300	—	—	—	—	0.57	0.61
Korea	M	200	+3.0**	−3.1**	—	—	0.37	0.34
	F	258	—	—	+2.1*	—	0.32	0.28
	M+F	458	+2.8**	−2.2*	—	—	0.37	0.33
Korea	M	200	+3.4***	−2.6**	—	—	0.46	0.46
(+heart rate)	F	258	+2.4*	—	+2.9**	—	0.41	0.44
	M+F	458	+4.1***	—	+2.6**	—	0.45	0.47
Belgium + Korea	M	333	+2.9**	−2.7**	—	—	0.44	0.42
	F	425	—	—	+2.0*	—	0.41	0.42
	M+F	758	+3.0**	−2.0*	+2.1*	—	0.45	0.47

Data reproduced from [2] with permission of editors
* $P < 0.05$; ** $P < 0.01$; *** $P < 0.001$
SBP systolic blood pressure, *DBP* diastolic blood pressure
[a] With the inclusion in the regression of age, height, weight, 24-h urinary sodium, potassium, and creatinine, region (Belgium, Korea), sex, and the interaction variables
[b] Multiple correlation coefficients of final regression model including all factors significant at the $P < 0.05$ level

the Korean population and the Belgian population, examined with the same methodology, are given in Table 1. In Table 2, the significance of the independent relationships of sodium and potassium with blood pressure in these populations is given. As can be seen from Table 3, with the exception of a borderline significant positive relationship of sodium and diastolic blood pressure in females, no significant relationship was found in Belgium between sodium, potassium, and blood pressure. In Korea, a significant positive relationship was found between

Table 3. Anthropometric and biological variables from an army survey in Belgium (means ± SD)

	Men ($n = 9321$)	Women ($n = 421$)
Age (years)	39.0 ± 11.5	27.7 ± 10.4
Height (cm)	174.2 ± 6.6	163.9 ± 6.6
Weight (kg)	77.3 ± 10.8	62.0 ± 9.7
SBP (mmHg)	130.4 ± 15.4	122.3 ± 15.3
DBP (mmHg)	80.5 ± 11.3	74.7 ± 11.3
Serum Ca (mmol/l)	2.42 ± 0.09	2.40 ± 0.09
Urinary Na (mmol/24 h)	162.0 ± 61.4	121.0 ± 50.9
Urinary K (mmol/24 h)	71.3 ± 24.2	56.8 ± 21.3
Urinary creatinine (g/24 h)	1.75 ± 0.60	1.43 ± 0.50
Heart rate (beats/min)	70.7 ± 10.3	76.8 ± 10.4
Log γ-GT (log U/l)	1.17 ± 0.26	0.95 ± 0.23

blood pressure and sodium and a negative one between blood pressure and potassium. For both of these cations, urinary 24-h excretion can be considered a reliable measure of intake. The maximum slope of sodium on blood pressure was 2.7 mmHg/100 mmol of 24-h urinary sodium and that of potassium was 9.8 mmHg/100 mmol of 24-h urinary potassium, both obtained in Korean male subjects. It can be stated that in Korea, per millimole, potassium was about three times more effective in lowering blood pressure than sodium was in raising it [1].

In a larger epidemiological study performed in Belgium, we were unable to demonstrate a positive effect of sodium or of the Na/K ratio on blood pressure [3]. The anthropometric characteristics of the population group are given in Table 3, the blood pressure data and the 24-h urinary excretion data of Na, K, and creatinine in Table 4. A negative independent relationship was found between the 24-h urinary Na/K ratio (expressed in millimoles) and blood pressure in male subjects [−0.536 mmHg ($P < 0.001$) for systolic blood pressure and −0.533 mmHg ($P < 0.001$) for diastolic blood pressure per unit change of the Na/K ratio].

Serum Calcium and Blood Pressure

In an epidemiological survey in Belgian male subjects (characteristics given in Table 3) a strong positive correlation was found between total serum calcium and blood pressure, by univariate and multivariate analysis. It was thus possible to demonstrate that the relation between total serum calcium and blood pressure was independent of height, weight, age, intake of sodium and potassium, heart rate, and gamma-glutamyl-transpeptidase, taken as an indicator of alcohol intake at the population level [4]. The slope of calcium on blood pressure obtained is given in Table 5. An interesting finding was that the slope of calcium on blood pressure was nearly identical to the slope published earlier in a study in which serum albumin was also included in the regression [5]. This positive correlation between total serum calcium and blood pressure has now been confirmed by several other studies [6, 7]. Another interesting finding was that the

Table 4. Blood pressure and 24-h urinary excretion of sodium, potassium, and creatinine in 9321 Belgian men by age (means ± SD)

	Age (years)			
	< 20	20–24	25–29	30–34
n	602	1045	893	838
SBP (mmHg)	126.1 ± 13.4	128.5 ± 13.0	129.4 ± 13.6	130.0 ± 14.8
DBP (mmHg)	72.2 ± 9.8	74.4 ± 10.1	77.2 ± 9.9	79.4 ± 10.9
Na (mmol/24 h)	154.9 ± 62.4	156.2 ± 61.8	156.0 ± 62.5	161.9 ± 60.4
K (mmol/24 h)	73.1 ± 28.8	71.0 ± 26.4	70.6 ± 24.1	70.1 ± 24.8
Creatinine (mg/24 h)	1680 ± 582	1797 ± 662	1811 ± 629	1740 ± 621
	35–39	40–44	45–49	≥ 50
n	817	1352	2044	1730
SBP (mmHg)	128.7 ± 14.3	129.4 ± 15.4	131.2 ± 16.4	134.6 ± 16.9
DBP (mmHg)	81.2 ± 10.4	82.0 ± 10.8	83.7 ± 10.8	84.3 ± 11.0
Na (mmol/24 h)	167.9 ± 64.9	166.3 ± 63.7	163.5 ± 58.0	163.6 ± 60.6
K (mmol/24 h)	72.9 ± 24.1	71.6 ± 23.7	77.9 ± 22.4	70.1 ± 23.1
Creatinine (mg/24 h)	1774 ± 599	1800 ± 595	1718 ± 563	1681 ± 569

Table 5. Relation between serum calcium (mmol/l) and blood pressure (mmHg) in Belgian men

	Age (years)		
	< 30 ($n = 2540$)	30–44 ($n = 3007$)	≥ 45 ($n = 3774$)
Slope SBP			
Univariate[a]	26.3	21.3	18.2
Multivariate[b]	23.8	19.0	15.9
Slope DBP			
Univariate[a]	12.2	8.3	9.8
Multivariate[b]	11.0	8.5	8.4
Slope pulse pressure			
Univariate[a]	14.1	13.0	8.4
Multivariate[b]	13.5	10.2	7.4

[a] All values significant at $P < 0.001$. The slope is given in mmHg/mmol/l serum calcium
[b] With the inclusion of age, height, weight, log γ-GT (gamma-glutamyl transpeptidase), 24-h urinary sodium, potassium, and creatinine, and heart rate; partial regression coefficeints were obtained from the final regression equation

slope of total serum calcium on blood pressure decreases with age, although the relevance of this is still not understood. Of great importance are the significant correlations between the serum calcium level and the level of the excretion of sodium and potassium: the higher the sodium excretion the lower the total serum calcium level; the reverse is true for potassium excretion [8]. As a result, the Na/K ratio shows a strong negative correlation with the total serum calcium level (Table

Table 6. Univariate relationship between serum calcium and 24-h urinary Na, K, and Na/K ratio in Belgian men

Slope serum Ca	24-h Na (mmol)	24-h K (mmol)	Na/K ratio
Total group ($n = 9321$)	−0.00012 (−7.57)	+0.00015 (3.74)	−0.0105 (−10.9)

The t-value of the slope is given in parentheses

6). This finding demonstrates that important interactions exist between different cations. These interactions should be taken into account whenever the effect of one cation on blood pressure is studied.

In a recent study of a population with high lipid and alcohol consumption, no relationship, or only a weak one, was found between serum calcium and blood pressure. However, a highly significant relationship existed between blood pressure and total serum protein. This significant relationship occurred in male and female subjects for systolic and diastolic blood pressure (Tables 7, 8).

Ionized Serum Calcium and Blood Pressure

Ionized serum calcium is biologically the most active part of total serum calcium. In epidemiological studies its determination is cumbersome, as in order to avoid deterioration, the measurements must be performed at the site of the survey. Results have been published demonstrating a lower ionized serum calcium value in subjects with hypertension than in normal controls [9]. However, in a fairly large population sample with a substantial variation in blood pressure, we were unable to find a positive correlation between ionized serum calcium and blood pressure in males or in females [10].

Urinary Calcium and Blood Pressure

The relationship in adults between calcium intake and urinary calcium is very complex. However, the urinary 24-h excretion of calcium can be readily measured. In Belgium and in Korea, a significant positive correlation was found between 24-h urinary calcium excretion and blood pressure, by univariate and multivariate analysis, with the inclusion of age, height, weight, urinary 24-h Na and K, and creatinine excretion [11]. In the People's Republic of China (PRC), however, a significant negative correlation was found between 24-h urinary calcium excretion and blood pressure, and the same was true for the Ca/Mg ratio. In the same multiple regression analysis the Na/K ratio always correlated positively with blood pressure. The urinary Na/K and Ca/Mg ratios were higher in South than in North China, both in male and in female subjects, although the absolute value of 24-h urinary Na excretion was higher in the North. Our studies

Table 7. Independent relationships[a] between blood pressure and serum calcium, total serum protein, and 24-h urinary Na and K in 3923 males

	S-Ca (mmol/l)	S-Prot (g/l)	U-Na (mmol/24 h)	U-K (mmol/24 h)	Na/K	R[b]
SBP	5.46 (2.38)	NI	NS	NS	NI	0.43
	5.46 (2.38)	NI	NI	NI	NS	0.43
	NS	0.349 (6.91)	NS	NS	NI	0.44
	NS	0.358 (7.07)	NI	NI	0.57 (2.19)	0.44
DBP	NS	NI	−0.0093 (−3.34)	NS	NI	0.54
	NS	NI	NI	NI	NS	0.53
	NS	0.179 (5.01)	−0.0061 (−2.44)	NS	NI	0.54
	NS	0.184 (5.16)	NI	NI	NS	0.54

Regression coefficients are given with t-values in parentheses
NS not significant, *NI* not included in the regression equation, *S-Ca* serum calcium, *S-Prot* serum protein, *U-Na* urinary sodium, *U-K* urinary potassium
[a] With the inclusion of age, height, weight, 24-h urinary creatinine, heart rate, and log γ-GT in the multiple regression analysis
[b] Multiple correlation coefficients of final regression model including all factors significant at the $P < 0.05$ level.

Table 8. Independent relationships between blood pressure and serum calcium, total serum protein, and 24-h urinary Na and K in 1592 females

	S-Ca (mmol/l)	S-Prot (g/l)	U-Na (mmol/24 h)	U-K (mmol/24 h)	Na/K	R
SBP	NS	NI	NS	−0.040 (−2.41)	NI	0.52
	NS	NI	NI	NI	0.80 (2.03)	0.52
	NS	0.367 (4.96)	NS	−0.039 (−2.40)	NI	0.53
	NS	0.378 (5.09)	NI	NI	0.90 (2.31)	0.53
DBP	8.06 (3.44)	NI	NS	−0.035 (−3.15)	NI	0.53
	7.72 (3.29)	NI	NI	NI	NS	0.53
	6.43 (2.73)	0.245 (4.89)	NS	−0.034 (−3.11)	NI	0.54
	6.09 (2.59)	0.247 (4.92)	NI	NI	NS	0.53

See notes to Table 7

in the PRC have also shown that the Ca/Mg ratio and the Na/K ratio are virtually independent of the completeness of the 24-h urine collection as judged from the 24-h creatinine excretion, much more so than the absolute values of the measured 24-h urine excretion of Na, K, Ca, and Mg. The slopes of the Ca/Mg and Na/K ratios in the PRC are given in Tables 9–11. Since important differences in electrolyte excretion exist between North China (Beijing region) and South China (Fuchow region) and between farmers and nonfarmers, region and occupation and their interaction with the other independent variables considered in the analysis, have been included.

Dietary Calcium and Blood Pressure

The major sources of calcium in Western countries are milk and other dairy products [12]. The calcium intake is generally much higher in Western countries than in Oriental populations. Both in Western and in Oriental populations, there has been a trend toward higher intake of calcium over the last 10 years. It has been claimed experimentally that a higher intake of calcium lowers blood pressure [13, 14] and that the higher the calcium intake, the lower the blood pressure [15]. Some population data showing a negative correlation between calcium intake and blood pressure have been claimed to be erroneous, and it has been stated that the results of the study do not show a significant relationship between calcium intake and blood pressure in any age, sex, or racial group in the USA. Epidemiological evidence, however, does not support the hypothesis that a higher calcium intake lowers blood pressure. In Finland, the calcium intake is one of the highest in the world [16], and Finnish mortality due to cerebrovascular disease is also one

Table 9. Multiple regression analysis[a] of blood pressure vs Na/K and Ca/Mg ratio in the People's Republic of China (by region)

Males ($n = 1002$)	Na/K	Na/K*Reg	Ca/Mg	Ca/Mg*Reg	R^b
SBP	+0.698	—	—	−7.048	0.43
	(3.78)			(−5.24)	
DBP-4	+0.336	—	—	−4.272	0.47
	(2.55)			(−4.15)	
DBP-5	—	—	—	−4.258	0.46
				(−3.51)	
Females ($n = 1006$)					
SBP	+0.806	—	—	−3.900	0.56
	(3.61)			(−2.45)	
DBP-4	—	+0.753	—	—	0.52
		(3.44)			
DBP-5	—	+0.739	—	—	0.52
		(3.28)			

Partial regression coefficients are given together with t-values in parentheses
[a] With inclusion of age, weight, height, heart rate, Na/K and Ca/Mg molar rates, region (North = 1; South = 0), and all interaction terms
[b] Multiple correlation coefficient with all significant ($P < 0.05$) factors included

Table 10. Multiple regression analysis[a] of blood pressure vs Na/K and Ca/Mg ratio in the People's Republic of China (by occupation)

Males (n = 1002)	Na/K	Na/K*Occ	Ca/Mg	Ca/Mg*Occ	R[b]
SBP	—	+0.952 (4.61)	−4.894 (−5.43)	—	0.43
DBP-4	−0.777 (−2.53)	+1.366 (4.02)	—	−3.622 (−5.32)	0.46
DBP-5	−0.779 (−2.13)	+1.203 (2.97)	—	−3.215 (−3.95)	0.45
Females (n = 1006)					
SBP	+0.863 (3.75)	—	−4.193 (−4.31)	—	0.53
DBP-4	—	+0.756 (3.57)	—	−3.059 (−3.94)	0.51
DBP-5	—	+0.622 (2.85)	−1.654 (−2.42)	—	0.50

Partial regression coefficients are given together with t-values in parentheses
[a] With inclusion of age, weight, height, heart rate, Na/K and Ca/Mg molar rates, occupation (nonfarmer = 1; farmer = 0), and all interaction terms
[b] Multiple correlation coefficient with all significant ($P < 0.05$) factors included

Table 11. Multiple regression analysis[a] of blood pressure vs Na/K and Ca/Mg ratio in the People's Republic of China (nonfarmers)

Males (n = 806)	Na/K	Na/K*Reg	Ca/Mg	Ca/Mg*Reg	R[b]
SBP	+0.870 (4.40)	—	—	−6.275 (−4.21)	0.46
DBP-4	+0.506 (3.62)	—	—	−4.517 (−4.29)	0.48
DBP-5	+0.369 (2.14)	—	—	−4.499 (−3.60)	0.45
Females (n = 646)					
SBP	—	+1.351 (3.21)	—	—	0.62
DBP-4	—	+1.143 (3.86)	—	—	0.57
DBP-5	—	+1.226 (3.91)	—	—	0.54

Partial regression coefficients are given together with t-values in parentheses
[a] With inclusion of age, weight, height, heart rate, Na/K and Ca/Mg molar rates, region (North = 1; South = 0), and all interaction terms
[b] Multiple correlation coefficient with all significant ($P < 0.05$) factors included

of the highest in the Western world, although it has been decreasing rapidly in recent years [17]. Compared with the extent of the differences in calcium intake between populations, the changes in calcium intake due to time trends within countries such as Belgium, the Netherlands, and Japan, are rather small [18], and cannot explain the large drop in cerebrovascular mortality with has occurred in these countries.

Calcium, Water Hardness, and Blood Pressure

Evidence exists of a significant negative relationship between hardness of drinking water and total, cardiovascular, and cerebrovascular death rates [19]. The most important determinant of water hardness is the amount of calcium and magnesium bicarbonate present in the water. In a recent review of all involved factors it was concluded that the available evidence favors magnesium as the protective factor in water, but that more evidence is needed before definite conclusions can be drawn [20].

This is underlined by the fact that in the PRC, 24-h urinary magnesium excretion correlates positively with blood pressure.

Magnesium and Blood Pressure

In Belgium a negative relationship was found between 24-h urinary magnesium excretion and blood pressure [3]. In the PRC, however, 24-h urinary magnesium correlated positively with blood pressure and a highly significant negative correlation was found between the Ca/Mg ratio and both systolic and diastolic pressure (Tables 9–11).

Discussion

In the past epidemiological evidence has often been considered "soft" evidence since it is difficult to control or to correct for all possible factors that could influence blood pressure levels in the population. However, it has been shown that mean population blood pressure levels can be measured accurately because the mean values obtained on different days are nearly identical [2]. Moreover, epidemiology is the only method to study the influence on blood pressrue, in individuals and in the population, of a given substance, e.g. sodium, consumed over a period of 40 or 50 years. In practice the study of such a relationship could not be duplicated by an experiment. The results of epidemiological studies should, of course, be compared with the results of experimental and human interventional studies but the reverse is equally true.

The relationship between sodium, potassium and blood pressure remains complex. In Eastern countries with a high sodium consumption (Japan, Korea and most of the PRC) a positive relationship of sodium with blood pressure and a negative one for potassium with blood pressure are generally found [1, 2, 21–23]. Besides a high sodium intake, these countries also have a low intake of potassium, calcium, and protein of animal origin. In Western countries the reverse holds true. In these countries, however, even large epidemiological surveys have been unable to demonstrate a positive correlation between sodium intake and blood pressure, or a negative one with potassium. The conclusion should be that at the present level of intake, and in combination with a high intake of potassium, calcium, magnesium, and animal protein, the role of sodium as a determinant of blood pressure appears to be minor in Western countries. Other factors, such as a higher alcohol intake in Western populations and a spontaneous reduction of sodium intake by subjects with high blood pressure or a family history of the disease should, however, also be taken into account [24].

There can be little doubt that total serum calcium correlates positively with blood pressure. This can be concluded from the strength of the association and from the fact that it was established in several studies. Some doubts, however, still persist on whether this effect is independent of serum albumin concentration. While this was the case in some studies, in others the slope of the effect of calcium on blood pressure was weakened when serum albumin was included in the multiple regression [16]. In a recent study performed by our department in a Belgian population sample with a high lipid and alcohol intake and with high levels of blood pressure, we were unable to confirm the relationship between serum calcium and blood pressure except in one subgroup. In this group total protein significantly correlates with blood pressure. If hypertension results in a reduction of blood volume and an increase in serum albumin, which is an important determinant of the level of total serum calcium, the increase in total serum calcium could be the result rather than the cause of arterial hypertension. The matter is even more complex, as total serum calcium correlates positively with potassium intake and negatively with sodium intake. No definite statement about the causality of the association between total serum calcium and blood pressure can be made at this moment. The relationship between ionized serum calcium and blood pressure also remains controversial.

In our opinion, until recently the strongest evidence pointed to a positive relationship between 24-h urinary excreted calcium and blood pressure, the correlation being positive in Belgium and Korea. Since in adults urinary excreted calcium is related to intake, this would point to a blood-pressure-raising effect of dietary calcium. The fact that in the PRC, however, 24-h urinary calcium correlates negatively with blood pressure undermines this assumption.

The evidence concerning the relationship between dietary calcium intake and blood pressure is also contradictory. It has been claimed that in experimental studies, the addition of calcium to the diet lowers blood pressure, but nutritional surveys have found no correlation between the individual level of calcium intake and blood pressure. Moreover, countries with a high calcium intake are not protected against cerebrovascular disease; on the contrary. The picture does not become clearer from studying the negative relationship between water hardness and cardiovascular and cerebrovascular death rates, as the evidence favors magnesium as the possible protective factor.

The facts remain, however, that intracellular vascular smooth muscle calcium plays an important role as a determinant of vascular tone [25] and that calcium antagonists lower blood pressure [26]. Whether blood pressure at the population level can be influenced by modulating the dietary intake of calcium remains to be established.

Summarizing, we can state that the relationship between cations and blood pressure as studied by epidemiological methods remains complex. Conflicting evidence exists about the role of most ions, and the situation is made even more complex by the significant interactions between cations. We can only make statements about the effect of cations at a certain level of intake. More epidemiological and interventional studies concerning the role of cations in blood pressure regulation are necessary in order to establish whether some general patterns can be recognized.

References

1. Kesteloot H, Park BC, Lee CS, Brems-Heyns E, Claessens J, Joossens JV (1980) A comparative study of blood pressure and sodium intake in Belgium and Korea. Eur J Cardiol 11:169–182
2. Kesteloot H, Park BC, Lee CS, Brems-Heyns E, Joossens JV (1980) A comparative study of blood pressure and sodium intake in Belgium and in Korea. In: Kesteloot H, Joossens JV (eds) Epidemiology of arterial blood pressure. Martinus Nijhoff, The Hague, pp 453–470
3. Kesteloot H (1984) Urinary cations and blood pressure—population studies. Ann Clin Res 16 (Suppl 43): 72–80
4. Kesteloot H, Geboers J (1982) Calcium and blood pressure. Lancet 1:813–815
5. Bulpitt CJ, Hodes C, Everitt MG (1976) The relationship between blood pressure and biochemical risk factors in a general population. Br J Prev Soc Med 30:158–162
6. Robinson D, Bailey AR, Williams PT (1982) Calcium and blood pressure. Lancet 2:1215
7. Sangal AK, Beevers DG (1982) Serum calcium and blood pressure. Lancet 2:493
8. Kesteloot H, Geboers J, Van Hoof R (1983) Epidemiological study of the relationship between calcium and blood pressure. Hypertension 5 (Suppl II): 52–56
9. McCarron DA (1982) Low serum concentration of ionized calcium in patients with hypertension. N Engl J Med 307:226–228
10. Kesteloot H, Van Schaftingen E, Van Hoof R, Geboers J (1983) Relationship between ionized serum calcium and blood pressure (abstract). Circulation 68:90
11. Kesteloot H (1984) Epidemiological studies on the relationship between sodium, potassium, calcium, and magnesium and arterial blood pressure. J Cardiovasc Pharmacol 6 (Suppl I): S192–S196
12. Block G, Dresser CM, Hartman AM, Carroll MD (1985) Nutrient sources in the American diet: quantitative data from the NHANES II survey. I. Vitamins and minerals. Am J Epidemiol 122:13–26
13. Ayachi S (1979) Increased dietary calcium lowers blood pressure in the spontaneously hypertensive rat. Metabolism 28:1234–1238
14. McCarron DA (1982) Calcium, magnesium, and phosphorus balance in human and experimental hypertension. Hypertension 4 (Suppl III): 27–33
15. McCarron DA, Morris CD, Cole C (1982) Dietary calcium in human hypertension. Science 217:267–269
16. Pietinen P, Dougherty R, Mutanen M, Leino U, Moisoi S, Iacono J, Puska P (1984) Dietary intervention study among 30 free living families in Finland. J Am Diet Ass 84:313–317
17. Tuomilehto J, Geboers J, Joossens JV, Salonen JT, Tanskanen A (1984) Trends in stomach cancer and stroke in Finland. Comparison to Northwest Europe and USA. Stroke 15:823–828
18. Tanaka H, Tanaka Y, Hayashi M, Ueda Y, Date C, Baba T, Shoji H, Horimoto T, Owada K (1982) Secular trends in mortality for cerebrovascular diseases in Japan, 1960 to 1979. Stroke 13:574–581
19. Masironi R (1970) Cardiovascular mortality in relation to radioactivity and hardness of local water supplies in the USA. Bull WHO 43:687–697
20. Kesteloot H (1985) Blood pressure, calcium and water hardness. In: Bulpitt CJ (ed) Epidemiology of hypertension. Handbook of hypertension, vol 6. Elsevier, Amsterdam, pp 216–229
21. Sasaki N (1980) Epidemiological studies on hypertension in Northeast Japan. In: Kesteloot H, Joossens JV (eds) Epidemiology of arterial blood pressure. Martinus Nijhoff, The Hague, pp 367–377
22. Komachi Y, Shimamoto T (1980) Salt intake and its relationship to blood pressure in Japan:

present and past. In: Kesteloot H, Joossens JV (eds) Epidemiology of arterial blood pressure. Martinus Nijhoff, The Hague, pp 395–400

23. Yamori Y, Nara Y, Kihara M, Horie R, Hoshima A (1981) Sodium and other dietary factors in experimental and human hypertension: the Japanese experience. In: Laragh JH, Buhler FE, Seldin DW (eds) Frontiers in hypertension research. Springer, New York Berlin Heidelberg, pp 46–48

24. Kesteloot H, Vuylsteke M, Costenoble A (1980) Relationship between blood pressure and sodium and potassium intake in a Belgian male population group. In: Kesteloot H, Joossens JV (eds) Epidemiology of arterial blood pressure. Martinus Nijhoff, The Hague, pp 345–351

25. Blaustein MP (1977) Sodium ions, calcium ions, blood pressure regulation and hypertension: a reassessment and a hypothesis. Am J Physiol 232:C165–C173

26. Aoki K, Kondo S, Mochizuki A, Yoshida T, Kato S, Kato K, Takikawa K (1978) Antihypertensive effects of cardiovascular calcium-antagonists in hypertensive patients in the presence and absence of beta-adrenergic blockade. Am Heart J 96:218–226

Hemodynamic Effects of Diltiazem in the Spontaneously Hypertensive Rat and in Human Essential Hypertension

E. D. Frohlich

Alton Ochsner Medical Foundation, New Orleans, LA 70121, USA

Summary. Hemodynamically, the elevated arterial pressure in both the patient with essential hypertension and in the experimental laboratory counterpart, the spontaneously hypertensive rat, is characterized by an increased total peripheral resistance that is more or less uniformly distributed throughout the various organ circulations. Cardiac output and organ blood flows are usually well maintained until severe adaptive hypertrophy of the left ventricle occurs and then heart failure supervenes unless antihypertensive therapy intervenes. Until recently, most forms of antihypertensive therapy that reduce arterial pressure through a reduced total peripheral resistance were associated with cardiac fluid retention or cardiac stimulation. Recent hemodynamic studies in both man and the rat demonstrate that the calcium entry-blocking agent diltiazem reduces arterial pressure through a fall in total peripheral resistance without reflexive cardiac stimulation or fluid retention with prolonged treatment. Further, this action is associated with renal vasodilation and, in man, a reduction in left ventricular mass.

Key words: Cardiac output—Organ blood flows—Essential hypertension—Spontaneously hypertensive rat (SHR)—Calcium entry blocking drugs

Over the past three decades, the field of hypertension has witnessed dramatic changes in the appreciation of the magnitude of the clinical problem and its impact on associated diseases, in its recognition in populations, in the evaluation of potential patients, and in its treatment. As a result, the awesome cardiovascular morbidity and mortality due to hypertensive disease has become eminently treatable and is no longer a uniformly fatal problem. Strokes have been reduced by over 40% in the United States. Congestive heart failure due to hypertension has been remarkably diminished. These outstanding advances have been attained by an increasingly sophisticated appreciation of the fundamental epidemiological, clinical, and therapeutic questions [1]. Obviously, behind these achievements has been a remarkable increase in our comprehension of the underlying fundamental mechanisms of the disease [2]. This has truly been the result of a multidisciplinary effort involving the anatomist, biochemist, cell biologist, immunologist, pharmacologist, physiologist, clinical scientist, and others.

No doubt, these clinical successes have been related directly to the development of major pharmacological entities; but it should be recognized that parallel with these contributions has been the understanding of basic disease mechanisms and their respective roles in the nature of the clinical disease. This discussion, then, relates to our present overall view of the most common form of the hypertensive diseases, essential hypertension, its hemodynamic characteristics, and a relatively new approach to its treatment with an agent that specifically attacks the hemodynamic abnormality.

Essential Hypertension and the Spontaneously Hypertensive Rat

Essential hypertension is that diagnostic grouping of the hypertensive diseases that affects over 95% of all patients with systemic arterial hypertension. In general, it has been considered a disease of unknown etiology. However, in recent years, more investigators of this disease have come to consider it a clinical problem that is produced by a dysregulation of the many mechanisms that serve to control arterial pressure [3]. Thus, there are a large number of factors that maintain arterial pressure and tissue perfusion at normal levels in the normotensive individual; among these are hemodynamic, neural, renal, renopressor, volume and electrolyte controlling, hormonal, and genetic mechanisms. Each mechanism is dependent upon the other; thus, Page offered his Mosaic Theory even before antihypertensive therapy was a reality [4].

There are certain characteristics of the patient with hypertension. There is no one cause of the disease. There is a certain genetic predisposition. The elevated arterial pressure seems to be associated with a faster heart rate. The patient population seems to be a heavier one compared with an age-, race-, and gendermatched normotensive population.

To provide an experimental laboratory counterpart for studying this disease, a number of experimental animal models have been developed. The rat provides a very logical counterpart since it is easy to breed, it is relatively cheap to obtain and maintain, it is very similar physiologically to man, and its life span is only 3 years. Over 20 years ago, Aoki developed by genetic inbreeding techniques a strain of Wistar rats that naturally and uniformly develops hypertension [5]. This rat model of genetic hypertension, the spontaneously hypertensive rat, has been [6] and still is [7] considered the best experimental model for human essential hypertension that is presently available.

General Hemodynamic Considerations

The hemodynamic hallmark of essential hypertension is an increased total peripheral resistance that, for the most part, is uniformly distributed throughout the organ circulations [8, 9]. As the disease progresses in severity, arterial pressure and total peripheral resistance increase *pari passu*, and the heart structurally adapts to this increasing afterload by the development of left ventricular hypertrophy [10–12]. The related biochemical consequence is increased myocardial oxygen consumption secondary to the increased arterial (i.e., systolic) pressure and the increased chamber diameter [2, 13, 14]. In addition to the cardiac structural changes are associated structural generalized arteriolar changes [15].

In addition to these pathophysiological changes that are related to the disease process, antihypertensive treatment may promote other physiological changes

[16, 17]. Thus, as arterial pressure is reduced pharmacologically, intravascular (plasma) volume tends to expand with most agents except for the diuretics, beta-adrenergic receptor blockers, and probably angiotensin coverting enzyme inhibitors and calcium entry-blocking drugs [18, 19]. Experience with these latter compounds most likely explains why they have been used as monotherapy in patients with hypertension and why the other classes of antihypertensive drugs, e.g., direct vascular smooth muscle relaxants and adrenergic inhibitors, are usually used with diuretics. Diuretics prevent volume expansion and the phenomenon of "pseudotolerance" and enhance the effectiveness of the other antihypertensive drugs. This explains why these have been used as first-step agents for the treatment of hypertension. A second important consideration in selecting antihypertensive therapy is the possibility that reflex cardiac stimulation may occur with those agents that do not inhibit adrenergic input to the cardiovascular system [16, 17, 20]. Recent reports indicate that cardiac stimulation does not occur as pressure is reduced also by the angiotensin converting enzyme inhibitors [21], angiotensin receptor inhibition [22], and possibly some of the calcium entry-blocking drugs [23, 24]. This concept is of major importance because reflex cardiac stimulation will increase myocardial metabolism and would therefore aggravate preexisting coronary arterial disease, cardiac decompensation, or aortic dissection.

It, therefore, follows that the ideal antihypertensive agent should reduce arterial pressure primarily by decreasing total peripheral resistance through a relatively uniform decline in vascular resistance in the major organ circulations of the body. The resultant arteriolar dilation should be produced in particular in the primary target organs of the disease—the kidneys heart, and brain. Further, the pressure reduction should be accomplished without secondary extracellular fluid retention or reflex cardiac stimulation. If there is some regression in the structural lesions of the heart and arterioles, this should be done without altering organ function. The discussion that follows will be concerned with whether the calcium entry-blocking drugs measure up to these criteria.

Experimental methods
In order to evaluate the hemodynamic effects of the calcium entry-blocking drug diltazem, we complemented our clinical studies in man with data obtained from normotensive Wistar-Kyoto (WKY) and age- and sex-matched spontaneously hypertensive (SHR) rats.

In brief, our protocol subjected WKY and SHR rats to a 3-week treatment period in a manner similar to that which we have reported for most of the antihypertensive drugs that we use, including methyldopa [25–27], clonidine [27], hydralazine [27], angiotensin converting enzyme inhibitors [28], prazosin [29], urapidil [29, 30], calcium entry-blocking drugs [24, 31], and others [32]. We have, therefore, developed a standardized bioassay (in effect, a long-term hemodynamic assay) for ascertaining the comparative effects of new antihypertensive compounds. Thus, at the end of a 3-week treatment period, with the animal under light ether anesthesia, catheters were placed through the femoral artery into the left ventricle, through the carotid artery, and into the femoral vein, and then exteriorized at the back of the neck. When the animal had fully recovered from this procedure, the microspheres were injected. Using the reference method, we determined cardiac output from the radioactive "envelope" of withdrawn arterial blood [33] and then measured radioactivity in all organs to determine the percentage distribution of cardiac output to each organ [34]. Then, by multiplying the ratio of radioactive counts in any organ to the total radioactivity injected by the cardiac output, we calculated a quantitative representation of blood flow to every organ of the body. Moreover, by recording arterial pressure directly, we were also able to calculate the changes in organ vascular resistances (as compared with control rats that were not given the drug). In each study, net organ weights were obtained in order to determine possible changes in organ mass with therapy and to obtain blood flow and vascular resistance indices.

Our clinical studies were conducted in patients with essential hypertension. In these studies, the systemic and regional hemodynamic effects of diltiazem and nitrendipine were determined using previously reported hemodynamic methods from our laboratory [35, 36]. In brief, all patients came to our laboratory in the morning after an overnight fast and after having not received antihypertensive drugs for at least 4 weeks. Polyethylene tubing was inserted into a brachial artery and antecubital vein to shoulder level for measurement of pressures, injection of dye or vasoactive agents, and withdrawal of arterial blood for inscription of the dye curves. Indocyanine green dye, injected centrally and through the vein, permitted calculation of cardiac output. Renal and splanchnic blood flows were determined by injection of radioiodinated para-amino-hippurate and indocyanine green dye, respectively. Hemodynamic indices were calculated by standard methods. Plasma renin activity, circulating norepinephrine levels, and plasma volume were determined by previously reported methods from our laboratory. M-mode echocardiographic techniques were likewise employed to determine structural and functional cardiac changes [37].

In all studies, in the rat or man, standard statistical techniques using Student's t-test for paired data analysis or the patient as his own control were employed.

Hemodynamic Effects of Diltiazem

Clinical studies
We have obtained preliminary hemodynamic measurements in seven patients with uncomplicated essential hypertension who first received intravenous diltiazem (0.24 mg/kg in divided doses) and were then treated with the oral formulation for 4 weeks. These seven patients, whose age averaged 47 years, included six men and one woman. Following logarithmically incremental doses (0.06, 0.06, and 0.12 mg/kg, i.v.), arterial pressure progressively fell from 118 to 101 mmHg within quite a short period of time. This was associated with a reflexive increase in heart rate, cardiac index, and left ventricular ejection rate index, as calculated total peripheral resistance declined (Table 1). When these same patients continued treatment for 4 weeks (60 mg b.i.d. to 120 mg b.i.d.), arterial (systolic/ diastolic) pressures fell from 165/95 to 149/86 mmHg, respectively, after 4 weeks. However, the reflexive increase in heart rate, cardiac index, and left ventricular ejection rate was no longer observed and total peripheral resistance

Table 1. Immediate hemodynamic effects of diltiazem (i.v.) in seven patients with essential hypertension

Index	Control	Dose (mg/kg)		
		0.06	0.06	0.12
Mean arterial pressure (mmHg)	118	107[a]	107[a]	101[a]
Heart rate (beats/min)	65	75[a]	78[a]	78[a]
Cardiac index (l/min/m^2)	3.1	4.0	4.3	5.0
Total peripheral resistance index (U/m^2)	40	28[a]	26[a]	23[a]
Left ventricular ejection rate index (ml/s/m^2)	153	175[a]	183[a]	194[a]

[a] Represents statistical significance at least at the $P < 0.05$ level

Table 2. Preliminary data from seven patients with essential hypertension treated for 4 weeks with diltiazem (60–120 mg BID)

Index	Control	Treatment
Mean arterial pressure (mmHg)	118	107[a]
Heart rate (beats/min)	65	62
Cardiac index (l/min/m^2)	3.1	3.0
Total peripheral resistance index (ml/s/m^2)	40	37[a]
Left ventricular ejection rate index (ml/s/m^2)	153	154
Left ventricular mass (g)	242	217[a]
Posterior wall thickness (cm)	1.1	1.1
Septal thickness (cm)	1.2	1.2
Ejection fraction (%)	62	62
Fractional fiber shortening (%)	33	34
Renal blood flow (ml/min/m^2)	390	479[a]
Renal vascular resistance (m/m^2)	0.167	0.12[a]
Glomerular filtration rate (ml/min)	134	120
Filtration fraction (%)	17.4	12.9[a]
Splanchnic blood flow (ml/min)	741	766
Splanchnic vascular resistance (U/m^2)	0.176	0.152

[a] Represents statistical significance at least at the $P < 0.05$ level

was further reduced. Echocardiographic measurements demonstrated reduced left ventricular mass although other structural and functional measurements remained unchanged [36] (Table 2). Thus, following the immediate reflexive stimulation with intravenous diltiazem, more prolonged therapy evoked either some form of baroreceptor "adaptation" or lesser adrenergic stimulation of the heart.

Rat studies
When the rats were treated with diltiazem (60 mg/day by gastric tube), no systemic hemodynamic changes were observed in the normotensive WKY; how-

Table 3. Effects of 3-week diltiazem treatment in normotensive (WKY) and spontaneously hypertensive (SHR) rats on organ hemodynamics

	Organ blood flow		Organ vascular resistance	
	WKY	SHR	WKY	SHR
Skin	Decrease	Decrease	Increase	No change
Skeletal muscle	No change	No change	No change	No change
Brain	No change	Increase	No change	Decrease
Heart	Increase	Decrease	Decrease	No change
Lung	Decrease	Decrease	Increase	No change
Kidneys	Decrease	Decrease	Increase	No change
Splanchnic organs	No change	Decrease	Increase	Decrease
Testes	No change	No change	Increase	No change

ever, this treatment produced a significant fall in arterial pressure that was associated with a fall in total peripheral resistance in SHR. These systemic hemodynamic changes were also associated with some slowing of heart rate and reduction in cardiac index that were not statistically significant. There were no changes in left ventricular mass or the weight ratio of the left ventricle to the total body. We also determined changes in organ hemodynamics in these WKY and SHR. In the normotensive WKY, vascular resistance increased in the skin, lungs, kidneys, splanchnic organs, and testes, but decreased in the heart. In contrast, vascular resistance decreased in the brain and the splanchnic organs of the SHR, but remained unchanged in the other organs (Table 3) [38]. These findings differed somewhat from our preliminary findings in man with essential hypertension [36].

References

1. Levy RI, Moskowitz J (1982) Cardiovascular research: Decades of progress, a decade of promise. Science 217:121
2. Frohlich ED, Messerli FH, Re RN, Dunn FG (1984) Mechanisms controlling arterial pressure. In: Frohlich ED (ed) Pathophysiology: Altered regulatory mechanisms in disease, 3rd edn. Lippincott, Philadelphia, p 45
3. Frohlich ED (1983) Mechanisms contributing to high blood pressure. Ann Intern Med 98:709
4. Page IH (1960) Mosaic theory of hypertension. In: Bode KD, Cottier PT (eds) Essential hypertension: An international symposium. Springer, Berlin Heidelberg New York, p 1
5. Okamoto K, Aoki K (1963) Development of a strain of spontaneously hypertensive rats. Jpn Circ J 27:282
6. Udenfriend S, Spector S (1972) Spontaneously hypertensive rat. Science 176:1155
7. Frohlich ED (in press) Is the SHR a model for human hypertension? J Hypertension
8. Frohlich ED (1977) Haemodynamics of hypertension. In: Genest J, Koiw E, Kuchel O (eds) Hypertension: Physiopathology and treatment. McGraw-Hill, New York, p 15
9. Frohlich ED (1982) Hemodynamic factors in the pathogenesis and maintenance of hypertension. Fed Proceed 41:2400
10. Frohlich ED, Tarazi RC, Dustan HP (1971) Clinical-physiological correlations in the development of hypertensive heart disease. Circulation 44:446
11. Frohlich ED (1983) The heart in hypertension. In: Genest J, Kuchel O, Hamet P, Cantin M

(eds) Hypertension: Physiopathology and treatment, 2nd edn. McGraw-Hill, New York, p 791

12. Frohlich ED (1983) Hemodynamics and other determinants in development of left ventricular hypertrophy: Conflicting factors in its regression. Fed Proceed 42:2709

13. Dunn FG, Frohlich ED (1978) Hypertension and angina pectoris. In: Yu PN, Goodwin JF (eds) Progress in cardiology, vol 7. Lea and Febiger, Philadelphia, p 163

14. Sarnoff SJ, Braunwald E, Welch GH Jr, Case RB, Stainsby WN, Macruz R (1958) Hemodynamic determinants of oxygen consumption of the heart with special reference to the tension time index. Am J Physiol 192:148

15. Folkow B, Hallback M, Lundgren Y, Sivertsson R, Weiss L (1973) Importance of adaptive changes in vascular design for establishment of primary hypertension studied in man and in spontaneously hypertensive rats. Circ Res 32 (I): 2

16. Frohlich ED (1978) Essential hypertension: Hemodynamics, pressor mechanisms, and mechanisms of drug action. In: Onesti G, Brest AN (eds) Hypertension: Mechanisms, diagnosis and treatment. Davis, Philadelphia, p 197

17. Frohlich ED (1984) Newer antihypertensive drugs. In: Yu PN, Goodwin JF (eds) Progress in cardiology, vol 12. Lea and Febiger, Philadelphia, p 265

18. Weil JV, Chidsey CA (1968) Plasma volume expansion resulting from interference with adrenergic function in normal man. Circulation 37:54

19. Dustan HP, Tarazi RC, Bravo EL (1973) Dependence of arterial pressure on intravascular volume in treated hypertensive patients. N Engl J Med 286:861

20. Bhatia S, Frohlich ED (1973) Hemodynamic comparison of agents useful in hypertensive emergencies. Am Heart J 85:367

21. Dunn FG, Oigman W, Ventura HO, Messerli FH, Kobrin I, Frohlich ED (1984) Enalapril improves systemic and renal hemodynamics and allows regression of left ventricular mass in essential hypertension. Am J Cardiol 53:105

22. De Carvalho JGR, Dunn FG, Kem DC, Chrysant SG, Frohlich ED (1978) Hemodynamic correlates of saralasin-induced arterial pressure changes. Circulation 57:373

23. Pegram BL, Kobrin I, Sesoko S, Frohlich ED (1984) Nitrendipine: Hemodynamic effects in conscious normotensive and spontaneously hypertensive rats. J Cardiovasc Pharmacol 6:S1016

24. Kobrin I, Sesoko S, Pegram BL, Frohlich ED (1984) Reduced cardiac mass by nitrendipine is dissociated from systemic or regional haemodynamic changes in rats. Cardiovasc Res 3:158

25. Kuwajima I, Kardon MB, Pegram BL, Sesoko S, Frohlich ED (1982) Regression of left ventricular hypertrophy in two-kidney, one clip Goldblatt hypertension. Hypertension 4 (II): 113

26. Ishise S, Pegram BL, Frohlich ED (1980) Disparate effects of methyldopa and clonidine on cardiac mass and haemodynamics in rats. Clin Sci 59 (Suppl 6): 449s

27. Pegram BL, Ishise S, Frohlich ED (1982) Effect of methyldopa, clonidine and hydralazine on cardiac mass and haemodynamics in Wistar-Kyoto and spontaneously hypertensive rats. Cardiovasc Res 16:40

28. Pegram BL, Frohlich ED (1982) Immediate systemic and regional hemodynamic effects of MK-421 converting enzyme inhibitor in conscious Wistar-Kyoto and spontaneously hypertensive rats. In: Rasher W, Clough D, Genton D (eds) Hypertensive mechanisms of the spontaneously hypertensive rat as a model for human hypertension. Schattauer, New York, p 677

29. Pegram BL, Kobrin I, Natsume T, Gallo AJ, Frohlich ED (1984) Systemic and regional hemodynamic effects of acute and prolonged treatment with urapidil or prazosin in normotensive and spontaneously hypertensive rats. Am J Med 77 (4A):64

30. Kobrin I, Gallo AJ, Pegram BL, Duckworth D, Frohlich ED (1984) Urapidil in normotensive and spontaneously hypertensive rats: Systemic and regional hemodynamics, cardiac mass and arterial baroreflex sensitivity. J Hypertension 2:317

31. Sesoko S, Pegram BL, Frohlich ED (1984) Systemic and regional hemodynamics in normotensive and spontaneously hypertensive rats after slow-channel calcium blocker nitrendipine. Clin Exper Hyper A6:979

32. Gallo A, Kobrin I, Pegram BL, Frohlich ED (1985) Hemodynamic effects of a new alpha- and

beta-adrenergic receptor inhibitor with calcium entry blocking effects (CGS 10078B) in WKY and SHR rats. Am J Med Sci 290:47

33. Tsuchiya M, Walsh GM, Frohlich ED (1977) Systemic hemodynamic effects of microspheres in conscious rats. Am J Physiol 233:H617

34. Ishise S, Pegram BL, Yamamoto J, Kitamura Y, Frohlich ED (1980) Reference sample microsphere method: cardiac output and blood flows in conscious rats. Am J Physiol 239:H443

35. Ventura HO, Messerli FH, Oigman W, Dunn FG, Reisin E, Frohlich ED (1983) Immediate hemodynamic effects of a new calcium-channel blocking agent (nitrendipine) in essential hypertension. Am J Cardiol 51:783

36. Amodeo C, Kobrin I, Ventura HO, Messerli FH, Frohlich ED (1986) Immediate and short-term hemodynamic effects of diltiazem in patients with hypertension. Circulation 73:108

37. Dunn FG, Chandraratna P, de Carvalho JGR, Basta LL, Frohlich ED (1977) Pathophysiological assessment of hypertensive heart disease with echocardiography. Am J Cardiol 39:789

38. Natsume T, Gallo A, Pegram BL, Frohlich ED (1985) Hemodynamic effects of prolonged treatment with diltiazem in conscious normotensive and spontaneously hypertensive rats. Clin Exper Hyper A7:1471

Hemodynamic Changes in Essential Hypertension and the Hemodynamic Effects of Calcium Antagonists

P. Lund-Johansen and P. Omvik

Cardiology Section, Medical Department A, University of Bergen, School of Medicine, Bergen, Norway

Summary. The cardinal hemodynamic disorder in essential hypertension is an increased total peripheral resistance. In young hypertensives, this is clearly seen during muscular exercise, although calculated resistance might be "normal" during rest. The purpose of the present study was to investigate the hemodynamic effects of three calcium-channel blockers (calcium antagonists)—verapamil, nifedipine, and nisoldipine—in patients with mild to moderate hypertension.

Forty-four patients aged 20–64 years with a pretreatment diastolic blood pressure of between 100 and 120 mmHg were studied at rest and during exercise on an ergometer bicycle. Blood pressure was recorded intra-arterially; cardiac output was measured by Cardiogreen. After the initial study, 10 patients were treated with verapamil (dose 40–80 mg three times daily), 15 with nifedipine (long-acting form, 20–80 mg daily), and 19 with nisoldipine (10–40 mg daily). After 1 year, the hemodynamic study was repeated. The immediate response to the first dose was studied in the nisoldipine series.

All drugs induced a reduction in blood pressure and in total peripheral resistance without any reduction in cardiac index. Heart rate was reduced on verapamil, particularly during exercise, but this was compensated by an increase in the stroke volume. Reflex tachycardia was seen in the first 2 h after the very first dose of nisoldipine. After 1 year (on nifedipine), heart rate was unchanged compared with the pretreatment level at rest as well as during exercise. The hemodynamic profile of the calcium-channel blockers clearly differs from the hemodynamic effects of beta blockers.

Key words: Hypertension—Hemodynamics—Calcium-channel blockers—Verapamil—Nifedipine—Nisoldipine—Cardiac output—Total peripheral resistance

It is generally accepted that the dominant hemodynamic disturbance in established essential hypertension is an increased total peripheral resistance. This is caused partly by functional, partly by structural changes and reflects increased arteriolar resistance in most vascular beds. The cardiac output during rest is normal or reduced, but during physical exercise it is generally lower than in age-matched normotensive controls [review—1].

In subjects with mild and borderline hypertension in their twenties or thirties, the cardiac output during rest is often increased, while calculated total peripheral resistance is numerically "normal" [2]. However, during muscular exercise total peripheral resistance is abnormally high and cardiac output is then subnormal [1]. When mild hypertension is left untreated over a long period (10–17 years), there is a gradual fall in cardiac index and stroke index and an increase in total peripheral resistance and blood pressure (Fig. 1) [3]. These are the spontaneously occurring changes in central hemodynamics that we would like to reverse by drug therapy.

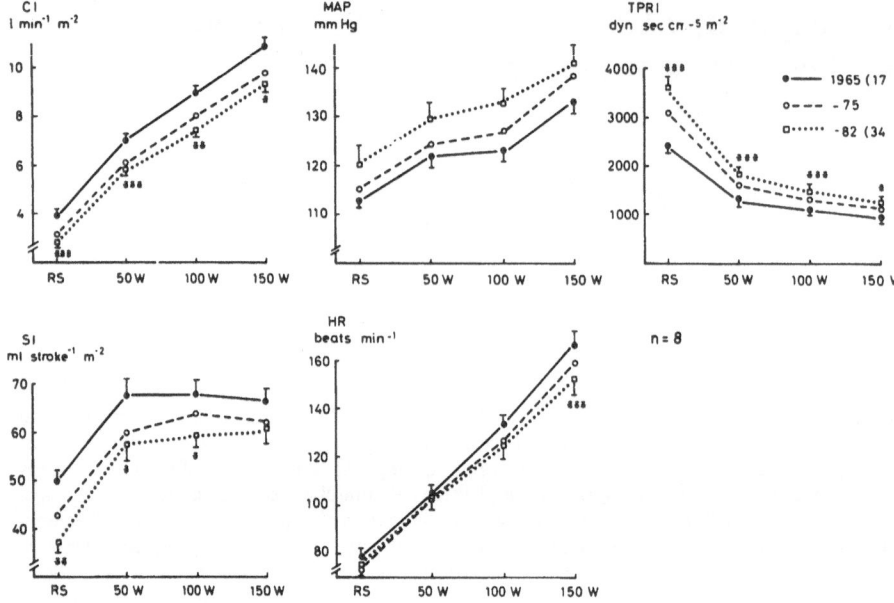

Fig. 1. Hemodynamic changes during a period of 17 years in untreated mild hypertension. *CI* cardiac index, *MAP* mean arterial pressure, *TPRI* total peripheral resistance index, *SI* stroke index, *HR* heart rate. ●——● first study, o------o second study, □······□ third study. Mean values and SEM. *$P < 0.05$, **$P < 0.01$, ***$P < 0.001$

Hemodynamic Effects of Calcium-Channel Blockers

Drugs able to reduce the increased total peripheral resistance without reducing the blood flow would seem to be of particular interest in the treatment of hypertension. Acute hemodynamic studies of the calcium-channel blockers (calcium antagonists) verapamil [4–6] and nifedipine [7–15] would seem to indicate such a hemodynamic profile and similar effects are expected from the newer drugs like nisoldipine. So far, there have been few hemodynamic studies including measurements during exercise.

The purpose of this paper is to review briefly our hemodynamic results at rest and during exercise with three different calcium-channel blockers, verapamil, nifedipine, and nisoldipine, in patients with mild to moderate essential hypertension. The results indicate that the blood pressure reduction is achieved through an acute as well as a chronic reduction in total peripheral resistance without any reduction in blood flow. The verapamil [16] and nifedipine [17] studies have been published previously, while the data from the nisoldipine study are preliminary (as the chronic part of the study is not yet completed).

Material and Methods

The studies included 44 patients (42 males and 2 females) with mild to moderate essential hypertension (diastolic pressure between 100 and 120 mmHg at rest during several visits). Secondary hypertension was excluded by the usual procedures. All but three patients (in the nisoldipine group) were previously untreated and in WHO stage I, actively working without other diseases. The washout period in the three treated patients was 8 weeks. Informed consent was obtained from all patients.

All hemodynamic studies were performed on an outpatient basis at the same time in the morning. Oxygen consumption (VO_2) was measured by the Douglas bag technique using the Beckman automatic gas analyzer for O_2 and CO_2. Blood pressure—systolic (SAP), diastolic (DAP), and mean (MAP)—was recorded continuously by a catheter in the brachial artery and cardiac output (CO) was measured by the dye-dilution technique (Cardiogreen). Duplicate measurements of CO were recorded in all situations. Heart rate (HR) was recorded continuously by electrocardiogram (ECG). Cardiac index (CI), stroke index (SI), and total peripheral resistance index (TPRI) were calculated using conventional formulae.

Procedure in the acute study on nisoldipine
Predrug studies were performed at supine rest, sitting, and during 100-W exercise. The patients ($n = 19$) then swallowed a 10-mg tablet of nisoldipine with one glass of water in the sitting position and rested supinely for 1 h. Hemodynamic recordings were then performed after 1 h, 2 h, and 3 h, all at supine rest. After 3 h and 15 min, measurements were carried out in the sitting position and during 100-W exercise. Thereafter, the patients entered the chronic study and received nisoldipine, 10–40 mg daily, aiming at a sitting blood pressure of 140/90 mmHg without side effects. After approximately 1 year, central hemodynamics were measured at supine rest, sitting, and during 100-W exercise (so far, only 12 of the 19 patients have completed the chronic study).

Procedure in the chronic studies on verapamil and nifedipine
In the predrug situation, the patients were studied at supine rest, sitting, and at three exercise levels (50, 100, and 150 W). Following the first hemodynamic study, the patients were treated with verapamil ($n = 10$), 40–80 mg three times daily, or with nifedipine (long-acting form ($n = 15$), starting with 20 mg twice daily with a gradual increase to 80 mg daily.

After a treatment period of about 1 year, the hemodynamic study was repeated. In the second study, the patients took their morning dose at 7:00 A.M. and the hemodynamic study was performed between 9:00 and 11:00 A.M.

Comparison between verapamil and nifedipine
After the second hemodynamic study, eight of the patients in the verapamil group (all but two on 240 mg daily) had their treatment changed to nifedipine (20–60 mg daily) and had a third hemodynamic study after 1 year on nifedipine long-acting form.

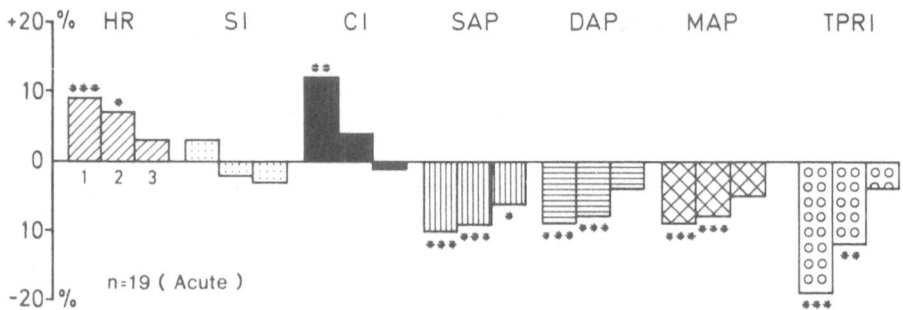

Fig. 2. Relative changes in central hemodynamics 1, 2, and 3 h after first dose of nisoldipine (10 mg) in rest supine, $n = 19$

Results

Nisoldipine group (acute study)

In the first hemodynamic study (before nisoldipine was given), all but one patient had increased total peripheral resistance. At sitting rest, the mean total peripheral resistance (TPRI) was 4055 dyn s cm^{-5} m^2. At the same time, the mean SAP/DAP was 177/109 mmHg, CI 2.66 1 min^{-1} m^{-2}, and HR 73 beats min^{-1}. These figures compare well with the results from other drug studies in our laboratory.

The major changes after the first dose of 10 mg nisoldipine are shown in Fig. 2. One hour after tablet intake, there was a marked decrease in TPRI of 19% ($P < 0.001$) associated with a compensatory increase in heart rate (HR) of 9% ($P < 0.001$) and in CI of +12% ($P < 0.01$). There was a significant reduction in SAP, DAP, and MAP of 9% ($P < 0.001$ for all parameters). During the following 2 h, the effect leveled off, and after 3 h the changes in TPRI, CI, and SAP were -4% (not significant, NS), -1% (NS), and -6% ($P < 0.05$), respectively.

After 3 h sitting at rest, the reductions in SAP, DAP, and MAP were -11%, -8% and -7%, respectively (all P values <0.001). During 100-W exercise, the reductions in the same parameters were -6%, -5%, and -7% (all P-values also <0.001). The reductions in TPRI at sitting rest and during exercise after 3 h were only -6% and -4%, respectively (NS). There were no significant changes in CI.

Since all nisoldipine patients have not yet performed the second hemodynamic study, the chronic results will not be discussed.

Verapamil group (chronic study)

In the first hemodynamic study, all patients had an increased TPRI, mean value 3848 dyn s cm^{-5} m^2, sitting at rest. At the same time, the mean SAP/DAP was 167/102 mmHg, CI 2.70 1 min^{-1} m^{-2}, and HR 73 beats min^{-1}. The results of the hemodynamic measurements before and after verapamil treatment are shown in Fig. 3 and Table 1. The oxygen consumption did not change. At supine and sitting rest, SAP, DAP, and MAP fell in all but one subject. This subject showed no fall in casual blood pressure or intra-arterial blood pressure, and this nonresponder was excluded from the statistical calculations.

On average, MAP fell by 11.7 mmHg (10%) at supine rest and by 13.3 mmHg

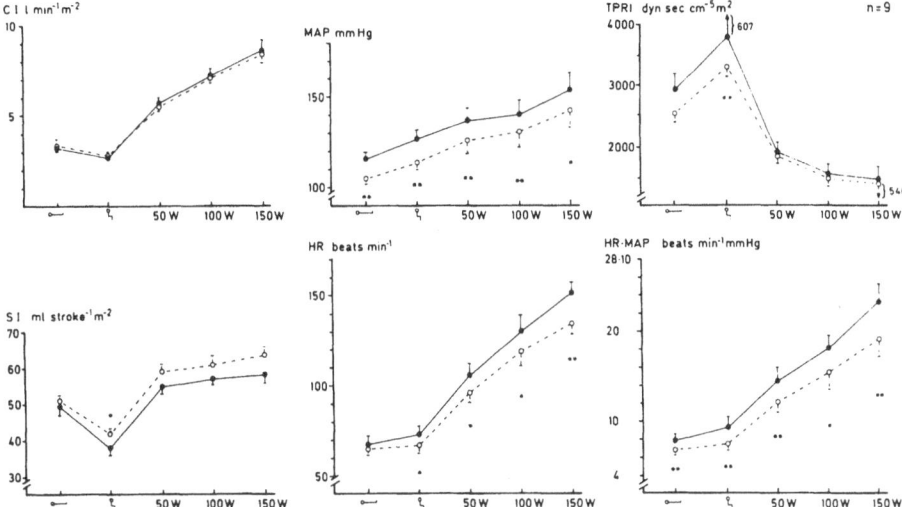

Fig. 3. Cardiac index (*CI*), mean arterial pressure (*MAP*), total peripheral resistance index (*TPRI*), stroke index (*SI*), heart rate (*HR*), and pressure heart rate product (*HR* × *MAP*) at rest and during exercise before (●————●) and after (○------○) verapamil treatment, $n = 9$. Mean values and SEM. * $P < 0.05$, ** $P < 0.01$, *** $P < 0.001$ [16]

(10%) at sitting rest. During exercise, the reductions were somewhat smaller— 10.9, 9.6, and 11.3 mmHg or 8%, 6%, and 7%, respectively (all changes statistically significant). At supine rest, HR showed a small decrease (3%, NS), at sitting rest 8% ($P < 0.05$). However, during exercise (when sympathetic tone is much greater than during rest), HR was significantly reduced at all three work levels— 10, 11, and 17 beats min^{-1}, or 9%, 8%, and 11%, respectively. This reduction in HR was compensated by an increase in SI and consequently the CI was practically unchanged in all situations at rest as well as during exercise.

The TPRI fell in all but one of the responders at rest and in all nine during exercise. The greatest reduction was seen at sitting rest—14% ($P < 0.01$).

Nifedipine group (chronic study)

The pretreatment hemodynamic data were very similar to the corresponding values in the verapamil group. Thus, in the first hemodynamic study, all but one subject had an increased TPRI, the mean value at sitting rest being 3870 dyn s cm^{-5} m^2. At the same time, the SAP/DAP was 166/103 mmHg, CI 2.80 1 min^{-1} m^{-2}, and HR 73 beats min^{-1}. Casual blood pressure fell in all patients. The pretreatment value was 160/104 mmHg; after 6 months the mean value was 140/94 mmHg. There was a slight, but not significant increase in HR from 74 to 77 beats min^{-1}.

The hemodynamic results are shown in Fig. 4 and Table 2.

There were no changes in the oxygen consumption. The reductions in SAP, DAP, and MAP were rather similar at rest as well as during exercise. At sitting

Table 1. Hemodynamic measurements before and after verapamil treatment

	Rest				Work					
	Supine		Sitting		50		100		150	
	1	2	1	2	1	2	1	2	1	2
VO_2 (ml min^{-1} m^{-2})										
Mean			177	163	587	522	887	791	1225	1129
SD			24	44	42	50	82	90	112	120
P		NS		NS		<0.01		<0.05		NS
CI (l min^{-1} m^{-2})										
Mean	3.30	3.32	2.70	2.79	5.69	5.47	7.20	7.10	8.62	8.41
SD	0.86	0.53	0.45	0.22	0.67	0.46	0.93	0.67	1.47	1.40
P		NS		NS		NS		NS		NS
SI (ml stroke^{-1} m^{-2})										
Mean	49.7	51.3	38.2	42.4	54.9	57.9	56.8	60.9	57.7	63.4
SD	13.5	7.2	10.1	6.0	9.2	9.1	11.3	11.1	12.5	12.5
P		NS		<0.05		NS		NS		NS
HR (beats min^{-1})										
Mean	67.3	65.3	72.7	67.0	105.6	96.1	129.9	119.4	151.3	134.4
SD	11.8	9.3	13.3	11.1	17.7	13.8	24.0	21.5	15.0	15.5
P		NS		<0.05		<0.02		<0.02		<0.001
SAP (mmHg)										
Mean	158.0	142.9	167.4	154.2	187.6	175.2	196.2	186.7	214.9	202.0
SD	12.5	8.8	16.3	15.2	26.0	24.0	29.6	31.3	28.1	31.0
P		<0.01		<0.01		<0.01		NS		<0.01
DAP (mmHg)										
Mean	89.8	80.6	102.4	90.3	100.9	92.6	101.2	93.7	111.4	100.3
SD	8.9	4.7	12.2	7.4	15.0	13.2	16.9	16.4	18.0	20.6
P		<0.01		<0.001		<0.01		<0.01		<0.01
MAP (mmHg)										
Mean	116.4	104.7	127.4	114.1	137.3	126.4	140.3	130.7	153.9	142.6
SD	9.0	7.0	14.2	9.1	19.3	17.0	22.6	24.1	27.0	26.0
P		<0.01		<0.01		<0.01		<0.01		<0.05
TPRI (dyn s^{-1} cm^{-5} m^2)										
Mean	2989	2565	3848	3292	1963	1859	1597	1488	1502	1421
SD	769	368	607	373	412	267	409	343	551	540
P		NS		<0.01		NS		NS		NS

VO_2 oxygen consumption, *CI* cardiac index, *SI* stroke index, *HR* heart rate, *SAP* systolic arterial pressure, *DAP* diastolic arterial pressure, *MAP* mean arterial pressure, *TPRI* total peripheral resistance index, *1* before verapamil treatment, *2* after verapamil treatment. With kind permission of Acta Medica Scandinavica

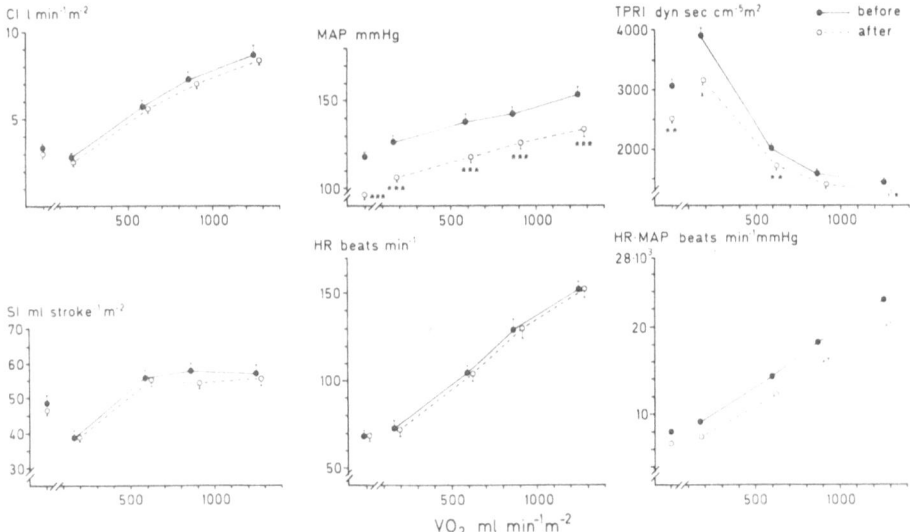

Fig. 4. Hemodynamic changes induced by chronic nifedipine treatment, $n = 14$. Legend as in Fig. 1. (With kind permission from Journal of Hypertension [17])

rest, the fall in SAP was 27.4 mmHg (17%) and in DAP 16.2 mmHg (17%). Only one subject demonstrated a fall in MAP of less than 10 mmHg (9 mmHg). During exercise at 50, 100, and 150 W, the reductions in MAP were 20.6, 15.9, and 19.0 mmHg (15%, 11%, and 12%, respectively). TPRI fell in all but three subjects at supine rest and in all but two at sitting rest.

Somewhat surprisingly, the HR values were unchanged at rest as well as during exercise. The mean values in the first and second studies were practically unchanged. In no situation were the changes greater than $\pm 2\%$. The stroke index and CI also showed only minor changes and all were statistically insignificant.

Verapamil versus nifedipine in the same patient

The major results from this study were as follows. The oxygen consumption did not show any statistically significant differences on any of the two drug regimes compared with pretreatment values. The blood pressure control was better on nifedipine (mean daily dose 52 mg) than on verapamil (mean daily dose 210 mg). At sitting rest and during 50-W exercise, all but one patient had lower SAP and DAP on nifedipine than on verapamil. At sitting rest, SAP was 163 ± 19 mmHg before therapy, 153 ± 16 mmHg on verapamil, and 138 ± 9 mmHg on nifedipine. The DAP was 101 ± 13 mmHg before treatment, 92 ± 9 mmHg on verapamil, and 85 ± 7 mmHg on nifedipine. The reductions in SAP/DAP at supine rest, sitting rest, and during exercise at 50, 100, and 150 W on verapamil were: $-12/-6$, $-10/-9$, $-5/-6$, $-5/-5$, and $-11/-9$ mmHg, respectively. On nifedipine, the corresponding values were: $-21/-11$, $-25/-16$, $-15/-9$, $-13/-6$, and $-14/-9$ mmHg.

There were no differences between the CI values on the two regimes, the CI

Table 2. Hemodynamic measurements before and after nifedipine treatment

| | Rest | | | | Workload (W) | | | | | |
| | Supine | | Sitting | | 50 | | 100 | | 150 | |
	1	2	1	2	1	2	1	2	1	2
VO$_2$ (ml/min/m^2)										
Mean			159	165	563	598	828	873	1205	1230
SD			29	14	84	51	114	71	141	84
P			NS		NS		NS		NS	
CI (l/min/m^2)										
Mean	3.28	3.15	2.80	2.67	5.72	5.60	7.31	6.97	8.63	8.33
SD	0.82	0.46	0.82	0.34	1.28	0.58	1.45	0.74	1.70	0.77
P	NS		NS		NS		NS		NS	
SI (ml/stroke/m^2)										
Mean	48.4	46.3	38.7	38.6	55.5	55.0	57.7	54.5	57.0	55.3
SD	8.5	4.9	7.1	6.3	9.1	7.1	9.8	6.8	8.9	7.6
P	NS		NS		NS		NS		NS	
HR (beats/min)										
Mean	68.1	68.9	72.5	70.9	103.6	103.6	128.5	130.0	151.6	152.4
SD	12.5	13.5	15.6	13.7	17.2	18.0	23.6	22.7	16.9	18.8
P	NS		NS		NS		NS		NS	
SAP (mmHg)										
Mean	157.0	129.6	165.6	138.2	186.0	162.5	196.6	174.9	211.3	189.6
SD	12.2	6.3	18.1	6.7	20.4	15.2	19.5	17.4	22.3	17.4
P	<0.001		<0.001		<0.001		<0.001		<0.001	
DAP (mmHg)										
Mean	93.7	77.4	102.6	86.4	104.5	88.6	105.6	93.6	113.0	100.3
SD	7.4	5.1	8.3	6.1	9.0	8.4	9.6	11.4	10.0	8.8
P	<0.001		<0.001		<0.001		<0.001		<0.001	
MAP (mmHg)										
Mean	117.7	97.4	126.4	105.5	138.4	117.8	141.6	125.7	152.9	133.9
SD	9.0	5.4	11.5	7.1	15.3	11.8	14.1	14.3	16.8	14.1
P	<0.001		<0.001		<0.001		<0.001		<0.001	
TPRI (dyn s/cm^5 m^2)										
Mean	3031	2516	3870	3215	2022	1701	1608	1450	1478	1299
SD	773	333	1129	477	499	253	372	167	389	213
P	<0.01		<0.05		<0.01		NS		<0.05	

Abbreviations, see Table 1
Fourteen patients were studied with kind permission of Journal of Hypertension

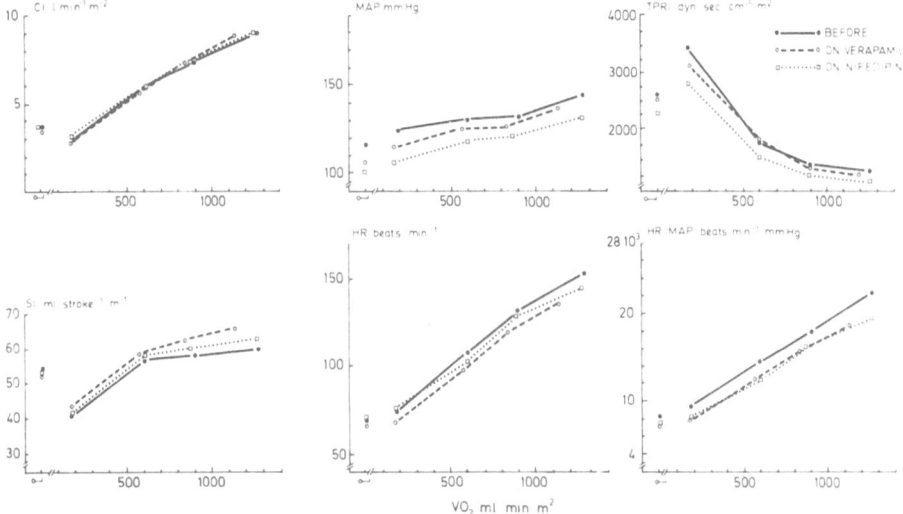

Fig. 5. Hemodynamic changes before treatment, after 1 year on verapamil, and then after 1 year on nifedipine ($n = 8$). Legend as in Fig. 1. Mean values only. Note that the effect on the MPA × HR product is the same on the two regimes. The reduction in MAP and TPRI is most pronounced on nifedipine

being practically unchanged compared with the pretreatment situation. The greater reduction in BP on nifedipine was due to a greater fall in TPRI. Thus, at supine and sitting rest, the TPRI was reduced by only 3% and 9% on verapamil in this group of patients versus 14% and 19% on nifedipine.

Figure 5 shows the mean values of the hemodynamic parameters before treatment, on verapamil, and on nifedipine. It is seen that the reduction in the pressure multiplied by the HR product was the same on both regimes, since verapamil induced some reduction in HR, compensating for the smaller reduction in the blood pressure.

Side effects
No orthostatic reactions were seen in any patients acutely or chronically. No side effects were seen in the patients with verapamil. In the nifedipine series, three patients complained of light flushing during the first 2 weeks after tablet intake, but the complaints disappeared after 2-3 weeks. One subject complained of a tendency to palpitations and the feeling of uneasiness, but after a premature second hemodynamic study a small dose of propranolol cured these complaints. In the nisoldipine series, no side effects were reported after the first dose, but pretibial or ankle edema was seen in three patients after 2-4 months, necessitating premature termination of the study in two of them.

Discussion

These hemodynamic studies have shown that the basic hemodynamic effect of the three calcium-channel blockers verapamil, nifedipine, and nisoldipine is a reduction in total peripheral resistance, without any reduction in CI. In previous studies of nifedipine in capsule form, other investigators have reported that there is a rapid fall in blood pressure associated with a reduction in TPRI associated with an increase in HR of about 10 beats min^{-1} [7–15]. In our acute study on nisoldipine, a similar reaction pattern was seen—the changes being most pronounced 1 h after tablet intake. The reduction in TPRI was then quite substantial (-19%). This marked fall in resistance seemed to have triggered a reflex tachycardia as the HR increased from 69.0 to 75.1 beats min^{-1} ($+9\%$, $P < 0.001$). There was also a slight increase in stroke index and consequently CI increased from 3.16 to 3.53 1 min^{-1} m^{-2} ($+12\%$, $P < 0.01$).

However, during long-term treatment, the reflex tachycardia seemed to vanish. This was clearly found in our nifedipine series, and at the 1-year follow-up the HR values were the same as before treatment at rest as well as during exercise. Figure 6 illustrates the difference between the acute and chronic effects of calcium blockade by nisoldipine and nifedipine. Preliminary clinical follow-ups from our nisoldipine series seem to indicate the same reaction pattern.

The HR response to verapamil differs from the response to nifedipine and nisoldipine. At the 1-year follow-up, verapamil tended to reduce HR, particularly during exercise. The reduction in HR was, however, compensated by an increase in SI and no reduction in cardiac output was seen.

The blood pressure reduction induced by verapamil in our series was modest, but is most likely due to the low dose used. In other reports, when verapamil has been used in higher doses (320–480 mg daily), a greater fall in blood pressure has been seen [18, 19]. The hemodynamic changes induced by verapamil agree well with what has been reported in other studies acutely as well as chronically [4–6].

Comparison with other antihypertensive agents (long-term use)

A reduction in TPRI may be achieved during chronic treatment with diuretics [20] and with alpha blockers like prazosin [21]. A fall in TPRI has also been demonstrated for the ACE inhibitors [22–24]. In contrast, in most patients with mild to moderate essential hypertension, chronic beta-blocker treatment is associated with a chronic reduction in cardiac index at sitting rest and, in particular, during exercise [25, 26]. The fall in CI on chronic beta blockade is compensated by an increase in the arteriovenous oxygen difference [25]. When beta-blocker treatment is induced, complaints due to the reduction in blood flow are quite common (heavy legs, reduction in physical working capacity), and during chronic treatment cold hands and feet are common complaints in cold climates. Such problems should hopefully be reduced with antihypertensive agents not inducing chronic reduction in blood flow.

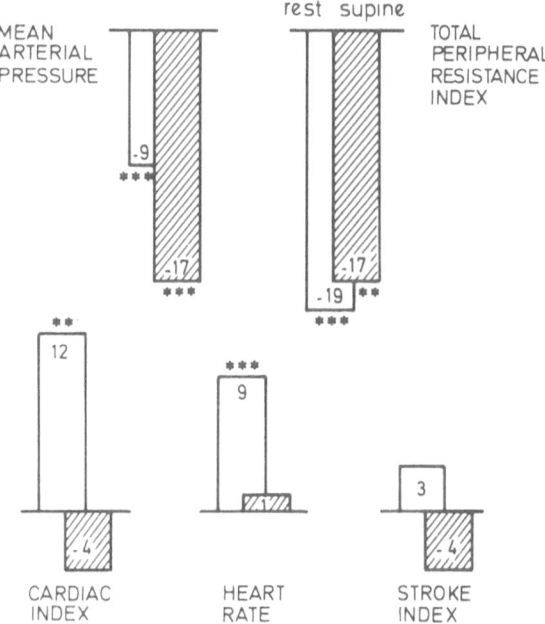

Fig. 6. Relative changes (%) in central hemodynamics induced by acute (1 h) calcium-channel blockade (nisoldipine, *open bars*) and by chronic therapy (1 year) (nifedipine, *hatched bars*). Note that no significant changes in CI or HR are seen on chronic therapy, in contrast to the immediate effect. *Asterisks* show level of statistical significance of difference from pretreatment levels

Conclusion

The calcium-channel blockers verapamil, nifedipine, and nisoldipine reduced blood pressure in the majority of patients with mild to moderate essential hypertension acutely as well as chronically [29–31]. During chronic therapy, verapamil should probably be given in a dose of 320 mg/day or sometimes more, while long-acting nifedipine seems to control blood pressure satisfactorily at a daily dose of 40–60 mg in most patients with mild hypertension. Preliminary results from our nisoldipine series indicate that most patients are well controlled on a daily dose of 20–40 mg.

With all these drugs, the fall in blood pressure is associated with a significant reduction in total peripheral resistance acutely as well as chronically. There is no acute or chronic depression in cardiac output, and during long-term treatment cardiac output is unchanged compared with pretreatment levels at rest as well as during exercise. When treatment with nifedipine or nisoldipine is started, a temporary increase in HR (reflex tachycardia) and in CI is usually seen.

The HR response to verapamil differs from the response to nifedipine and nisoldipine. At supine rest, there is a slight fall in HR, but this more marked when the sympathetic tone is higher, as in the sitting position and during muscular exercise. However, the reduction is only in the order of 10% (in contrast to 25% on many beta blockers without intrinsic sympathicomimetic activity (ISA). The HR reduction is fully compensated by an increase in SI and thus cardiac output is also not reduced on verapamil.

The hemodynamic profile of these calcium-channel blockers clearly differs from the hemodynamic profile of most beta blockers. The changes are more similar to what is induced by chronic use of alpha blockers, angiotensin converting enzyme (ACE)-inhibitors, or thiazide diuretics.

At present, the place of the calcium-channel blockers in the treatment of mild to moderate essential hypertension is not established. However, the antihypertensive effect is well documented and the hemodynamic profile and relatively few side effects should make them an important alternative to our presently available antihypertensive agents [27–31].

References

1. Lund-Johansen P (1983) The hemodynamics of essential hypertension. In: Robertson JIS (ed) Clinical aspects of essential hypertension. Handbook of hypertension, vol 1. Elsevier, Amsterdam, pp 151–173
2. Frohlich ED, Kozyl VJ, Tarazi RC, Dustan HP (1970) Physiological comparison of labile and essential hypertension. Circ Res (Suppl 1): 55–69
3. Lund-Johansen P (1983) Haemodynamic changes in the elderly hypertensives. Acta Med Scand (Suppl 676): 86–102
4. Muiesan G, Agabiti-Rosei E, Alicandri C, et al (1981) Influence of verapamil on catecholamines, renin and aldosterone in essential hypertensive patients. In: Zanchetti A, Krikler DM (eds) Calcium antagonism in cardiovascular therapy. Experience with verapamil. Excerpta Medical, Amsterdam, p 238
5. Lewis GRJ (1980) Verapamil in the management of chronic hypertension. Clin Invest Med 3: 175–177
6. deLeeuw PW, Smout AJPM, Willemse PJ, Birkenhäger WH (1981) Effects of verapamil in hypertensive patients. In: Zanchetti A, Krikler DM (eds) Calcium antagonism in cardiovascular therapy. Experience with verapamil. Excerpta Medica, Amsterdam, p 233
7. Olivari MT, Bartorelli C, Polese A, Fiorentini C, Moruzzi P, Guazzi M (1979) Treatment of hypertension with nifedipine, a calcium antagonist agent. Circulation 59: 1056–1062
8. Aoki K, Sato K, Kawaguchi Y, Yamamoto M (1982) Acute and long-term hypotensive effects and plasma concentrations of nifedipine in patients with essential hypertension. Eur J Pharmacol 23: 197–201
9. Corea L, Alunni G, Bentiviglio M, Boschetti E, Cosmi F, Giaimo MD, Miele N, Motolese M (1980) Acute and long-term effects of nifedipine on plasma renin activity and plasma catecholamines in controls and hypertensive patients before and after metoprolol. Acta Ther 6: 177–189
10. Corea L, Bentiviglio M, Cosmi F, Alunni G, Carnovali M (1981) Nifedipine versus prazosin in essential hypertension: a double blind study. Cur Ther Res 30: 708–717
11. Ekelund L-G, Ekelund C, Rossner S (1982) Antihypertensive effects at rest and during exercise of a calcium blocker, nifedipine, alone and in combination with metoprolol. Acta Med Scand 212: 71–75
12. Kuwajima I, Ueda K, Kamta C, Matsushita S, Kuramoto K, Murakami M, Hada Y (1978) A study on the effects of nifedipine in hypertensive crises and severe hypertension. Jap Heart J 19: 455–467
13. Lederballe Pedersen O, Christensen NJ, Ramsch KD (1980) Comparison of acute effects of nifedipine in normotensive and hypertensive man. J Cardiovasc Pharmacol 2: 357–366

14. Maeda K, Tanaka C, Tsukano Y, Minamikawa H, Komatsu H, Kotsumi K, Inoue E (1982) Antihypertensive effects of the calcium antagonist agent nifedipine. Drug Res 32:267–271
15. Thibonnier M, Bonnet F, Corvol P (1980) Antihypertensive effects of fractionated sublingual administration of nifedipine in moderate essential hypertension. Eur J Pharmacol 17:161–164
16. Lund-Johansen P (1984) Hemodynamic long-term effects of verapamil in essential hypertension at rest and during exercise. Acta Med Scand (Suppl 681): 109–115
17. Lund-Johansen P, Omvik P (1983) Haemodynamic effects of nifedipine in essential hypertension at rest and during exercise. J Hypertension 1:159–163
18. Doyle AE, Anavekar SN, Oliver LE (1981) A clinical trial of verapamil in the treatment of hypertension. In: Zanchetti A, Krikler DS (eds) Calcium antagonism in cardiovascular therapy. Excerpta Medica, Amsterdam, p 252
19. Midtbø K, Hals O (1980) Verapamil in the treatment of hypertension. Curr Ter Res 27: 830–838
20. Lund-Johansen P (1970) Hemodynamic changes in long-term diuretic therapy of essential hypertension. Acta Med Scand 187:509–518
21. Lund-Johansen P (1974) Hemodynamic changes at rest and during exercise in long-term prazosin therapy of essential hypertension. In: Cotton DWK (ed) Prazosin–Evaluation of a new anti-hypertensive agent. Proceedings of a symposium. Excerpta Medica, Amsterdam, p 43
22. Dunn FG, Oigman W, Ventura HO, Messerli FA, Kobrin I, Frohlich ED (1983) Enalapril improves systemic and renal hemodynamics and allows regression of left ventricular mass in essential hypertension. Am J Cardiol 53:195–108
23. Fouad FM, Tarazi RC, Bravo EL (1983) Cardiac and haemodynamic effects of enalapril. J Hypertension 1 (Suppl 1): 135–142
24. Lund-Johansen P, Omvik P (1984) Long-term haemodynamic effects of enalapril (alone and in combination with hydrochlorothiazide) at rest and during exercise in essential hypertension. J Hypertension 2 (Suppl 2): 49–56
25. Lund-Johansen P (1983) Central haemodynamic effects of beta-blockers in hypertension. A comparison between atenolol, metoprolol, timolol, penbutolol, atenolol, pindolol and bunitrolol. Eur Heart J 4 (Suppl D): 1–12
26. Lund-Johansen P (1976) Hemodynamic long-term effects of timolol at rest and during exercise in essential hypertension. Acta Med Scand 199:263–267
27. Bühler FR, Hulthen UL (1982) Calcium channel blockers: a pathophysiologically treatment concept for the future? Eur J Clin Invest 12:1–3
28. Bühler FR, Bolli P, Hulthen UL (1984) Calcium-influx dependent vasoconstrictor mechanisms in essential hypertension. In Opie LH, Krebs R (eds) Calcium antagonists and cardiovascular disease. Raven, New York, p 313
29. Aoki K, Yoshida T, Kato S, Tazumi K, Sato I, Takikawa K, Hotta K. (1976) Hypotensive action and increased plasma renin activity by Ca^{2+} antagonist (nifedipine) in hypertensive patients. Jpn Heart J 17:479
30. Aoki K, Kondo S, Mochizuki A, Yoshida T, Kato S, Kato K, Takikawa K (1978) Antihypertensvie effect of cardiovascular Ca^{2+}-antagonist in hypertensive patients in the absence and presence of beta-adrenergic blockade. Am Heart J 96:218
31. Aoki K, Sato K, Kondo S, Yamamoto M (1983) Hypotensive effects of diltiazem to normals and essential hypertensives. Eur J Clin Pharmacol 25:475

Comparative Efficacy of Calcium Antagonists and Beta Blockers in Essential Hypertension

A. E. Doyle

Department of Medicine, University of Melbourne, Austin Hospital,
Heidelberg, Victoria, 3084, Australia

Summary. The calcium antagonist drug verapamil was compared in double-blind, double-dummy crossover studies with two beta-adrenoceptor blocking drugs, pindolol and labetalol. All were equally effective as antihypertensive drugs in patients with mild to moderate hypertension. Verapamil caused a fall in blood pressure by reducing total peripheral resistance; since cardiac output rose slightly as judged by echocardiographic studies, verapamil had no adverse effects on airways resistance in patients with obstructive airways disease. The favourable haemodynamic effects and absence of serious side effects suggest that verapamil may represent an important advance in the treatment of mild to moderate hypertension.

Key words: Echocardiography—Lung function—Verapamil—Blood pressure

Beta blockers have been widely acknowledged to be very effective antihypertensive agents. Originally introduced for the treatment of angina pectoris, the antihypertensive properties of propranolol were described by Prichard and Gillam [1], since when many drugs with similar properties have become available. Although these drugs differ in other pharmacological properties, such as partial agonist activity, membrane stabilizing actions and relative affinity for the beta-1 receptor, their relative efficacy as antihypertensive drugs seems little different in equivalent doses [2, 3]. The extent of the antihypertensive effects relates closely to the magnitude of the receptor blockade induced.

Verapamil, which diminishes Ca^{2+}-dependent contractile force of the heart muscle without a major change in action potential, reduces Ca^{2+}-dependent high-energy phosphate utilization of the heart and reduces oxygen consumption in parallel with the reduction in contractile activity [4]. These actions are reversed by an increasing calcium concentration, by beta adrenoceptor agonists and by cardiac glycosides. Isolated sarcolemmal membranes can be depleted of calcium by verapamil by the inhibition of low-affinity calcium binding [5] so that the availability of calcium for passage through the slow calcium channels is reduced. The end results of calcium antagonism by verapamil and of beta adrenoceptor blockade are very similar in the heart. Verapamil has been extensively used in the treatment of angina and superventricular tachyarrythmias. During a comparison of oral verapamil with propranolol in the treatment of angina, verapamil was noticed to reduce blood pressure [6] and Lewis and his colleagues [7] have reported that verapamil is often an effective antihypertensive agent. The present paper reports a comparison of the effects of verapamil and the beta-blocking drug pindolol in a group of patients with mild to moderate hypertension and a comparison of the effects of verapamil and labetalol in patients with hypertension who also had chronic obstructive airways disease.

Methods

Comparison of verapamil and pindolol
Six male and eleven female patients aged 30–60 years with essential hypertension were studied. Patients with congestive heart failure, heart block, obstructive airways disease, peripheral vascular disease and clinically evident gout were excluded from the trial; all had normal blood urea and plasma creatinine.

All patients had been receiving antihypertensive therapy before the study began. Previous antihypertensive drugs included thiazide diuretics, amiloride, beta-blocking agents, alpha methyldopa and prazosin. In 14 patients the blood pressures had been satisfactorily controlled but in three patients basal diastolic blood pressure was still greater than 100 mmHg. On entering the study, patients were weighed, urinalysis and full blood examination were performed and serum sodium, potassium, urea, creatinine, bicarbonate, uric acid, antinuclear factor and DNA binding were measured. These observations were repeated at regular intervals. Plasma renin concentration was measured. After an initial observation period of 3 weeks all antihypertensive drugs except diuretics were replaced by placebo tablets. The patients were then assigned to treatment in a double-blind, randomized fashion.

Patients were treated with a fixed dose of 120 mg verapamil three times daily or 7.5 mg pindolol twice daily. During active treatment with verapamil, placebo pindolo tablets were used, and placebo verapamil tablets were given during the active pindolol treatment. In the placebo periods, placebos for both drugs were used.

The dose of thiazide diuretics was kept constant throughout the study and sodium intake remained unchanged. Patients were seen at regular intervals and blood pressures were measured by the auscultatory method by the same two observers.

Echocardiographic measurements
Echocardiography was performed in eight patients at the end of placebo and each active treatment period with the patients semi-recumbent. A commercially available echograph (Ekoline 20, Smith-Kline Instruments) with a 1.27-cm diameter 2.25-mHz transducer and a repetition rate of 1000/s was used. The tracings were displayed and recorded on a fibre optic recorder (Model 1856, Honeywell Corporation). Particular care was taken to standardize the position of the patient and the pathway of the ultrasonic beam through the left ventricle, so that comparable views could be obtained during serial recordings. Efforts were made to obtain echoes form the endocardial surfaces of the interventricular septum and posterior left ventricular wall, which were as complete as possible. No patients had known coronary artery disease or segmental abnormalities of ventricular contraction.

The following measurements were made from the echocardiographic record.

Left ventricular end-diastolic (LVIDd) and end-systolic (LVIDs) dimensions.
These were measured from the endocardial surfaces of the interventricular septum and posterobasal left ventricular wall at the peak of the R-wave and at the point of maximal approximation of the structures, respectively.

Systolic ejection time (EjT). This was measured from the first deflection of the QRS complex of the simultaneously recorded electrocardiogram to the time that the smallest end-systolic internal dimension was reached; 50 ms was subtracted for the pre-ejection time in all patients.

Heart rate. The following values were derived from echocardiographic measurements.

Echocardiographic fractional shortening (FS) was calculated as the difference between LVIDd and LVIDs normalized for end-diastolic dimensions [8]:

$$FS = \frac{LVIDd - LVIDs}{LVIDd} \times 100\%$$

Mean velocity of circumferential fibre shortening (mVcF) was derived from the left ventricular dimensions and ejection time [9]:

$$mVcF = \frac{LVIDd - LVIDs}{LVIDd \times EjT}.$$

Left ventricular volumes in end systole and end diastole were calculated by methods previously described [10]. Echocardiography provides a reliable means for determining left ventricular endocardial dimensions, which have been shown to be closely related to left ventricular volume. The calculated volumes provided an estimate of stroke volume (LVSV):

$$LVSV = LVEDV = LVESV.$$

Systemic vascular resistance was computed as the quotient of mean arterial pressure/cardiac output multiplied by a conversion factor of 80 to obtain dyne.s.cm^{-5}:

$$PVE = \frac{MBP}{CO \ (l/min)} \times 80 \ (dyne.s.cm^{-5})$$

Measurements taken at the end of each placebo period and at 6 weeks of active treatment periods were compared using paired student's t-test.

Comparison of verapamil and labetalol
Nine male patients between the age of 50 and 65 years were studied. They had both essential hypertension and chronic obstructive airways disease [defined as a forced expiratory volume at 1 s (FEV$_1$) between 30%–60% of the forced vital capacity (FVC)]. None had congestive heart failure, heart block, peripheral vascular disease or clinically evident gout and all patients had normal renal function.

All patients had been receiving antihypertensive therapy before the study began, the duration of treatment being from 2 to 18 years. Previous antihypertensive drugs included a thiazide diuretic, frusemide, methyldopa and prazosin. The bronchodilator drugs included salbutamol, betamethasone inhalations and theophylline, and three patients were also taking prednisolone. In five patients blood pressures had been satisfactorily controlled with existing medication, but in four patients the basal diastolic blood pressure was persistently above 100 mmHg. On entering the study, the patients were weighed, urinalysis and full blood examination were performed and serum sodium, potassium urea, creatinine, bicarbonate, uric acid, antinuclear factor, DNA binding and respiratory function tests (FEV$_1$ and FVC) were measured. These observations were repeated at regular intervals. After an initial observational period of 4 weeks, all antihypertensive drugs except diuretics were replaced by placebo tablets. The patients were then assigned to treatment in a double-blind, randomized fashion according to the study design described for the previous study.

The doses of thiazide diuretic and bronchodilator drugs were kept constant throughout the study and sodium intake remained unchanged. Patients were seen at regular intervals and blood pressures were measured by the auscultatory method by the same two observers.

Measurements taken at the end of each placebo period and at the end of 6 weeks of active treatment were compared using a paired student's t-test.

Plasma levels of verapamil
In both studies venous blood samples were obtained at 3 and 6 weeks of verapamil therapy 3–4 h after the patients had taken their morning dose. Plasma concentrations of verapamil and its metabolites were measured by using rapid high-pressure liquid chromatographic analysis [11].

Results

Verapamil and pindolol
Both recumbent systolic and diastolic blood pressures were increased when existing antihypertensive medications were replaced by placebo tablets. The effects of active treatment on recumbent blood pressure are shown in Table 1. Both verapamil and pindolol significantly reduced the mean systolic (paired $t = 2.54$, $P < 0.01$ for verapamil; $t = 4.20$, $P < 0.005$ for pindolol) and diastolic ($t = 4.81$, $P < 0.005$ for verapamil; $t = 5.35$, $P < 0.005$ for pindolol) blood pressure levels compared with the preceding placebo period. Placebo treatment for 2 weeks before the crossover treatment resulted in a rise in blood pressure to initial placebo treatment levels. Verapamil reduced diastolic blood pressure to below 90 mmHg in 12 patients. In the remaining five patients, a diastolic blood pressure of 95–100 mmHg was attained. Pindolol produced good blood pressure control in 11 patients and a satisfactory response in five patients. One patient on pindolol had a diastolic blood pressure of > 100 mmHg. Both verapamil and pindolol satisfactorily controlled blood pressure in the three patients who were not well controlled on their previous antihypertensive regimen before entering the study. Neither drug produced any carryover effect on blood pressure.

There were no significant differences in the blood pressure responses between the two compounds ($t = 0.02$, $P > 0.5$ for systolic; $t = 0.123$, $P > 0.45$ for diasto-

Table 1. Mean ($\pm$SD) levels of body weight, pulse, systolic and diastolic blood pressure during verapamil and pindolol treatment

Parameter	Previous treatment	Placebo	Verapamil (6 weeks)	Placebo	Pindolol (6 weeks)
Body weight (kg)	75.7 $\pm$ 12.0	77.3 $\pm$ 12.1	75.9 $\pm$ 10.6	75.9 $\pm$ 12.1	74.3 $\pm$ 20.1
Pulse/min	74.0 $\pm$ 12.4	80.7 $\pm$ 10.9	79.8 $\pm$ 10.2	84.4 $\pm$ 12.5	75.4 $\pm$ 9.2*
SBP (mmHg)	168.8 $\pm$ 22.2	172.1 $\pm$ 2.3	158.5 $\pm$ 11.9**	175.1 $\pm$ 20.5	160.1 $\pm$ 19.3**
DBP (mmHg)	94.8 $\pm$ 9.5	98.2 $\pm$ 8.1	87.8 $\pm$ 6.9**	101.5 $\pm$ 7.4	91.1 $\pm$ 8.2**

SBP systolic blood pressure, *DBP* diastolic blood pressure
* $P < 0.05$ compared with corresponding placebo period
** $P < 0.01$ compared with corresponding placebo period

lic blood pressure). There were similar reductions in the blood pressure levels with both compounds after the patients had been standing for 3 min, and neither drug produced any symptoms of postural hypotension. Neither drug had significant effects on weight. Verapamil had no significant effect on pulse rate ($t = 0.59$, $P > 0.35$); pindolol significantly reduced the pulse rate ($t = 2.40$, $P < 0.025$).

Neither drug had significant effects on the serum levels of sodium, potassium, bicarbonate, creatinine or uric acid. There was a slight but statistically insignificant reduction in plasma renin concentration with pindolol ($t = 1.77$, 0.1, $P > 0.05$); verapamil had no significant effect on plasma renin concentration ($t = 0.13$, $P > 0.45$). Other laboratory determinations, including full blood examination, antinuclear factor and DNA binding, remained unchanged throughout the study.

Three patients reported minor side effects with pindolol, which included tiredness, vivid dreams and muscle cramps. Two patients reported mild constipation with verapamil.

Neither drug had significant effects on fractional shortening, mean velocity of circumferential shortening and cardiac output measured by echocardiography (Table 2). Pindolol produced no significant effect on peripheral vascular resistance compared with placebo ($t = 1.69$, $P > 0.05$). Verapamil produced a slight but significant reduction in the peripheral vascular resistance ($t = 1.95$, $P < 0.05$).

Verapamil and labetalol
Both recumbent systolic and diastolic blood pressures were increased when existing antihypertensive medications were replaced by placebo tablets.

Both drugs significantly reduced the mean pulse rate ($t = 2.43$, $P < 0.01$ for verapamil; $t = 5.31$, $P < 0.005$ for labetalol), systolic ($t = 4.08$, $P < 0.0025$ for verapamil; $t = 2.1$, $P < 0.05$ for labetalol) and diastolic ($t = 5.76$, $P < 0.0005$ for verapamil; $t = 2.83$, $P < 0.01$ for labetalol) blood pressure levels compared with the preceding placebo periods. Placebo treatment for 2 weeks before the crossover treatment resulted in a rise in blood pressure to the initial placebo treatment levels. Verapamil produced a good blood pressure response (diastolic blood pressure < 90 mmHg) in six patients. In the remaining three patients the diastolic blood pressure ranged from 95 to 100 mmHg. Labetalol produced good blood pressure control in five patients, three patients had diastolic blood pressure between 95 and 100 mmHg and in one patient the diastolic pressure remained at 110 mmHg. Neither drug produced any carryover effect on blood pressure.

There were no significant differences in blood pressure responses between the two compounds ($t = 0.42$, $P > 0.10$ for systolic blood pressure; $t = 0.93$, $P > 0.10$ for diastolic blood pressure). There were similar reductions in the blood pressure levels after the patients had been standing for 3 min and neither drug produced any symptoms of postural hypotension.

The effects of both verapamil and labetalol on respiratory function (FEV_1 and FVC) before and after salbutamol inhalation are shown in Table 3. Verapamil had no significant effect on either FEV_1 or FVC before and after salbutamol inhalation in these patients compared with the corresponding placebo period. Both FEV_1 ($t = 4.02$, $P < 0.0025$ before salbutamol; $t = 2.39$, $P < 0.025$ after salbutamol) and FVC ($t = 1.98$, $P < 0.05$ before salbutamol; $t = 3.49$, $P < 0.005$ after salbutamol) were significantly reduced with labetalol compared with the corresponding placebo periods.

Neither drug had significant effects on sodium, potassium, bicarbonate, creatinine, uric acid or blood glucose levels. Other laboratory determinations, including full blood examination, antinuclear factor and DNA binding, remained unchanged throughout the study.

Two patients, one taking verapamil and the other labetalol complained of slight worsening of their respiratory symptoms, which included increased dysp-

Table 2. Haemodynamic variables and indices of myocardial performance derived from echocardiography (mean ± SD)

Parameter	Placebo	Verapamil	Pindolol
Fractional shortening (%)	36.3 ± 7.0	35.43 ± 5.98	35.40 ± 5.04
Velocity of circumferential fibre shortening (circ/s)	0.97 ± 20.0	1.02 ± 0.20	0.94 ± 0.11
Cardiac output (ml/min)	4717.75 ± 1487.61	5218.00 ± 1538.64	4724.60 ± 976.02
Peripheral vascular resistance (dyne.s.cm^{-5})	2288.13 ± 665.16	1787.25 ± 585.29*	1948.57 ± 520.42

* $P < 0.05$ compared with placebo period

Table 3. Effects of verapamil and labetalol on respiratory function tests

	Placebo	Verapamil	Placebo	Labetalol
Mean (± SE) level of FEV_1/l/BTPS				
Before salbutamol	1.39 ± 0.25	1.46 ± 0.19	1.46 ± 0.23	1.18 ± 0.18*
After salbutamol	1.43 ± 0.25	1.58 ± 0.20	1.57 ± 0.23	1.32 ± 0.18*
Mean (± SE) levels of FVC/l/BTPS				
Before salbutamol	2.88 ± 0.32	2.98 ± 0.23	3.26 ± 0.29	2.69 ± 0.27*
After slbutamol	3.17 ± 0.34	3.26 ± 0.23	3.43 ± 0.26	2.93 ± 0.20*

* $P < 0.025$

noea on exertion and cough during the study. These symptoms were trivial in nature and did not necessitate any change in the bronchodilator therapy. Three patients reported minor side effects with labetalol, which included tiredness and muscle cramps. Two patients reported mild constipation, and one mild tremor with verapamil.

Plasma levels of verapamil and metabolites
There was a wide variation in the plasma concentrations of verapamil and nor-verapamil in individual patients. The plasma concentrations of verapamil and nor-verapamil, however, were similar. There was no correlation between either the verapamil or nor-verapamil concentrations and blood pressure response.

Discussion

The studies presented here indicate that in patients with mild to moderately severe hypertension verapamil is as effective in reducing blood pressure as either pindolol or labetalol. As might be expected from its pharmacological properties, verapamil appears to reduce blood pressure mainly by inducing a fall in peripheral resistance, but unlike the effects of vasodilator drugs, such as hydralazine or minoxidil, the fall in peripheral resistance was not associated with reflex tachycardia or a rise in plasma renin concentration. In this respect the effect of verapamil also differs from that of nifedipine, which has been reported to induce both tachycardia and a rise in RPA [12–15]. The haemodynamic effects of verapamil more closely resemble the actions of alpha-methyl dopa than those of any other available anti-hypertensive drug, although the apparent mechanism of action of these two drugs is widely different. It has been suggested that the lack of reflex tachycardia when blood pressure is lowered by verapamil is because reflex sympathetic action is dampened by the action of verapamil or transmitter release at the sympathetic nerve endings [16], a process which is known to be calcium dependent [17]; but such an explanation does not account for why a similar effect is not seen with nifedipine. It is possible that verapamil may, like alpha-methyl dopa, have an action on the central sympathetic nervous system, although this is speculative. It is more probable that the action of verapamil on cardiac muscle may prevent the heart responding to reflex sympathetic stimulation, but this should not interfere with the effect on plasma renin.

Whatever the mechanism of action may be, it appears that verapamil has a desirable haemodynamic profile in reversing the haemodynamic pattern usually seen in hypertension.

From the present studies it appears that verapamil may be a particularly useful drug in patients with hypertension and co-existing obstructive airways disease. Beta-adrenoceptor blocking drugs may indicate worsening of airways obstruction and are usually not considered safe to use in patients who have this problem. It is of interest that labetalol, a drug combining alpha and beta-adrenoceptor properties, also induces a reduction in forced expiratory volume in some patients.

Verapamil appears to have substantial theoretical advantages over most other types of antihypertensive agents in that it reduces blood pressure mainly by reducing peripheral resistance without compensatory tachycardia and without reducing cardiac output. Moreover, the absence of side effects related to interference with peripheral or central sympathetic mechanisms is also an advantage. The major side effect induced by verapamil appears to be constipation, due to a reduction of contractions in intestinal smooth muscle. While occasionally severe, this symptom is usually well tolerated.

Although the use of verapamil in the spectrum of antihypertensive drugs is not finally established, it appears to have major advantages and may prove to be the drug of first choice in many patients with mild to moderate hypertension.

References

1. Prichard BNC, Gillam PMS (1964) Use of propranolol in the treatment of hypertension. Brit Med J 2:275
2. Morgan TO, Sabto J, Anavekar SN, Louis WJ, Doyle AE (1974) A comparison of beta adrenergic blocking drugs in the treatment of hypertension. Postgrad Med J 50:253
3. Ligman P, Amery A, dePlane JF, Fagard R, Reybruck T (1976) Hyporeninaemia and hypotensive effect of a cardioselective and a non cardioselective beta blocker. In: Saxona PR, Forsyth RP (eds) Beta adrenoceptor blocking agents. North Holland, Amsterdam, p 229
4. Fleckenstein A, Tritthart H, Fleckenstein B (1969) A new group of competitive Ca-antagonists (iproveratril, DbOO, prenylamine) with highly potent inhibitory effects on excitation-contraction coupling in mammalian myocardium. Pflugers Arch Ges Physiol 307:R25
5. Nayler WG, Szeto J (1972) Effect of verapamil on contractility, oxygen utilization and calcium exchangeability in mammalian heart muscle. Cardiovasc Res 6:120
6. Livesley B, Catley PF, Campbell RC, Oram S (1973) Double blind evaluation of verapamil, propranolol and isosorbide nitrate against a placebo in the treatment of angina pectons. Brit Med J i:375
7. Lewis GR, Morley KD, Maslowski AH, Bones PJ (1979) Verapamil in the management of hypertensive patients. Aust NZ J Med 9:62
8. McDonald IG, Feigenbaum H, Chang S (1972) Analysis of left ventricular wall motion by reflected ultrasound: application to assessment of myocardial function. Circulation 46:14
9. Cooper RH, O'Rourke RA, Karliner JS (1972) Comparison of ultrasound and cineangiographic measurement of the mean rate of circumferential fiber shortening. Circulation 96:914
10. Teicholz LE, Krenlen T, Herman MV, Gorlin R (1976) Problems in echocardiographic volume determination: echocardiographic-angiographic correlations in the presence or absence of synergy. Amer J Card 37:7
11. Harapat SR, Kates RE (1979) Rapid high pressure liquid chromatographic analysis of verapamil in blood and plasma. J Chromatog 170:385
12. Olivari MT, Bartonelli C, Polese A, Fiorantini C, Monuzzi P, Guozzi MD (1979) Treatment of hypertension with nifedipide, a calcium antagonist agent. Circulation 59:1056
13. Aoki K, Yoshida T; Kato S, Tazumi K, Sato I, Takikawa K, Hotta K (1976) Hypotensive action and increased plasma renin activity by Ca^{2+} antagonist (nifedipine) in hypertensive patients. Jpn Heart J 17:479
14. Aoki K, Kondo S, Mochizuki A, Yoshida T, Kato S, Kato K, Takikawa K (1978) Antihypertensvie effect of cardiovascular Ca^{2+}-antagonist in hypertensive patients in the absence and presence of beta-adrenergic blockade. Am Heart J 96:218
15. Aoki K, Sato K, Kawaguchi Y, Yamamoto M (1982) Acute and long-term hypotensive effects and plasma concentrations of nifedipine in patients with essential hypertension. Eur J Clin Pharmacol 23:197
16. Zanchetti A (1981) Perspectives in antihypertensive treatment. In: Zanchetti A, Kribler DM (eds) Calcium antagonism in cardiovascular therapy. Excerpta Medica, Amsterdam, p 292
17. Burn JH, Gibbons WR (1965) The release of noradrenaline from sympathetic nerve fibres in relation to calcium concentration. J Physiol (Lond) 187:214

Etiology of Hypertension

Calcium Membrane Theory of Essential Hypertension

K. Aoki

Second Department of Internal Medicine, Nagoya City University Medical School, Mizuho-ku, Nagoya, 467 Japan

Summary. Essential hypertension (major gene hypertension, arterial hypertension) develops and persists by an inappropriate increase in total peripheral vascular resistance. The significant elevation of vascular resistance is observed in both early and established stages of essential hypertension after 1-hour supine resting, but a rise in cardiac output is not observed. The elevation of vascular resistance can result from an abnormal increase in active tension in the vascular smooth muscle and this may arise from an increased contractility of arterial smooth muscle by the membrane abnormalities. Reduced calcium binding and uptake by the cell membrane and sarcoplasmic reticulum membrane brings about depolarization on the membrane, which results in activation of voltage-dependent calcium channels. The channel activation leads to calcium influx, which induces calcium release from the membrane storage sites. In addition, an increased inhibitory effect of calcium antagonists on agonist-induced contraction of arterial smooth muscle suggests an increased number of calcium channels in the cell membrane of arterial smooth muscle. The increased number of calcium channels brings about an increase in calcium influx. A decrease in the number of binding sites and/or an increase in the number of calcium channels leads to calcium influx and release, which results in a rise in the concentration in the cytosol of arterial smooth muscle, causing contraction of the muscle. The increase in calcium concentration leads to overcontraction and incomplete relaxation, which result in thickening of the arterial wall, bringing about a reduction of the arterial lumen. Any reduction of the arterial lumen causes increased total peripheral vascular resistance, which results in hypertension. Thus, abnormality of the calcium-handling properties of the membrane causes hypertension. In conclusion, the calcium membrane theory of essential hypertension is proposed as a mechanism for the development and persistence of high blood pressure in humans and animals in essential hypertension.

Key words: Calcium membrane theory—Essential hypertension—Membrane abnormality—Calcium handling abnormality—Overcontraction—Incomplete relaxation

In essential hypertension (major gene hypertension, arterial hypertension), total peripheral vascular resistance is abnormally elevated [1–5]. Since total peripheral vascular resistance is regulated by vascular smooth muscle, the abnormal elevation of total peripheral vascular resistance results from an increase in active contraction in the vascular smooth muscle [6–9]. For this reason, arterial smooth muscle may be abnormal in arterial hypertension.

Many investigators [4, 5] in hypertension have attempted to identify the elevation of total peripheral vascular resistance in the early phase of essential hypertension. The small rise in blood pressure is associated with a small elevation of vascular resistance, thus it is difficult, but not impossible, to demonstrate a significant elevation of vascular resistance in the earliest phase of essential hypertension. One of the purposes of the present paper is to review our studies which demonstrate a progressive elevation of total peripheral vascular resistance, resulting in a gradual rise in blood pressure in patients with essential hypertension.

The abnormal vascular resistance resulting from both structural and functional changes in the arterial wall has been investigated as the possible etiology of hypertension. Folkow [10, 11] has reviewed the evidence for the increased vascular resistance seen in hypertension being accounted for by an increased wall thickness. If structural changes in the wall thickness of blood vessels are physiological adaptations to an increase in blood pressure, then functional changes must be held accountable for the genesis of elevated blood pressure. Functional changes in the arterial smooth muscle in Aoki spontaneously hypertensive rats (SHR) [12] have been demonstrated; they consisted of isolated arterial vessels from SHR displaying a reduced threshold and ED_{50} to vasoactive stimuli [13], abnormal vascular responses preceding the development of high blood pressure [14, 15], and increased sensitivity of vascular smooth muscle to agonists occurring without high blood pressure [8, 9, 13–16]. We have demonstrated that in calcium-containing solution, noradrenaline-induced contraction of vascular smooth muscle is smaller in SHR than in normotensive control rats, and after washing the vascular strips with calcium-free ethyleneglycol-bis (β-aminoethyl ether) N,N,N',N'-tetraacetic acid (EGTA), vascular contraction developed by the addition of calcium was greater in SHR than in normotensive controls [17]. Functional changes in vascular smooth muscle to calcium agonists and antagonists is reviewed as related to the cause of hypertension in the present paper.

The degree of contraction or relaxation of arterial smooth muscle is controlled by the level of calcium concentration in the cytosol. The calcium concentration is regulated by the activity of the cell membrane and sarcoplasmic reticulum. It has been reported that the ability of the sarcoplasmic reticulum [18–23] and cell membrane [24–26] of arterial smooth muscle to retain and accumulate calcium is reduced in SHR.

Calcium ions determine the initiation and termination of excitation-contraction coupling in arterial smooth muscle cells. The threshold for initiation of contraction is of the order of 10^{-7} M and full contraction occurs at about a $10^{-5}M$ intracellular free calcium concentration. The gradient across the membrane amounts to a 10 000-fold concentration and there is a 60-mV potential gradient between outside and inside the cell membrane. The low permeability of the cell membrane to calcium makes it possible for this large calcium gradient to be maintained. The upstroke of the action potential induces calcium influx through voltage-dependent calcium channels. An agonist-induced activation of receptors leads to calcium influx through receptor-operated channels [27, 28]. Calcium is released from the cell membrane and sarcoplasmic reticulum by a calcium-induced mechanism, and this raises the concentration of intracellular free calcium [29–31]. Thus, the concentration of intracellular free calcium is regulated by the membrane function, which is dependent on calcium channels and calcium uptake abilities. Abnormal activities and handling properties of calcium in the membrane in hypertension will be presented in this paper.

Several inorganic chemical compounds block actions of the calcium channels; these compounds are termed calcium antagonists (calcium entry blockers). They strongly inhibit potassium-induced contraction, while their inhibitory effect on noradrenaline-induced contraction is less [32–34]. These compounds, nifedipine, verapamil, and diltiazem, have a therapeutic effect on cardiac arrhythmia, coronary spasm, and hypertension [1–3, 15, 35–44]. The effect of calcium antagonists suggests that calcium channels may be genetically abnormal in essential hypertension.

Over the past 15 years, evidence has accumulated of primary abnormalities in the membrane handling of calcium in arterial smooth muscle in hypertension [39–47]. The membrane abnormalities may contribute in causing an increased contractile response of the muscle and an elevated total peripheral vascular resistance in patients and animals with essential hypertension. The calcium membrane theory of essential hypertension has been proposed as a mechanism of hypertension [1–3, 15, 40–44]. This theory is based on the fact that patients with essential hypertension are subject to a type of membrane abnormality which leads to abnormal handling of calcium; this may cause the increased concentration of intracellular free calcium and bring about overcontraction and incomplete relaxation of arterial smooth muscle. The abnormal contraction induces a reduction of the arterial lumen, which results in an elevation of the total peripheral vascular resistance and this develops and produces persistent high blood pressure in patients and animals with essential hypertension. Finally, the calcium membrane theory of essential hypertension [1, 2] will be discussed in this paper.

Hemodynamics of Essential Hypertension

The level of blood pressure is dependent upon two fundamental factors—the cardiac output and the total peripheral vascular resistance. The relationship of pressure with the fluid flow volume and flow resistance was described in 1835 by Poiseuille [48, 49]. On the basis of his experiments, the pressure is determined by four factors—the flow volume, flow resistance (the radius of the tubing), length of the tube, and viscosity of the fluid. In the closed blood circulating system in humans and animals, we consider the length of the tube and the viscosity of the fluid to be the same in normotension and essential hypertension. The flow volume is equal to the cardiac output and flow resistance is equal to the total peripheral vascular resistance. Therefore, we may translate the mathematical Poiseuille's formula into the generally used formula in medical science as follows: MBP = CO × TPR; where MBP represents the mean blood pressure in mmHg, CO the cardiac output in l/min, and TPR the total peripheral vascular resistance in mmHg/l/min [4, 5, 48, 49].

An inappropriate increase in either the cardiac output or the total peripheral vascular resistance results in hypertension. To demonstrate an elevated total peripheral vascular resistance in patients with essential hypertension, we [3, 43] determined the blood pressure, heart rate, cardiac output, and calculated total peripheral vascular resistance in subjects with normotension and patients with early stage of essential hypertension. Normotensive men with a resting blood pressure of $111 \pm 4/64 \pm 5$ mmHg, heart rate of 61 ± 7 beats/min, and aged 29 ± 4 years ($n = 6$; values = mean $\pm$ SD) and hypertensive men with $131 \pm$

6/85 ± 5 mmHg, 59 ± 6 beats/min, and 41 ± 4 years ($n = 10$) were investigated for hemodynamic data before and after 1-h rest in the supine position [43]. The blood pressure of the upper right arm was measured by auscultation, using a mercury manometer. The heart rate was continuously measured with a heart rate monitor. Cardiac output was determined by the earpiece dye dilution method, using a bedside cardiac computer (Erma Dyemac EW 90-A). A bolus of 5 mg indocyanine green dye in 10 ml 5% glucose solution was intravenously administered [3, 43].

The hemodynamic indices were calculated as follows: MBP = $\frac{1}{3}$ (SBP − DBP), MBP = CO × TPR, MBP = CI × TPRI, SV = CO/HR, CI = CO/body surface area, SI = CI/HR, TPRI = MBP/CO × body surface area; where MBP represents mean blood pressure, SBP systolic blood pressure, DBP diastolic blood pressure, HR heart rate, CO cardiac output, SV stroke volume, TPR total peripheral vascular resistance, CI cardiac index, SI stroke volume index, and TPRI total peripheral vascular resistance index.

Supine resting significantly decreased blood pressure, heart rate, stroke volume, and cardiac output in subjects with both normotension and hypertension. Conversely, the resting supine position elevated total peripheral vascular resistance. Blood pressure and vascular resistance were greater in patients with hypertension than in the subjects with normotension [43] (Fig. 1).

To prove a positive correlation between blood pressure and total peripheral vascular resistance, we [3] measured the blood pressure, heart rate, and cardiac

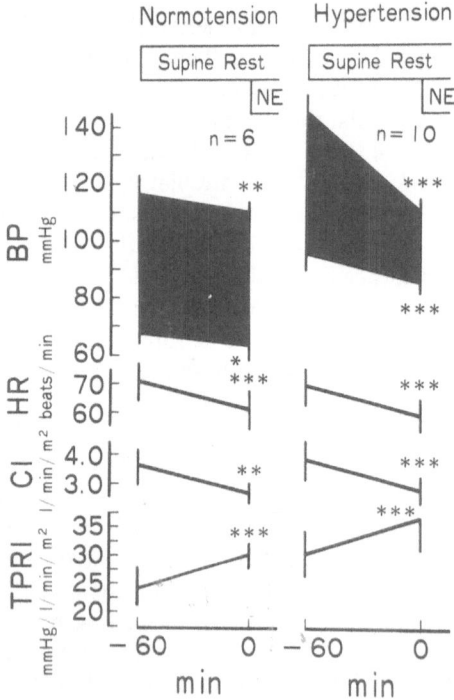

Fig. 1. Effect of supine rest on hemodynamic data in subjects with normotension and patients with essential hypertension. Supine rest diminishes blood pressure (*BP*), heart rate (*HR*), and cardiac output (*CI*), whereas it elevates total peripheral vascular resistance (*TPRI*) in both groups. Values shown are means ± SD. *P* compared with values before rest (−60 min): * *P* < 0.05, ** *P* < 0.01, *** *P* < 0.001. After Aoki et al. [43]

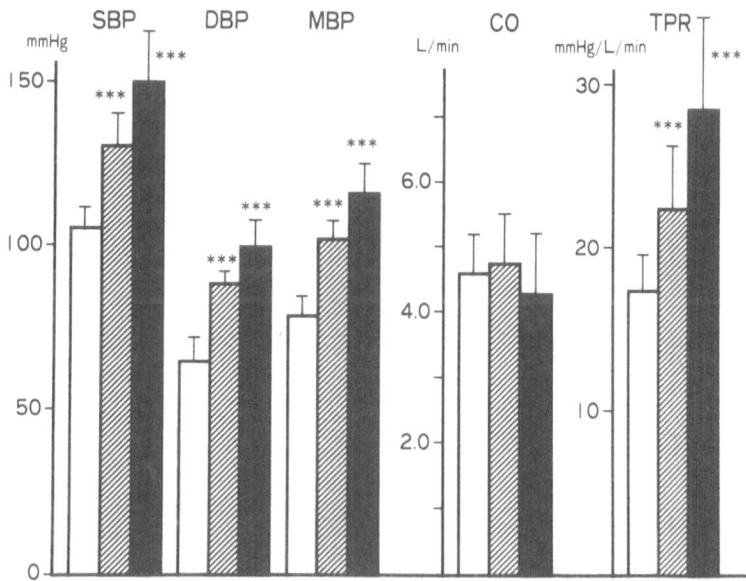

Fig. 2. Hemodynamic data in subjects with normotension and patients with essential hypertension after 1-h supine rest. Systolic blood pressure (*SBP*), diastolic blood pressure (*DBP*), and mean blood pressure (*MBP*) are greater in the borderline phase (▨) and established phase (■) of essential hypertension than in normotension (□). Cardiac output (*CO*) does not differ between normotension and both phases of essential hypertension. In contrast to cardiac output, the total peripheral vascular resistance (*TPR*) is greater in both phases of essential hypertension than in normotension. Values shown are mean ± SD. *P* compared with values of normotension: *** $P < 0.001$

output after 1-h rest in the supine position in 45 male subjects, including normotensives with a blood pressure of $105 \pm 6/65 \pm 7$ mmHg, heart rate of 58 ± 6 beats/min, and aged 33 ± 4 years ($n = 12$), subjects in the borderline phase of essential hypertension with $130 \pm 10/88 \pm 4$ mmHg, 61 ± 4 beats/min, and 46 ± 7 years ($n = 11$), and patients in the established phase of essential hypertension with $150 \pm 16/100 \pm 8$ mmHg, 60 ± 6 beats/min, and 46 ± 6 years ($n = 22$). After 1 h of supine resting, the blood pressure and vascular resistance in the patients with hypertension were higher than in the subjects with normotension (Fig. 2). Blood pressure was positively correlated with vascular resistance ($y = 0.261 \times -2.94$, $r = 0.710$, $n = 45$, $P < 0.001$) [3] (Fig. 3). Blood pressure was not correlated with cardiac output [3]. The elevated vascular resistance may indicate that the radius of the tubing of the circulating blood is decreased in patients with essential hypertension. The radius of the tubing corresponds to the radius of the arterial lumen in humans and animals.

Lund-Johansen [4, 5] reported that recent studies using noninvasive methods for measurement of blood pressure and cardiac output in children and adolescents with hypertensive parents would seem to indicate that the raised blood pressure is due to an elevated total peripheral vascular resistance in the resting

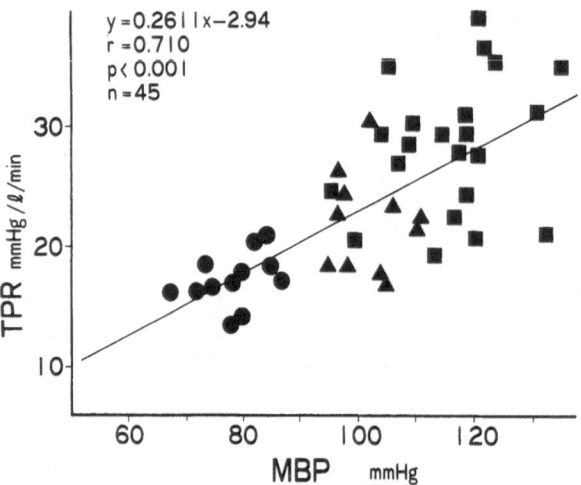

Fig. 3. Correlation of mean blood pressure and total peripheral vascular resistance. Mean blood pressure (*MBP*) increases with elevation of total peripheral vascular resistance (*TPR*) in subjects with normotension (•) and the borderline phase (▲) and established phase (■) of essential hypertension. After Aoki et al. [43]

supine position but not due to an increased cardiac output. Our observed findings of a reduction in cardiac output and elevation of vascular resistance induced by the 1-h supine rest suggest that some inadequate condition increases the cardiac output and diminishes vascular resistance. Both the increase in cardiac output and decrease in vascular resistance under mentally and physically restless conditions, combine to abolish an elevated vascular resistance and there is no correlation of blood pressure and total peripheral vascular resistance in patients with essential hypertension. Therefore, after the subject rested in the supine position for 1 h, it could clearly be demonstrated that the vascular resistance was greater in the early stage of essential hypertension and the blood pressure was positively correlated with the vascular resistance [3]. This evidence suggests that an elevation of vascular resistance results in an increase in blood pressure in patients with essential hypertension.

The progressive elevation of the vascular resistance is associated with the increase in blood pressure over a period of 50 years from the normotensive stage to the borderline hypertensive stage and established stage of essential hypertension. It may be concluded that the increase in blood pressure is induced by the abnormal elevation of vascular resistance in patients with essential hypertension (Fig. 4).

Contractile Responses of Arterial Smooth Muscle

The elevated arterial blood pressure in patients with essential hypertension is caused by increased total peripheral vascular resistance [3–5]. Total peripheral

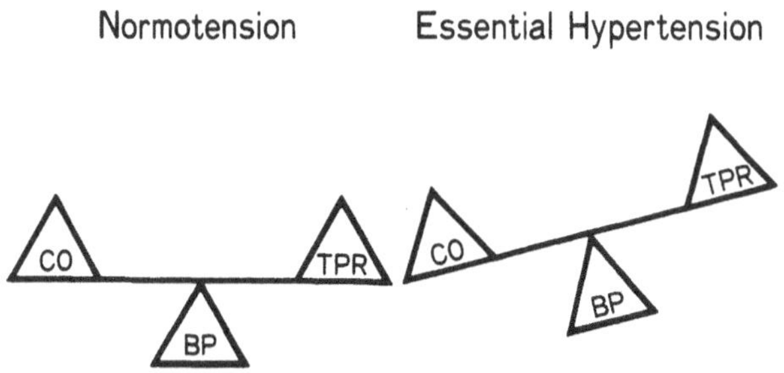

Normotension   Essential Hypertension

Fig. 4. Schema of hemodynamic factors in subjects with normotension and essential hypertension. Elevated total peripheral vascular resistance (*TPR*) increases the blood pressure (*BP*) but not the cardiac output (*CO*) in subjects with essential hypertension

vascular resistance (TPR) is regulated by changes in the size of the lumen of arteries as follows:

$$TPR = \frac{(\text{cardiac output}) \times (\text{length of arteries})}{(\text{radius of arterial lumen})^4} \times 8\pi$$

This formula indicates that vascular resistance is markedly affected by relatively small changes in the radius of the arterial lumen. Therefore, the elevated blood pressure in patients with essential hypertension is the result of a change in the arterial lumen, either structual or functional. Folkow [10, 11] in reviews showed that the increased vascular resistance in hypertension can be accounted for by an increased wall thickness by media hypertrophy of arterial vessels. The hypertrophy in hypertension consists of both hyperplasia and hypertrophy of the arterial smooth muscle, which can increase the bulk of the wall so that it encroaches upon the lumen of the arteries. A rise in pressure for the arterial wall results in thickening of the wall by muscle hypertrophy through physiological adaptation, which is a structural wall thickening. An other mechanism is then needed to account for the increased thickness of the arterial wall, which may be a functional alteration of arterial smooth muscle. Contraction of arterial smooth muscle results in shortening of the circumference of the arterial lumen and contraction of the muscle brings about the increase in thickening of the arterial media [50, 51] (Fig. 5).

An increased contraction of arterial smooth muscle may originate from an abnormality of the contractile properties in the muscle cells themselves. Functional changes in the contractile activity of the muscle can be demonstrated from the increased contractile response to vasoconstrictive agents. We [13–15, 17, 40] have attempted to demonstrate an increased contractile response to agonists in the muscle from SHR. The contractile responses were measured by the calcium-induced tension development of the muscle in the presence and absence of potassium or noradrenaline.

Arterial strips from 6-week-old male SHR and age- and sex-matched normotensive Wistar Kyoto rats (WKY) were studied [12]. The blood pressure was 130 ± 5 and 110 ± 5 (mean $\pm$ SD) mmHg in SHR and WKY, respectively. He-

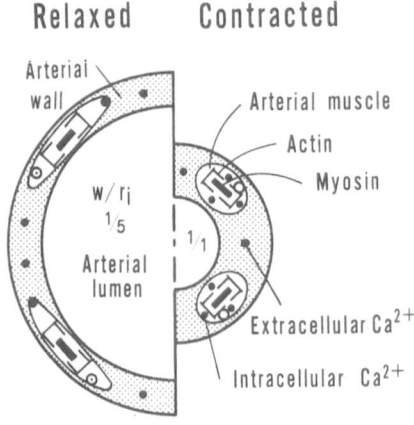

Relaxed   Contracted

Arterial wall

Arterial muscle

Actin

Myosin

W/r_i $\frac{1}{5}$

$\frac{1}{1}$

Arterial lumen

Extracellular Ca^{2+}

Intracellular Ca^{2+}

Fig. 5. Schema of an arterial cross section. Arterial smooth muscle is subject to contraction and relaxation. Contraction is induced by a rise of the calcium concentration in the cytosol, which leads to shortening and widening of the arterial smooth muscle through overlapping of the actin and myosin filaments. Contraction of arterial muscle brings about thickening and widening of the arterial wall, which results in wall thickening of the arterial vessels and reduction of the arterial lumen. Wall thickening and lumen reduction bring about an increase in the wall-lumen ratio. W/r_i thickness of wall/radius of arterial lumen

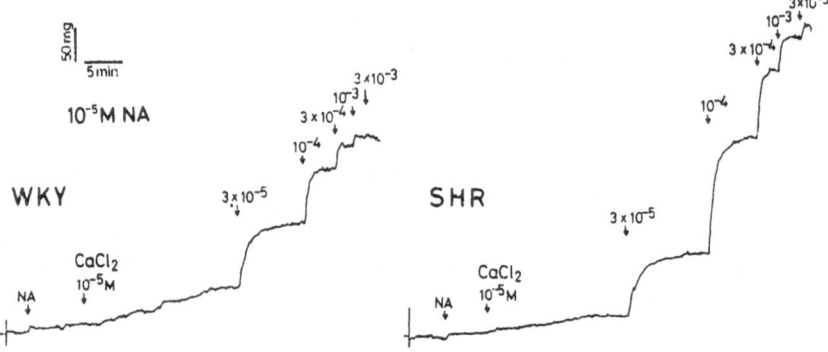

Fig. 6. Increase in calcium-induced contraction of arterial smooth muscle from SHR compared with that from normotensive WKY. The calcium-induced contraction of arterial smooth muscle of the mesenteric artery from SHR is greater than in that from WKY. Contraction is induced by the cumulative addition of $CaCl_2$ to Ca^{2+}-free solution in the presence of 10^{-5} M noradrenaline (NA) after removal of intra- and extracellular calcium by washing the tissue with PSS containing EGTA

lical strips of the superior mesenteric artery were mounted vertically between hooks in a muscle bath containing physiological salt solution (PSS). The strips were placed in calcium-free PSS containing 10^{-5} M noradrenaline for 15 min for the extrusion of calcium from the intracellular storage and binding sites. The strips were then equilibrated in calcium-free PSS containing 0.5 mM EGTA for 60 min. After they had been washed out in calcium-free PSS, some strips were immersed in calcium-free PSS containing a high level of potassium (121 mM K$^+$) to open the voltage-dependent calcium channels, while others were immersed in calcium-free PSS containing noradrenaline (10^{-5} M) to open the receptor-operated calcium channels. Dose-response curves for calcium-induced tension were obtained by a cumulative stepwise increase in the concentration of calcium (Fig. 6).

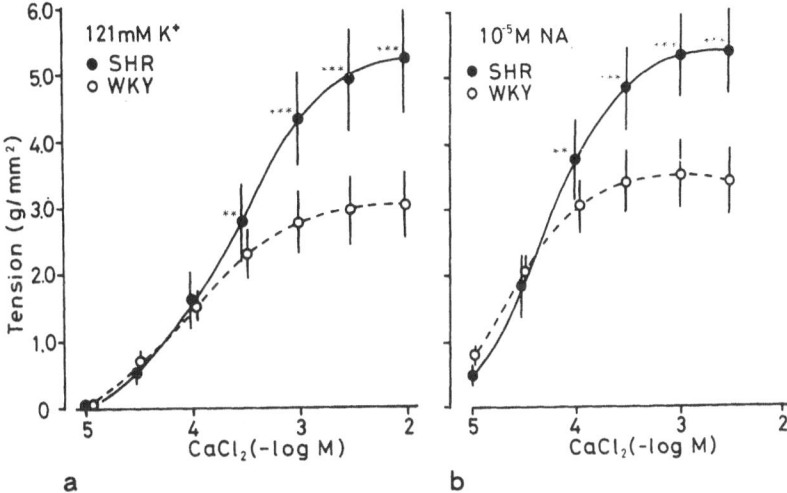

Fig. 7a b. Dose-response curves of calcium-induced contraction of mesenteric arterial smooth muscle. Calcium-induced tension development of mesenteric arterial strips from SHR (●) is greater than in those from WKY (o) **a** in the presence of potassium (121 mM K) and **b** noradrenaline (10^{-5} M NA). After Aoki et al. [15]

Absolute tension per unit of cross-sectional area was calculated using the wet weight of the strips, which was expressed as g/mm^2. The calcium-induced tension was significantly greater in the SHR than in the WKY strips in the presence of high levels of potassium (Fig. 7a) and noradrenaline (Fig. 7b). The observed increased calcium-induced tension of the SHR strips means that, in contrast to WKY, contraction of arterial smooth muscle of SHR is enhanced by an increase in the available calcium to the contractile apparatus. Thus, the cell membrane and sarcoplasmic reticulum membrane of arterial smooth muscle of SHR may increase calcium permeability as calcium influx through calcium channels by either voltage-dependent or noradrenaline receptor-operated channels.

The calcium-handling properties of the cell membrane and sarcoplasmic reticulum membrane regulate the level of intracellular free calcium concentration in arterial smooth muscle. Therefore, alterations in the function of the cellular membranes, such as calcium influx, calcium release, and calcium-binding ability, may be essential factors for the regulation of the intracellular calcium concentration, which determines the level of contraction of arterial smooth muscle. Calcium binding by isolated fragments of the cell membrane and sarcoplasmic reticulum from arterial smooth muscle of SHR is significantly decreased compared with that of normotensive controls [18–21]. A reduction in the amount of calcium bound to the cellular membranes leads to partial membrane depolarization, which increases the membrane permeability of calcium ions. The deficient calcium binding to the cell membrane in SHR can account for a greater membrane lability and an increased sensitivity to vasoconstrictive agents [6–9, 13–17].

It has been observed that the calcium concentration required to cause relaxation of a contractile response in isolated arterial strips from SHR is higher than that in arteries from normotensive controls [7] and that the fast component of the contraction is steeper in arteries from SHR than in those from normotensive rats [7, 17]. These findings suggest that alterations in membrane permeability to ions in arteries from SHR may result from a decrease in the binding by calcium in the cell membrane and sarcoplasmic reticulum [7].

Contractile Proteins, Cell Membrane, and Sarcoplasmic Reticulum Membrane in Arterial Smooth Muscle

Contraction and relaxation operate in arterial smooth muscle, which is similar to the skeletal muscle system in its basic arrangement. In 1954, Huxley and Niedergerke [52], Huxley and Simmons [53], and Huxley [54, 55] proposed that shortening of striated muscle is the result of a relative sliding between two sets of filaments—thick (myosin) and thin (actin) filaments. The filaments are arranged in a regular array. The change in muscle length is achieved by a variation in the amount of overlap between the actin and myosin filaments. The filaments do not alter in length during shortening (Fig. 5). In the contracted state, this actin and myosin interaction is responsible for shortening or isometric tension development [56–58]. In vascular smooth muscle, the process of the basic contractile machinery is controlled by a component of the head of the myosin molecule, the myosin light chain. The velocity of shortening of the vascular smooth muscle is determined by the degree of phosphorylation of the myosin light chain. This phosphorylation is produced by the enzyme myosin light-chain kinase, which is activated by the calcium-calmodulin complex.

The increase in calcium concentration in the myoplasm initiates the interaction of myosin with actin. The threshold for mechanical activation of the contractile proteins is of the order of 10^{-7} M intracellular free calcium concentration. The full activation of contraction occurs at about 10^{-5} M [27, 58–61]. Since the concentration of the extracellular fluid is greater than 10^{-3} M, the cell membrane constitutes a barrier that is capable of maintaining this 10 000-fold concentration gradient of calcium. An increase of intracellular calcium in smooth muscle can be obtained either by increasing the calcium influx across the cell membrane and calcium release from membrane calcium storage sites or by decreasing the calcium extrusion. The inward current responsible for the upstroke of the action potential is mainly due to the influx of calcium ions through potential-dependent calcium channels [27, 28]. Activation of a receptor by an agonist noradrenaline can induce an increase in the calcium influx and release. This pathway uses calcium entering the cell and is termed a receptor-operated calcium channel [27, 28]. The other mechanism of the calcium-induced calcium-release mechanism triggers the contraction, i.e., calcium entering through the cell membrane may not directly increase the free calcium in the myoplasm but may be accumulated at a storage site. After a certain amount of calcium has been stored, the release of calcium is started [29–31]. The sarcoplasmic reticulum can store enough calcium to activate contraction and induce maximal contraction of arterial smooth muscle [31, 58].

To demonstrate alteration of the calcium-handling properties of the cell membrane and sarcoplasmic reticulum membrane, we [18–21] investigated calcium binding with isolated fragmented membrane fractions from the arterial smooth muscle of SHR and compared them with those from normotensive control rats. The subcellular membrane fractions were prepared by the method of Fitzpatrick et al. [62] with slight modifications, i.e., successive centrifugation of homogenates of small pieces of arterial tissue in 0.25 M mannital, 5 mM histidine, and 1 mM dithiothreitol. A major part of the membrane fraction was sarcoplasmic reticulum. Measurement of calcium uptake and ATPase activity were performed in 0.1 M KCl, 3 mM ATP and MgCl$_2$, and 10 mM tris-HCl (pH 7.4) containing 0.5 μCi ^{45}Ca [20, 21]. The bound and free calcium were separated using a Millipore filter and measured utilizing a liquid scintillation counter (Packard tricub). The maximum uptake and apparent binding constants were estimated by double reciprocal plots of free and bound calcium to the subcellular membrane fraction of sarcoplasmic reticulum. For measurement of the calcium content, the sample was hydrolyzed in perchloric acid and concentrated nitric acid at 120°C for 7 h, then diluted with 5 ml water. Calcium was measured using an atomic absorption spectrometer (Hitachi-208).

The ATPase activity of the sarcoplasmic reticulum showed no significant difference between SHR and normotensive control rats. The calcium uptake of the sarcoplasmic reticulum was significantly lower in SHR than in normotensive control rats (Fig. 8a). The maximal calcium uptake was 17.28 ± 0.30 and 22.16 ± 1.81 nmol/mg protein in SHR and normotensive control rats, respectively (Fig.

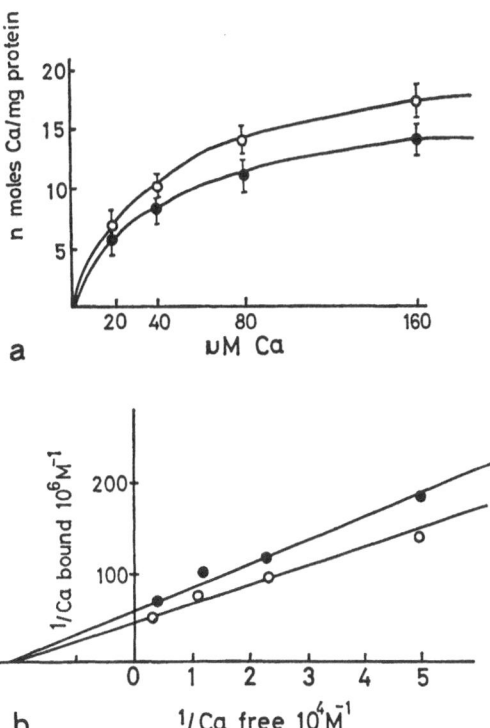

Fig. 8a, b. ATP-dependent Ca^{2+} accumulation by the sarcoplasmic reticulum from arteries. **a** The calcium accumulation is smaller in the sarcoplasmic reticulum from SHR (●) than in that from WKY (o) in the medium containing 0.1 M KCl, 3 mM MgCl$_2$, 3 mM ATP in 1 mM tris-HCl (pH 7.4) at 37°C for 10 min. **b** Double reciprocal plot of bound and free Ca^{2+} obtained from the values of calcium accumulation. The maximum binding is greater in SHR than in WKY, but the binding constant is not different. Values shown are means ± SD. After Aoki et al. [19, 21]

Table 1. Mobilizable and unmobilizable calcium content of sarcoplasmic reticulum of arteries from SHR and normotensive rats

	Calcium content 10^{-8} mol/mg	
	Normotension	Hypertension
Sample in standard buffer[a]	2.43 ± 0.22	2.72 ± 0.28
Sample washed with buffer containing ATP, Mg, and EGTA[b]	1.87 ± 0.23	1.83 ± 0.30
Sample washed with buffer containing EGTA (unmobilizable calcium)[c]	1.20 ± 0.22	1.47 ± 0.30
ATP-dependent mobilizable calcium (a−b)	0.56	0.89
ATP-independent mobilizable calcium (a−c)	1.23	1.25
ATP-dependent uptake calcium (b−c)	0.70	0.40

[a] Sample prepared by standard buffer containing 3 mM ATP, 3 mM Mg
[b] Sample was washed with buffer containing 3 mM ATP, 3 mM Mg, and 5 mM EGTA
[c] Sample was washed with buffer containing 5 mM EGTA without ATP and Mg

8b). The maximum calcium uptake of the sarcoplasmic reticulum was significantly lower in SHR than in normotensive control rats; the apparent binding constant was 2.22 ± 0.08 and $2.07 \pm 0.16 \times 10^{-4}$ M^{-1}, respectively (Fig. 8b). The calcium-binding constant did not differ between SHR and the control. The SHR sarcoplasmic reticulum always showed a greater calcium content than did that of the normotensive control. After washing with buffer solution containing 5 mM EGTA, the calcium content was reduced to approximately half that of the prewashing level. When ATP, 3 mM Mg, and 6 mM EGTA were present in the washing medium, the washing treatment reduced calcium in the sarcoplasmic reticulum, which became less effective. Mobilizable (exchangeable) calcium in the sarcoplasmic reticulum from SHR was greater than that from normotensive controls [20, 21] (Table 1). The obtained results [20, 21] of a decrease in both the calcium uptake and binding sites by the sarcoplasmic reticulum and an increase in the membrane mobilizable calcium suggest that the available calcium for the contractile machinery may be greater in SHR than in normotensive controls in the calcium-containing medium. This is supported by an increase in the contractile response of arterial smooth muscle to calcium and other vasoconstrictive stimuli such as noradrenaline [14] and Bay k 8644 [13]. Impairment of ATP-dependent calcium accumulation and defective calcium binding by the cell membrane and sarcoplasmic reticulum may be a primary genetic mechanism for essential hypertension. It is suggested that a genetic mechanism operates to induce the impairment and defective calcium-handling properties of the cellular membrane of arterial smooth muscle as a primary cause of essential hypertension in humans and animals.

Calcium Antagonist in Hypertension

Genetically altered activity of the arterial smooth muscle is considered a major cause of essential hypertension [1–3, 13–26]. Muscle function is controlled by the intracellular ionic environment, especially the distribution of calcium in the cell. Noradrenaline acts on α-receptors in the cell membrane and induces calcium influx and release, which induces a rise in the intracellular free calcium. This rise brings about the contraction of arterial smooth muscle and elevates the blood pressure, which is a pressure response to noradrenaline. We [3, 43] have investigated the pressor responses to noradrenaline in patients with essential hypertension compared with those in normotensives. The stepwise increase in the intravenous noradrenaline infusion, over 5 min from 0.1 to 0.2 and 0.3 μg/kg/min, cumulatively elevated blood pressure and total peripheral vascular resistance, and the infusion decreased heart rate, stroke volume, and cardiac output. The elevation of blood pressure in patients with essential hypertension was greater than that in normotensives [3, 43] (Fig. 9).

Calcium antagonists (calcium channel blockers) inhibit influx through the cell membrane and release of calcium from the sarcoplasmic reticulum and cell membrane. They antagonize the calcium function which are responsible for excitation and contraction in the electromechanical coupling. Thus, calcium antagonists block contraction of arterial smooth muscle cells and induce relaxation. The actions of calcium antagonists bring about arterial vasodilation, which can be expected to lower elevated vascular resistance and then lower arterial blood pressure.

The calcium antagonists nifedipine [35–38] and diltiazem [39] were studied in normotensive volunteers and patients with essential hypertension as to their hypotensive action and hemodynamic effects. Nifedipine decreased blood pressure and total peripheral vascular resistance, while increasing heart rate, stroke volume, and cardiac output. The decrease in blood pressure and vascular resistance and increase in cardiac output in the patients with essential hypertension were greater than in normotensives [3, 43]. In the presence of nifedipine (1 h after nifedipine administration), the intravenous norepinephrine infusion, over 5 min from 0.1 to 0.2 and 0.3 μg/kg/min, did not increase the total peripheral vascular resistance either in hypertensives or normotensives. The presence of nifedipine partly inhibited the increase in blood pressure by noradrenaline in the patients with essential hypertension, but it did not inhibit the blood pressure increase in the normotensive subjects. The norepinephrine did not change cardiac output in the presence of nifedipine in both groups [3, 43] (Fig. 9).

The subsequent administration of propranolol elevated both diastolic blood pressure and vascular resistance and it diminished heart rate and cardiac output in the presence of nifedipine. In the presence of nifedipine and propranolol, the noradrenaline infusion increased blood pressure and vascular resistance, but it decreased cardiac output in both groups. The norepinephrine infusion diminished heart rate and stroke volume in the normotensive subjects, but it did not change in the hypertensives [3, 43] (Fig. 9).

The calcium antagonist nifedipine induces a significant decrease in both blood pressure and vascular resistance, but it increases the cardiac output. The observed fall in blood pressure results from arterial vasodilation. Nifedipine reaches the arterial smooth muscle and inhibits calcium infux and release. The inhibition induces relaxation of arterial smooth muscle, which leads to widening of the arterial lumen and reduction of the total peripheral vascular resistance. The reduction results in a decrease in blood pressure in hypertension [3, 43] (Fig. 10).

236

K. Aoki

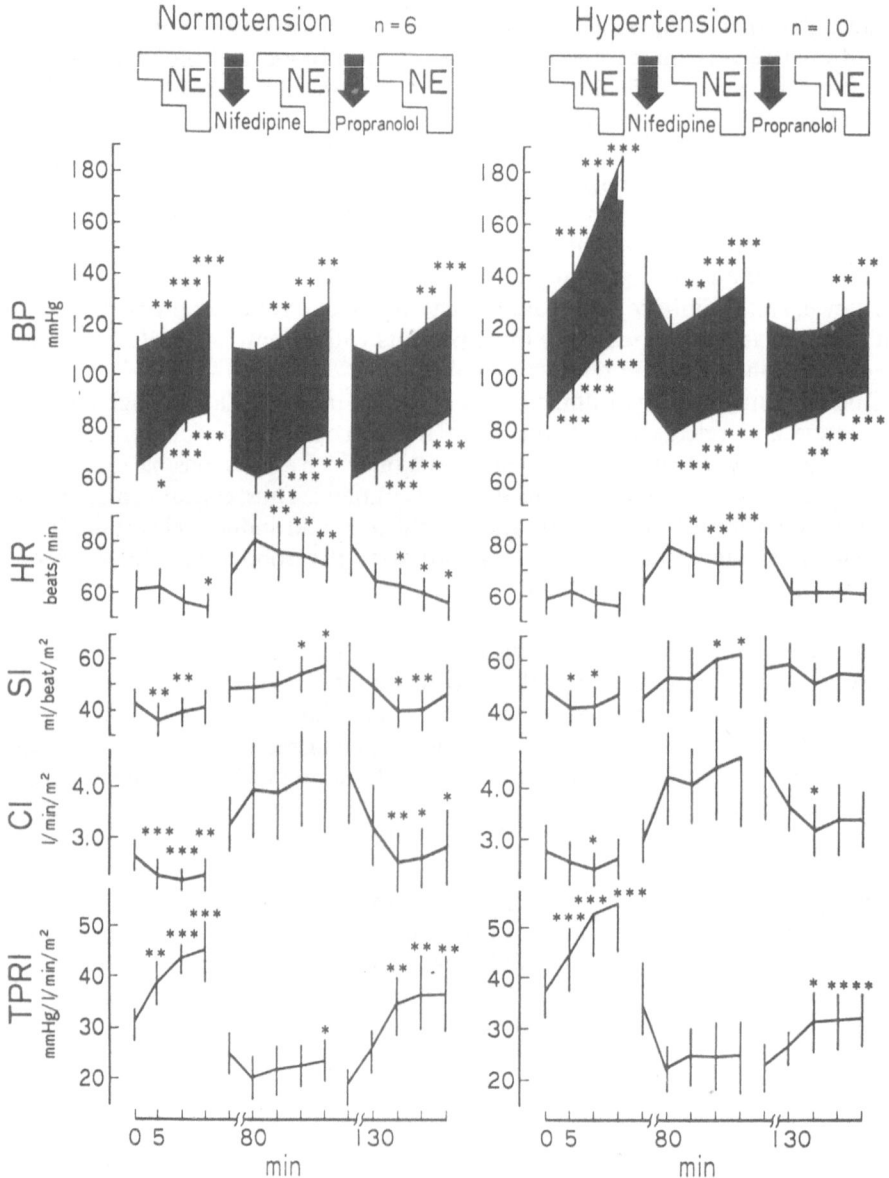

Fig. 9. Effects of noradrenaline infusion on hemodynamic data in the presence and absence of the calcium antagonist nifedipine and the beta-blocker propranolol in subjects with normotension or essential hypertension. Intravenous noradrenaline (*NE*) infusion of 0.1–0.3 μg/kg/min increases the blood pressure (*BP*) and total peripheral vascular resistance (*TPRI*), while decreasing the heart rate (*HR*), stroke volume (*SI*), and cardiac output (*CO*) in both groups. Administration of nifedipine (10 mg Adalat) reduces BP and TPR, while it increases HR, SI, and CI. Nifedipine reduces the noradrenaline-dependent increases in BP evident in hypertensives, while having little or no effect in normotensives. In the presence of nifedipine, noradrenaline does not elevate TPRI in hypertensives, and it only slightly elevates TPRI in normotensives. Propranolol (10 mg i.v.) raises BP and TPRI, and it reduces HR, SI, and CI. Thirty minutes after propranolol administration, noradrenaline increases BP and TPRI and reduces CI in both groups. P compared between prenoradrenaline and noradrenaline * $P < 0.05$, ** $P < 0.01$, *** $P < 0.001$. After Aoki and Sato [3]

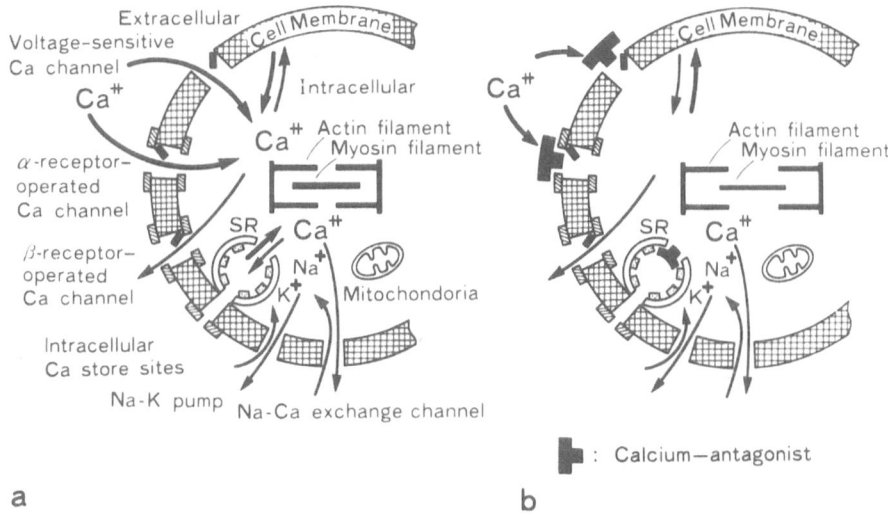

Fig. 10a, b. Schema of membranes and their cellular and molecular functions of arterial smooth muscle. **a** A characteristic of the cell membrane is a barrier between the internal and external environment which regulates the cell's activities. This may exist as a complex cell-surface structure. There are voltage-dependent (sensitive) and receptor-operated calcium channels, sodium-calcium exchange channels, and sodium-potassium pump channels. Depolarization opens the voltage-dependent calcium channels, which leads to calcium influx. Noradrenaline acts on the α-receptor-operated calcium channels and induces influx and release of calcium. Within the cell, the sarcoplasmic reticulum binds and accumulates calcium. Noradrenaline affects the sarcoplasmic reticulum and releases calcium from the membrane storage sites. The concentration of intracellular free calcium is mainly regulated by the amount of the calcium influx and release. **b** The calcium antagonist blocks the calcium channels, both voltage dependent and α-receptor operated, and this inhibits calcium influx. The drug may act on calcium-storage sites of the cell membrane and the sarcoplasmic reticulum and inhibit calcium release. These effects depress a rise in the intracellular free calcium, which blocks the overlapping of the actin and myosin filaments. Thus, the calcium antagonist inhibits contraction of the muscle. *SR* sarcoplasmic reticulum, surface vesicle, or caveole. ▶ calcium antagonist. After Aoki et al. [43]

Calcium Membrane Theory of Essential Hypertension

Reports from several independent groups [18–26] have attested to defective ATP-dependent calcium accumulation and defective calcium binding with membrane preparations from vascular smooth muscle obtained from SHR. Calcium acts on the cell membrane in that potassium conduction is increased with resultant hyperpolarization of the cell. Therefore, impaired calcium binding would favor depolarization with consequent activation of voltage-dependent calcium channels, which leads to calcium influx. The increased calcium influx induces the release of calcium from the sarcoplasmic reticulum and cell membrane and results in an increase in calcium concentration in the cytosol.

In other studies, the calcium antagonist exerts a more pronounced relaxation of arterial smooth muscle from SHR contracted with or without noradrenaline than in muscle from normotensive rats [13, 63, 64]. In addition, we have demonstrated that: (1) the noradrenaline-induced increase in blood pressure and vascular resistance in patients with essential hypertension is greater than in subjects with normotension [3, 43], and (2) the inhibitory effect of the calcium antagonist on elevation of blood pressure and vascular resistance induced by noradrenaline in hypertension is greater than in normotension [3, 43]. These observations suggest that α-receptor-operated calcium channels are abnormal and that the abnormality induces increased calcium permeability. This may result from an increase in the number of calcium channels in the cell membrane in patients with essential hypertension.

Impaired calcium-binding sites, calcium-accumulation sites, and abnormality of calcium channels in the membrane, either singly or combined, cause an increase in the calcium concentration of the cytosol. The increase in calcium concentration induces an increase in overlap of the actin and myosin filaments, which results in overcontraction and incomplete relaxation. The abnormal contraction brings about shortening of the long diameter and widening of the short diameter of arterial vessels. These changes in the muscle induce a reduction of the arterial lumen, which increases the total peripheral vascular resistance and elevates the blood pressure, causing hypertension to develop and persist in patients and animals with essential hypertension (Fig. 11).

The mechanism of elevation of blood pressure in essential hypertension is as follows:

In arterial smooth muscle:

Genetic abnormalities of cell membrane
and sarcoplasmic reticulum
↓
Increase in calcium influx and release
↓
Increase in calcium concentration in cytosol
↓
Increase in overlapping of actin and myosin filaments
(Overcontraction and incomplete relaxation)
↓
Shortening of long diameter,
widening of short diameter
↓
Reduction of arterial lumen
↓
Rise in total peripheral vascular resistance
↓
Elevation of blood pressure

In conclusion patients with essential hypertension are subject to a disorder of membrane function in arterial smooth muscle. The membrane abnormality leads to altered handling of calcium. The abnormalities occur in the cell membrane and sarcoplasmic reticulum membrane, which increase calcium influx and release, causing the increase in calcium concentration in the cytosol. The raised concentration of calcium induces an excess of overlapping of actin and myosin filaments,

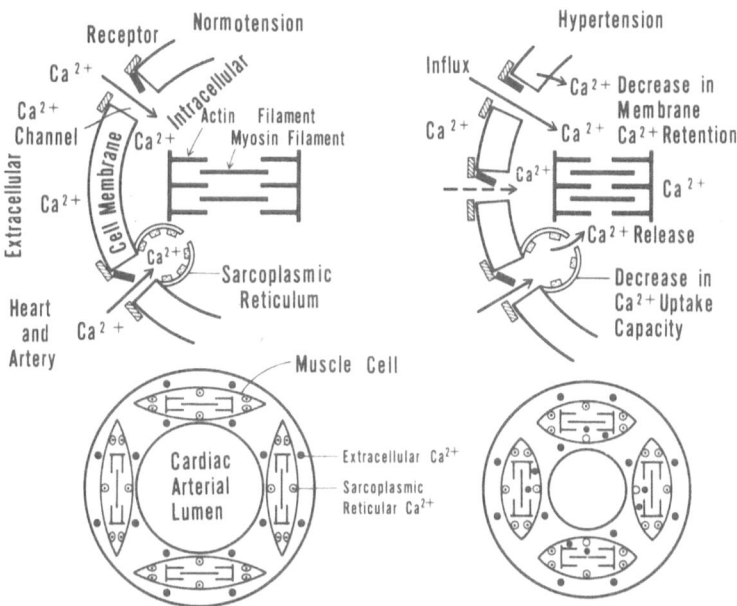

Fig. 11. Schema of the calcium membrane theory of essential hypertension. There is an abnormality of the membrane calcium handling in arterial smooth muscle in patients with essential hypertension. An increase in the number of calcium channels as an abnormality in the cell membrane is a possible mechanism of increasing the calcium influx. A decrease in calcium-binding and storage sites in the cell membrane and sarcoplasmic reticulum increases calcium release. Increases in both calcium influx and release lead to raised calcium concentration in the cytosol, which induces overcontraction and incomplete relaxation of arterial smooth muscle. The abnormal contraction of arterial smooth muscle brings about a raised total peripheral vascular resistance, which causes an elevation of blood pressure in patients with essential hypertension. After Aoki [1]

producing overcontraction and incomplete relaxation. Overcontraction brings about shortening of the long diameter and widening of the short diameter of arterial smooth muscle, which leads to encroachment upon the arterial lumen, causing reduction. Reduction of the arterial lumen results in a rise in the total peripheral vascular resistance, which elevates blood pressure and brings about the development and persistence of hypertension in patients with essential hypertension [1]. Therefore, I propose that membrane abnormality of the membrane calcium-handling properties leads to hypertension in both patients with essential hypertention and SHR, which is the calcium membrane theory of essential hypertension [1–3, 41–44].

References

1. Aoki K (1982) Hypertensiology, Essential and Secondary Hypertension, Concepts, Nature, Diagnosis, and Treatment (in Japanese). Shinkoh Igaku Shuppan, Tokyo, pp 4–20

2. Aoki K (1982) Hypertensiology, Essential and Secondary Hypertension, Concepts, Nature, Diagnosis, and Treatment (in Japanese). Shinkoh Igaku Shuppan, Tokyo, pp 20–29
3. Aoki K, Sato K (1985) Pathophysiological background for the use of calcium antagonists. J Cardiovasc Pharmacol 7 (Suppl 4): S28–S32
4. Lund-Johansen P (1983) Haemodynamics in early essential hypertension—still an area of controversy. J Hypertension 1: 209–213
5. Lund-Johansen P (1983) The hemodynamics of essential hypertension. In: Robertson JIS (ed) Clinical aspects of essential hypertension. Handbook of hypertension, vol 1. Elsevier, Amsterdam, pp 151–173
6. Bohr DF (1973) Vascular smooth muscle updated. Circ Res 32: 665–672
7. Bohr DF, Webb RC (1984) Vascular smooth muscle function and its changes in hypertension. Am J Med 77 (4A): 3–16
8. Winquist RJ, Webb RC, Bohr DF (1982) Vascular smooth muscle in hypertension. Federation Proc 41: 2387–2393
9. Webb RC, Bohr DF (1981) Recent advances in the pathogenesis of hypertension: Consideration of structural, functional, and metabolic vascular abnormalities resulting in elevated arterial resistance. Am Heart J 102: 251–264
10. Folkow B (1978) Cardiovascular structural adaptation: its role in the initiation and maintenance of primary hypertension. Clin Sci Mol Med 55: 3s–22s
11. Folkow B (1982) Physiological aspects of primary hypertension. Physiol Rev 62: 347–504
12. Okamoto K, Aoki K (1963) Development of a strain of spontaneously hypertensive rats. Jpn Circ J 27: 282–293
13. Aoki K, Asano M (1986) Effects of Bay k 8644 and nifedipine on femoral arteries of spontaneously hypertensive rats. Brit J Pharmacol 88: 221–230
14. Asano M, Aoki K, Matsuda T (1984) Quantitative changes of maximum contractile response to norepinephrine in mesenteric arteries from spontaneously hypertensive rats during the development of hypertension. J Cardiovasc Pharmacol 6: 727–731
15. Aoki K, Kawaguchi Y, Sato K, Kondo S, Yamamoto M (1982) Clinical and pharmacological properties of calcium antagonists in essential hypertension in humans and spontaneously hypertensive rat. J Cardiovasc Pharmacol 4: S298–S302
16. Hansen TR, Bohr DF (1975) Hypertension, transmural pressure, and vascular smooth muscle response in rats. Circ Res 36: 590–598
17. Aoki K, Mochizuki A, Hotta K (1981) Noradrenaline and calcium induced tension in aortic strips of normotensive and spontaneously hypertensive rats. Jpn Circ J 45: 547–551
18. Aoki K, Ikeda N, Hotta K (1972) Cardiac myofibrillar adenosine triphosphatase activity and calcium binding of microsome in the spontaneously hypertensive rat. In: Okamoto K (ed) Spontaneous hypertension, its pathogenesis and complications. Igaku Shoin, Tokyo, pp 173–175
19. Aoki K, Ikeda N, Yamashita K, Tazumi K, Sato I, Hotta K (1974) Cardiovascular contraction in spontaneously hypertensive rat: Ca^{2+} interaction of myofibrils and subcellular membrane of heart and arterial smooth muscle. Jpn Circ J 38: 1115–1121
20. Aoki K, Ikeda N, Yamashita K, Hotta K (1974) ATPase activity and Ca^{2+} interaction of myofibrils and sarcoplasmic reticulum isolated from the heart of spontaneously hypertensive rats. Jpn Heart J 15: 475–484
21. Aoki K, Yamashita K, Hotta K (1976) Calcium uptake by subcellular membranes from vascular smooth muscle of spontaneously hypertensive rats. Jpn J Pharmacol 26: 624–627
22. Moore L, Hurwitz L, Davenport GR, Landon EJ (1975) Energy-dependent calcium uptake activity of microsomes from the aorta of normal and hypertensive rats. Biochim Biophysic Acta 413: 432–443
23. Wei JW, Janis RA, Daniel EE (1976) Calcium accumulation and enzymatic activities of subcellular fractions from aortae and ventricles of genetically hypertensive rats. Circ Res 39: 133–140
24. Wei JW, Janis RA, Daniel EE (1977) Alterations in calcium transport and binding by the plasma membrane of mesenteric arteries from spontaneously hypertensive rats. Blood Vessels 14: 55–64

25. Kwan CY, Daniel EE (1982) Arterial muscle membrane abnormalities of hydralazine-treated spontaneously hypertensive rats. Eur J Pharmacol 92:187–190
26. Kwan CY, Belbeck L, Daniel EE (1979) Abnormal biochemistry of vascular smooth muscle plasma membrane as an important factor in the initiation and maintenance of hypertension in rats. Blood Vessels 16:259–268
27. Droogmans F, Himpens B, Casteels R (1985) Ca-exchange, Ca-channels and Ca-antagonists. Experientia 41:895–900
28. Bolton TB (1979) Mechanisms of action of transmitters and other substances on smooth muscle. Physiol Rev 59:606–718
29. Endo M (1977) Calcium release from the sarcoplasmic reticulum. Physiol Rev 57:71–108
30. Endo M, Tanaka M, Ogawa Y (1970) Calcium induced release of calcium from the sarcoplasmic reticulum of skinned skeletal muscle fibers. Nature (Lond) 228:34–36
31. Itoh T, Ueno H, Kuriyama H (1985) Calcium-induced calcium release mechanism in vascular smooth muscles—assessments based on contractions evoked in intact and saponin-treated skinned muscles. Experientia 41:989–996
32. Fleckenstein A (1983) Calcium antagonism in heart and smooth muscle. Wiley, New York
33. Cauvin C, Loutzenhiser R, van Breemen C (1983) Mechanisms of calcium antagonist-induced vasodilation. Ann Rev Pharmac Toxic 23:373–396
34. van Breemen C, Lukeman S, Cauvin C (1984) Atheoretic consideration on the use of calcium antagonists in the treatment of hypertension. Am J M 77 (4A):26–30
35. Aoki K, Yoshida T, Kato S, Tazumi K, Sato I, Takikawa, K, Hotta K (1976) Hypotensive action and increased plasma renin activity by Ca^{2+} antagonist (nifedipine) in hypertensive patients. Jpn Heart J 17:479–484
36. Aoki K, Kondo S, Mochizuki A, Yoshida T, Kato S, Kato K, Takikawa K (1978) Antihypertensive effect of cardiovascular Ca^{2+}-antagonist in hypertensive patients in the absence and presence of beta-adrenergic blockade. Am Heart J 96:218–226
37. Aoki K, Kondo S, Sato K, Kato K, Kawaguchi Y, Mochizuki A, Yamamoto M (1981) Hypotensive action of nifedipine (Ca^{2+}-antagonist) and propranolol in acute trials and its long-term therapy of hypertensive coronary heart disease patients. Jpn Heart J 22:575–584
38. Aoki K, Sato K, Kawaguchi Y, Yamamoto M (1982) Acute and long-term hypotensive effects and plasma concentrations of nifedipine in patients with essential hypertension. Eur J Clin Pharmacol 23:197–201
39. Aoki K, Sato K, Yamamoto M (1983) Hypotensive effects of diltiazem to normals and essential hypertensives. Eur J Clin Pharmacol 25:475–480
40. Mochizuki A, Aoki K, Kondo S, Mizuno T, Hotta K (1979) Specificity of tension development and calcium flux of the arterial smooth muscle in SHR. Jpn Heart J 20 (Suppl 1):225–227
41. Aoki K, Kondo S, Mochizuki A, Sato K, Yoshida T, Kato S, Kato K (1979) Ca^{2+}-antagonist therapy for hypertension in combination with beta-blockade: A new concept of essential hypertension. In: Yamori Y, Lovenberg W, Freis ED (eds) Prophylactic approach to hypertensive disease. Raven Press, New York, pp 377–386
42. Aoki K, Asano M, Sato K, Kondo S, Mochizuki A, Kawaguchi Y, Yamamoto M (1983) Calcium antagonists on the vascular smooth muscle of spontaneously hypertensive rat and human essential hypertension: A calcium membrane theory of essential hypertension. In: Beven JA, et al (eds) Vascular neuroeffector mechanisms: 4th International Symposium. Raven Press, New York, pp 295–299
43. Aoki K, Sato K, Kawaguchi Y (1985) Increased cardiovascular responses to norepinephrine and calcium antagonists in essential hypertension compared with normotensive in humans. J Cardiovasc Pharmacol 7:S182–S186
44. Aoki K (1985) Essential hypertension and secondary hypertension in humans and rats. Asian Med J 28:529–548
45. Robinson BF (1984) Altered calcium handling as a cause of primary hypertension. J Hypertension 2:453–460
46. Postnov YV, Orlov SN (1984) Cell membrane alteration as a source of primary hypertension. J Hypertension 2:1–6
47. Lau K, Eby B (1985) The role of calcium in genetic hypertension. Hypertension 7:657–667

48. Frohlich ED (1977) Hemodynamics of hypertension. In: Genest J, Koiw E, Kuchel O (eds) Hypertension, physiopathology and treatment. McGraw-Hill, New York, pp 15–48
49. Tarazi RC (1983) The hemodynamics of hypertension. In: Genest J, Kuchel O, Hamet P, Cantin M (eds) Hypertension, physiopathology and treatment, 2nd ed. McGraw-Hill, New York, pp 15–41
50. Mulvany MJ, Halpern W (1977) Contractile properties of small arterial resistance vessels in spontaneously hypertensive and normotensive rats. Circ Res 41:19–26
51. Mulvany MJ, Aalkjaer C, Christensen J (1980) Changes in noradrenaline sensitivity and morphology of arterial resistance vessels during development of high blood pressure in spontaneously hypertensive rats. Hypertension 2:664–671
52. Huxley AF, Niedergerke R (1954) Structural changes in muscle during contraction. Nature 173:971–973
53. Huxley AF, Simmons RM (1971) Proposed mechanism of force generation in striated muscle. Nature 233:533–538
54. Huxley AF (1974) Muscle contraction. J Physiol (Lond) 243:1–43
55. Huxley HE (1963) Electron microscope studies on the structure of natural and synthetic protein filaments from striated muscle. J Mol Biol 7:281–308
56. Somlyo AP, Wasserman AJ, Katazawa T, Bond M, Shuman H, Somlyo AV (1985) Calcium and sodium distribution and movements in smooth muscle. Experientia 41:981–988
57. Somlyo AP, Somlyo AV (1983) Calcium, magnesium, and vascular smooth muscle function. In: Genest J, Kuchel O, Hamet P, Cantin M (eds) Hypertension, physiopathology and treatment, 2nd ed. McGraw-Hill, New York, pp 441–457
58. Somlyo AP: (1985) Excitation-contraction coupling and the ultrastructure of smooth muscle. Circ Res 57:497–507
59. Ebashi S, Endo M (1968) Calcium ion and muscular contraction. Prog Biophy Mol Biol 18:123–183
60. Filo RS, Bohr DF, Ruegg JC (1965) Glycerinated skeletal and smooth muscle: calcium and magnesium dependence. Science 147:1581–1583
61. Saida K, Nonomura Y (1978) Characteristics of Ca- and Mg-induced tension development in chemically skinned smooth muscle fibers. J Gen Physiol 72:1–14
62. Fitzpatrick EJ, Landon EJ, Debbas G, Hurwitz L (1972) A calcium pump in vascular smooth muscle. Science 176:305–306
63. Lederballe Pedersen O (1979) Role of extracellular calcium in isometric contractions of the SHR aorta. Influence of age and antihypertensive treatment. Arch Int Pharmacodyn Ther 239:208–220
64. Lederballe Pedersen O, Mikkelsen E, Anderson KE (1978) Effects of extracellular calcium on potassium and noradrenaline induced contractions in the aorta of spontaneously hypertensive rats—increased sensitivity to nifedipine. Acta Pharmacol Toxicol 43:137–144

Index of Key Words